When Disease Came to This Country

Twentieth-century circumpolar epidemics shaped historical interpretations of disease in European imperialism throughout the Americas and beyond. In this revisionist history of epidemic disease as experienced by northern peoples, Liza Piper illuminates the ecological, spatial, and colonial relationships that allowed diseases – influenza, measles, and tuberculosis in particular – to flourish between 1860 and 1940 along the Mackenzie and Yukon rivers. Making detailed use of Indigenous oral histories alongside English- and French-language archives and emphasizing environmental as well as social and cultural factors, *When Disease Came to This Country* shows how colonial ideas about northern Indigenous immunity to disease were rooted in the racialized structures of colonialism that transformed northern Indigenous lives and lands and shaped mid-twentieth-century biomedical research.

LIZA PIPER is Professor of History at the University of Alberta whose previous work includes *The Industrial Transformation of Subarctic Canada* (2009).

Global Health Histories

Series editor:

Sanjoy Bhattacharya, University of York

Global Health Histories aims to publish outstanding and innovative scholarship on the history of public health, medicine and science worldwide. By studying the many ways in which the impact of ideas of health and well-being on society were measured and described in different global, international, regional, national and local contexts, books in the series reconceptualise the nature of empire, the nation state, extra-state actors and different forms of globalisation. The series showcases new approaches to writing about the connected histories of health and medicine, humanitarianism, and global economic and social development.

When Disease Came to This Country

Epidemics and Colonialism in Northern North America

Liza Piper

University of Alberta

CAMBRIDGE
UNIVERSITY PRESS

CAMBRIDGE
UNIVERSITY PRESS

Shaftesbury Road, Cambridge CB2 8EA, United Kingdom

One Liberty Plaza, 20th Floor, New York, NY 10006, USA

477 Williamstown Road, Port Melbourne, VIC 3207, Australia

314–321, 3rd Floor, Plot 3, Splendor Forum, Jasola District Centre, New Delhi – 110025, India

103 Penang Road, #05–06/07, Visioncrest Commercial, Singapore 238467

Cambridge University Press is part of Cambridge University Press & Assessment, a department of the University of Cambridge.

We share the University's mission to contribute to society through the pursuit of education, learning and research at the highest international levels of excellence.

www.cambridge.org
Information on this title: www.cambridge.org/9781009320870

DOI: 10.1017/9781009320924

First published 2023

A catalogue record for this publication is available from the British Library.

ISBN 978-1-009-32087-0 Hardback

This book is dedicated to caregivers, everywhere.

Contents

Figures

Maps

Tables

Acknowledgements

I gratefully acknowledge the Gwich'in Tribal Council Department of Culture and Heritage, the Inuvialuit Cultural Centre, and the Tr'ondëk Hwëch'in Heritage Department for granting access to unpublished interview transcripts with Elders for this research project and for permission to reproduce quotations found in this book. Royalties from the book will be shared among these heritage organizations.

The research for this project was funded originally by a Killam postdoctoral research fellowship and a SSHRC postdoctoral fellowship at the University of British Columbia in 2005–7. My involvement in the SSHRC-funded Northern Exposures project (2014–22) provided the means to study the longer history of food hazards and nutrition in the north. I am grateful for the financial support and to my Northern Exposures colleagues – Arn Keeling, Stephen Bocking, Matt Farish, Lianne Leddy, and John Sandlos.

My involvement with the Ganahghootr'onatan project in Teetł'it Zheh has taught me much about Gwich'in history, language, and culture. In particular, I wish to say *hai choo*, thank you, to Joanne Snowshoe and Bernice Francis for sharing their knowledge and wisdom, and to Gladys Alexie for doing likewise and for giving me a copy of *Jijuu*, which has been indispensable. I am also grateful to Elaine Alexie and Adam Gaudry for making that project happen.

I have reached out to many people for assistance, sometimes with very detailed questions. Others generously shared their time, enthusiasm, and expertise. I wish to thank all of them. Invaluable research assistance was provided at different stages by Samantha Blais, Elizabeth Briggs, Merissa Daborn, Krystal Isbister, and Erik Lizée. Access to the Canadian Circumpolar Library collection at the University of Alberta was essential to this project. Morgan Hite of Hesperus Arts, Smithers, BC, made the maps with exceptional thoughtfulness and attention to detail.

A northern discussion group organized several years ago, as well as many subsequent conversations with Crystal Fraser, Heather Green, Sara Komarnisky, and Hereward Longley, has shaped my understanding of the history of colonialism in northern places.

David Neufeld and Joy Waters opened their home to our family on a trip to Yukon when my children were small. On that visit, and others, I learned a lot from David. He was always generous with his knowledge and his time, guiding me in valuable directions and sharing archival materials. David and Joy both passed away in 2020, and I am sad that I was not able to share with them the final outcome of this work.

This book was written on Treaty 6 and 7 lands, where I am thankful to live and work. Kristi Benson, Sarah Carter, David Piper, and Zac Robinson, as well as the anonymous referees, gave feedback on drafts of the manuscript that helped refine the analysis, improve the writing and figures, and focus the ideas. My children, Michael and Sacha, didn't make the research or writing any easier, and for that I am also endlessly grateful. All errors are my own.

Place Names

Many languages were spoken on the lands that are the subject of this book. Places had names in more than one language. This list provides a reference for places named in this book and shown on the maps. This list is intended to be neither definitive nor comprehensive and draws on sources found in the Bibliography. There are different orthographies preferred by different people and communities, and names for places in languages and dialects that have not been included here. Some places have more than one official name (in bold) in the present. Official names are used to provide consistency in the text, with the exception of names used in primary sources or oral histories, which retain their original form. All errors are the responsibility of the author.

Akłarvik (I)	**Aklavik**		
Áa Tlein (TL)	**Atlin Lake** (E)		
Rae-Edzo (E)	**Behchokǫ̀** (T)	Fort Rae (E)[1]	
Tth’oh Zraii Njik (G)	**Blackstone River** (E)		
Iqaluktuuttiaq (IN)	**Cambridge Bay** (E)		
Sha Dhäla Ghą (ST)	**Champagne** (E)		
K’áhbamį̨túé (S)	**Colville Lake** (E)		
	Dawson (E)		
Fort Franklin (E)	**Délı̨nę** (S)		
	Fort Chipewyan (E)		
Tthebatthi (DS)	**Fort Fitzgerald** (E)	Ttthembatthie (DZ)	Smith’s Landing (E)
Rádeyı̨lı̨kóé (S)	**Fort Good Hope** (E)		

(*cont.*)

Echaot'į̨e Kų́ę́ (DZ)	**Fort Liard** (E)	Fort aux Liards (F)		
Teetł'it Zheh (G)	**Fort McPherson** (E)	Peel River Post (E)		
Zhahti Kų́ę́ (DZ)	**Fort Providence** (E)			
Deninu Kų́ę́ (DZ)	**Fort Resolution** (E)			
	Fort Selkirk (E)			
Łíídlį̨ Kų́ę́ (DZ)	**Fort Simpson** (E)	Fort of the Forks (E)		
Tthebacha (DS)	**Fort Smith** (E)			
Gwichyaa Zhee (G)	**Fort Yukon** (E)	Fort Youcon (E)		
Sahtú (DZ)	**Great Bear Lake** (E)	Sahtì (T)	Sáhtu (S)	
Sahtúdé (S)	**Great Bear River** (E)			
Tį̨į̨ndee (T)	**Great Slave Lake** (E)	Tucho (DZ)	Tindeè (W)	Tu Nedhé (DS)
Dakwä̀kä̀da (ST)	**Haines Junction** (E)			
Xátł'odehchee (DZ)	**Hay River** (E)			
Qikiqtaryuk (I)	**Herschel Island** (E)			
Inuuvik (I)	**Inuvik**			
Kitigaaryuit (I)	**Kittigazuit**	Kittigaryuit (I)		
Coppermine (E)	**Kugluktuk** (IN)			
	Lake Athabasca (E)			
Zheh Gwitsal (G)	**Lapierre House** (E)	LaPierre's House (E)		
Łútsę̨lk'é (DZ)	**Łutselk'e**	Snowdrift (E)		
Dehcho (DZ) **Deho** (S)	**Mackenzie River** (E)	**Nagwichoonjik** (G)	**Kuukpak** (I)	**Fleuve Mackenzie** (F) **Grande Rivière** (M)
	Moosehide (E)			

(*cont.*)

Tłegǫ́htı̨ (S)	**Norman Wells** (E)		
	Old Crow (E)		
Chahnjik (G)	**Old Crow River** (E)		
Nishì (T)	**Old Fort Rae** (E)[2]		
Paulatuuq (I)	**Paulatuk**		
Teetł'it Gwinjik (G)	**Peel River** (E)		
Ts'ekínyäk Chú (NT)	**Pelly River** (E)		
Ch'oodèenjik (G)	**Porcupine River** (E)		
Gindèh Chik (G)	**Rampart House (E)**		
Tache (DS)	**Reliance** (E)	Dechı̨ Húle Ndeé K'é (DS)	
Tapqaq (I)	**Shingle Point** (E)		
Des Nedhé (DS)	**Slave River** (E)	Deh Ndeé (DZ)	
Tsiigehtshik (G)	**Tsiigehtchic**	Arctic Red River (E)	
Tuktuuyaqtuuq (I)	**Tuktoyaktuk**		
Tulít'a (S)	**Tulita**	Tułít'a (DZ, DS)	Fort Norman (E)
Kwänlin (ST)	**Whitehorse** (E)		
Pedzéh Kı̨ (DZ)	**Wrigley** (E)	Fort Wrigley (E)	
Sǫ̀mbak'è (DZ)	**Yellowknife** (E)		
Wiiliìdeh (W)	**Yellowknife River** (E)	Beghúldes (DS)	
Chu kon' dëk (H)	**Yukon River** (E)	Tágà Shäw (ST)	Tàgé Cho (NT)

Languages and abbreviations: Dëne Sųłiné Yatıé/Chipewyan (DS); Dene Zhatıé/South Slavey (DZ); Dinji Zhu' Ginjik/Gwich'in (G); English (E); French (F); Hän (H); Inuinnaqtun (IN); Inuvialuktun (I); Michif (M); Sahtúot'ı̨nę Yatı̨́/North Slavey (S); Northern Tutchone (NT); Southern Tutchone (ST); Tłı̨chǫ Yatıì (T); Tlingit (TL); Wiiliìdeh dialect of Tłı̨chǫ (W)

1 Fort Rae and a second community, Edzo, created in the mid-1960s, combined to become Rae-Edzo, later officially renamed Behchokǫ̀.

2 Before 1909, Fort Rae in the text refers to Old Fort Rae. After 1909, I use Behchokǫ̀.

Abbreviations

APRCA	Alaska and Polar Regions Collections and Archives
DIA	Department of Indian Affairs
GM	Glenbow Museum and Archives, Calgary
GSA	General Synod Archives, Anglican Church of Canada, Toronto
GSCI	Gwich'in Social and Cultural Institute
HBC	Hudson's Bay Company
HBCA	Hudson's Bay Company Archives, Winnipeg
LAC	Library and Archives Canada, Ottawa
MHO	Medical Health Officer (or Medical Officer of Health)
MVPI	Mackenzie Valley Pipeline Inquiry
NT	Northern Trading Company
NWMP	North West Mounted Police (1873–1904)
NWT	Northwest Territories
NWTA	Northwest Territories Archives, Yellowknife
OMI	Oblates of Mary Immaculate
PAA	Provincial Archives of Alberta, Edmonton
RCMP	Royal Canadian Mounted Police (after 1920)
RNWMP	Royal North West Mounted Police (1904–20)
TRC	Truth and Reconciliation Commission of Canada
UAA	University of Alberta Archives
YA	Yukon Archives, Whitehorse

1 Introduction

> There was one or two flu epidemics and a lot of his relatives and friends passed away. But he's telling you this story and he is at the moment kind of leery of saying any more or carrying on because he thinks that maybe some of you think that he is not – he's just telling you a story because he is all alone now and no old person here to say that he is telling you the truth.
>
> Philip Simba's testimony to the Mackenzie Valley Pipeline Inquiry, speaking through an interpreter, Kakisa Lake, 17 July 1976

In the summer of 1928, epidemic influenza tore through villages and camps along the length of Dehcho (the Mackenzie River), out along the shores of the large lakes to the east – Sahtú (Great Bear Lake) and Tı̨ı̨ndee (Great Slave Lake) – north to the delta and along the coast of the Beaufort Sea. Observers estimated that one in ten people across the region perished in two short months. There were camps with only a handful of survivors. The 1928 epidemic was devastating and world-changing for Dene, Gwich'in, Inuvialuit, and Métis families. Stories about 1928 continue to be shared in the North a century later, whether told out on the land or published in collected histories.[1] In Dene Elder George Blondin's three books, the 1928 epidemic marks a major historical transition heralding the loss of Dene medicine power in the modern world.

In 1942, a research associate working at Toronto's Connaught Laboratories, Ronald Hare, wrote to Roy A. Gibson, a top government official responsible for Canada's northern territories, asking for information about the 1928 influenza epidemic.[2] Hare was looking for records, and Gibson had few to offer; an ironic response given that I found this correspondence at the end of a thick file about the epidemic preserved in Canada's national archives.[3] Although deputy

[1] Elizabeth Yakeleya, Sarah Simon, and other Sahtu and Gwich'in Elders, *We Remember the Coming of the White Man = Gahnaaandaih unjoo kat degehnoo dai anahgoogwaandak* (Calgary: Durvile & UpRoute Books, 2020); Leslie McCartney and Gwich'in Tribal Council, *Our Whole Gwich'in Way of Life Has Changed = Gwich'in K'yuu Gwiidandài' Tthak Ejuk Gòonlih: Stories from the People of the Land* (Edmonton: Polynya Press, 2020).

[2] R. Hare, to The Director, 13 Mar. 1942, RG 85 C-1-a vol. 789 file 6099 [hereafter file 6099], LAC.

[3] But characteristic of Gibson, see Matthew D. Evenden, 'Harold Innis, the Arctic Survey, and the Politics of Social Science during the Second World War', *Canadian Historical Review* 79, no. 1 (1998): 36–67 (pp. 56, 63).

commissioner of the Northwest Territories when the influenza struck, Gibson responded cursorily to Hare, offering little insight into the epidemic. Meanwhile, along the shores of the northern lakes and rivers there were hundreds of men and women who, as children, had lost parents and grandparents in that awful epidemic fifteen years previously. For them, 1928 was etched as an indelible memory, even as the federal bureaucracy chose to obscure and forget.

Ronald Hare, along with Laurella McClelland, directed influenza virus studies at the lab in Toronto. He was smack in the centre of a cohort of biomedical researchers who at mid-century turned their sights north, participating in a larger programme of what Joanna Radin has described as 'biomedical prospecting efforts'.[4] These Canadian researchers corresponded with international colleagues, most notably Yale epidemiologist John Rodman Paul, whose work would shape the World Health Organization's program of 'serological surveillance'.[5] This research imagined northern Indigenous people – Inuit in particular but not exclusively – as 'isolated' and 'pristine', and thereby potential subject populations for cutting-edge immunology and epidemiology. To imagine northern peoples in this fashion involved sharing a set of assumptions about them and entailed a process of forgetting epidemics like the 1928 influenza, and other influenza, scarlet fever, and measles epidemics that had come before.

The assumptions shared by Hare, Paul, and other biomedical researchers in Canada and globally during the post-war decades were built on anthropological constructions. As Jenny Reardon and Kim TallBear write, these imaginaries saw Indigenous peoples in the Americas as representing 'an earlier period in human evolution', who could thus 'help modern humans understand themselves'.[6] Researchers targeted northern Indigenous peoples and other populations because their perceived geographic and cultural isolation made them, in Radin's analysis, 'portals into the human past'.[7] Reardon, TallBear, Radin, and others examine the role of frozen blood samples and Indigenous DNA in shaping the study of population genetics and biological anthropology. These biomedical constructions, held by Hare and colleagues McClelland, C. E. Van Rooyen, A. J. Rhodes, Fred Nagler, and Arthur F. W. Peart in Toronto and Ottawa, also shaped the interpretation of 'virgin soil epidemics' used by historians to understand the impact of introduced pathogens in the process of European colonization.

[4] Joanna Radin, *Life on Ice: A History of New Uses for Cold Blood* (Chicago: University of Chicago Press, 2017), 63.

[5] Radin, *Life on Ice*, 6.

[6] Jenny Reardon and Kim TallBear, '"Your DNA Is *Our* History": Genomics, Anthropology, and the Construction of Whiteness as Property', *Current Anthropology* 53, suppl. 5 (2012): S233–45 (S237); see also Johannes Fabian, *Time and the Other: How Anthropology Makes Its Object* (New York: Columbia University Press, 2002); Jane Buikstra to June Helm, 8 Jul. 1983, file 'Fort Norman Deaths 1927–65', box 1, N-2002–012, June Helm Fonds, NWTA.

[7] Joanna Radin, 'Latent Life: Concepts and Practices of Human Tissue Preservation in the International Biological Program', *Social Studies of Science* 43, no. 4 (2013): 484–508 (p. 494).

The biomedical research undertaken in the 1940s and 1950s came after the histories of disease and colonialism that are the subject of this study. I begin at the end because constructions and considerations of *time* are central to the analysis in this book. The timing of smallpox, scarlet fever, and influenza epidemics shaped their history in northern North America – *not* because they came so late that they encountered 'isolated' and 'pristine' Indigenous populations, but because sometimes the delay (the ten years, for instance, between 1918 and 1928) influenced the course and consequences of an epidemic. This is a theme that will be explored in the chapters to come. For Alfred Crosby, though, a handful of twentieth-century northern epidemics served as models that could be projected backwards to understand the role of ecological relationships in European imperialism.[8] In so doing, Crosby collapsed the distance between Inuit along the Arctic Coast in the 1940s and the effects of smallpox at the sixteenth-century siege of Tenochtitlán. He created a portal to the past as described by Radin. This book, by following the path of northern epidemics between 1860 and 1940, seeking out stories shared in community oral histories, and using the colonial archive to hold government officials, traders, and missionaries to account for their roles in and responses to these epidemics, aims to reassert the distance between Tenochtitlán in 1521 and Tuktoyaktuk in 1940; to create a space within the academic literature to learn more about the experiences of these epidemics and their historical significance from those who survived; to assess how colonial ecologies shaped the history of northern disease; and to call on those who persist in using 'virgin soils' to understand the history of disease, to dispense with this distorted lens permanently.

Settler colonialism in the North involved diverse Indigenous peoples, settlers, and sojourners coming together and moving apart, an ebb and flow that involved pathogens and which increased in frequency and intensity between 1860 and 1940. There were epidemics before and after, but infectious diseases caused great mortality in this period. Throughout this book, *outbreak* refers to a disease with local effects; *epidemic* to a disease with regional effects; and *pandemic* to a disease that crossed continents. Tracing outbreaks, epidemics, and pandemics means following experiences of ill health, medicine, and dying, but in the process this history shows the relationships forged by colonialism: the new geographies and ecologies that emerged, the new identities including racial categories by which people and difference came to be defined, and the changed relationships of care that underpin persistent disparities in Indigenous and settler, northern and southern, health care in Canada.

The urgency and significance of these issues came to the fore in 2020 with the onset of the COVID-19 pandemic. Everything old became new again.

[8] Alfred W. Crosby, 'Virgin Soil Epidemics as a Factor in the Aboriginal Depopulation in America', *The William and Mary Quarterly* 33, no. 2 (1976): 289–99 (pp. 293–7).

In these pages, there are quarantines, vaccination mandates, and those who opposed them. There are Medical Health Officers who made poor decisions rooted in politics that enabled pathogens to spread with devastating effect. There are *syndemics* (when two or more diseases interact in a population, leading to worse health outcomes) that deepened mortality.[9] There is the role of nutrition, built environments, sanitation, and power in shaping vulnerability to disease. There are people who cared for and nursed family, friends, and community members and helped them in their time of need. These are themes common to the history of disease. Throughout the COVID-19 pandemic, I was attuned to the tensions between diverse local events and responses and the larger collective experience. From the desire to come to terms with the scale and scope of our most recent pandemic, there is a flattening of experiences. This book considers the importance of those instances when the history of epidemic disease in the North diverged from the main historical patterns elsewhere: in the absence of smallpox epidemics with high mortality or the appearance of influenza in 1928, these divergent episodes are not just outliers but illuminate important changes in diseases over time and shaped northern experiences of epidemics and colonialism.

Places and People

Two great rivers and their tributaries run through this history (Map 1.1). The lands rise to peaks in the northern reaches of the Rocky Mountains. Between 1860 and 1940, waters normally froze by November, with the first new ice appearing as early as September. The land thawed in May, although waterways might not be free of ice until June or July. August was at once the height of summer and the arrival of fall. Into the twenty-first century, lands and waters are frozen for more than half the year.

Dehcho, the Dene Zhatıé name for what came to be called the Mackenzie River, translates as 'big river'. Along with the Inuvialuktun name, Kuukpak, meaning 'great river', and the Gwich'in name, Nagwichoonjik, 'river flowing through a big country', each captures the importance of the river, its great size, and its role as a 'highway' for northern peoples.[10] The river threads through the land, carrying waters from two enormous lakes, Tı̨ı̨ndee/Tucho/Tu Nedhé/Great Slave Lake, and Sahtú/Sahtì/Great Bear Lake, the latter via Sahtúdé or the Great Bear River. The lands and waters of these lakes were home to many different Dene: Dënesųłıné (Chipewyan), Tłı̨chǫ (Dogrib), Dehcho (South

[9] Timothy P. Newfield, 'Syndemics and the History of Disease: Towards a New Engagement', *Social Science & Medicine* 295 (2022) http://doi.org/10.1016/j.socscimed.2021.114454.

[10] Gabe Andre in M. Heine, A. Andre, I. Kritsch, A. Cardinal, and the Elders of Tsiigehtshik, *Gwichya Gwich'in Googwandak: The History and Stories of the Gwichya Gwich'in, As Told by the Elders of Tsiigehtshik* (Tsiigehtshik, NT: Gwich'in Social and Cultural Institute, 2007), 61.

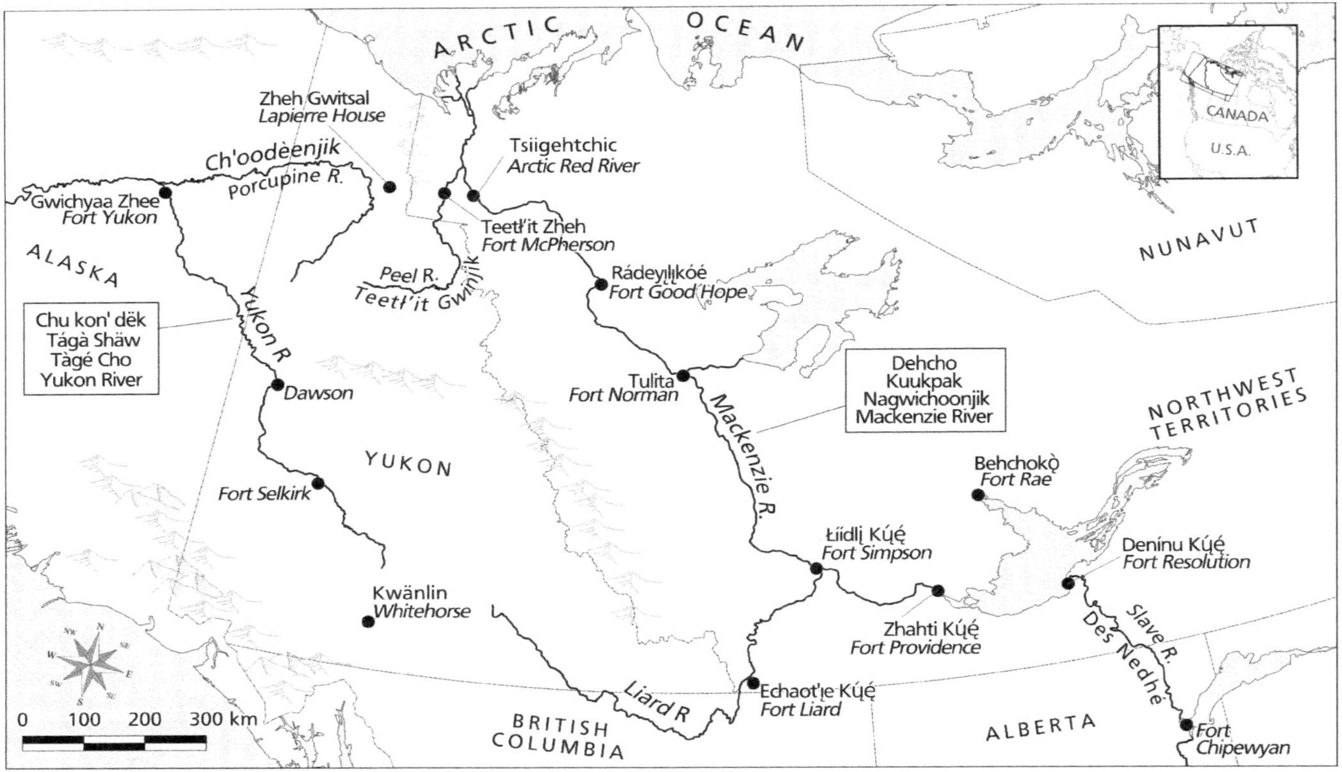

Map 1.1 Map of northern North America.

Slavey), Tetsǫt'ıné (Yellowknives) and their descendants the Wìılìıdeh Yellowknives Dene, K'áhshó Got'ıne̜ (Hare), Sahtúot'ine (Bearlake), K'áalǫ Gotine (Willow Lake), and Shita Got'ine (Mountain).[11]

Dehcho flowed north to the delta, a flat coastal plain connecting the lands along the river to the coast and ocean beyond. Teetł'it Gwinjik, or the Peel River, joins with the main stem of Dehcho in the delta. Gwich'in, Inuvialuit, Métis, and many others met and mixed on these lands. Among the Dinjii Zhuh or Gwich'in (who are also Dene) who appear in this book, the Van Tat Gwich'in (Vuntut Gwitchin), Teetł'it Gwich'in, and Gwichya Gwich'in figure most prominently.[12] Along the coast lived Inuvialuit, Inupiat from the west, and Inuinnait to the east. Van Tat (or Crow Flats), to the west of the delta, was a place used by both Van Tat Gwich'in and Inuit.[13] Inuvialuit and Gwich'in traditional territories overlapped in places that both groups used at different times of the year.[14] Relations between these two northern peoples shifted in the decades and centuries preceding the arrival of Europeans. According to Gwich'in Elders, the 'age of the great travellers and leaders [ts'ii dę̨į̨ days – the long-ago time] was followed by a time when fights with the [Inuit] occurred more frequently'.[15] Before that, Gwich'in had fewer conflicts with Inuit but had fought more with Dene to the south. Ishmael Alunik emphasized that Inuit and Gwich'in conflicts took place in the delta, where they competed for hunting areas. He noted that 'long ago Inupiat or Inuvialuit never travelled too far into the delta areas because the [Gwich'in] lived there'.[16]

The Yukon River is called Chu kon' dëk in Hän, meaning 'sparkling water river'.[17] In Northern Tutchone and Southern Tutchone, the names Tàgé Cho and Tágà Shäw respectively both translate to 'great river', like its counterpart to the east.[18] Chu kon' dëk, runs from its source in Áa Tlein (Atlin Lake)

[11] James Auld and Robert Kershaw, *The Sahtu Atlas: Maps and Stories from the Sahtu Settlement Area in Canada's Northwest Territories* (Norman Wells: Sahtu GIS Project, 2005), 5, 9; Yellowknives Dene First Nation and Prince of Wales Northern Heritage Centre, *This Land Is Our Home: Wìılìıdeh Yellowknives Dene* (Yellowknife: Prince of Wales Northern Heritage Centre, 2015), www.nwtexhibits.ca/navigator/ykdene/index-en.html.

[12] For the Van Tat Gwich'in, I follow the conventions set out in Vuntut Gwitchin First Nation and Shirleen Smith, *People of the Lakes: Stories of Our Van Tat Gwich'in Elders* (Edmonton: University of Alberta Press, 2009), xx.

[13] Vuntut Gwitchin First Nation and Smith, *People of the Lakes*, 106.

[14] Ishmael Alunik, *Call Me Ishmael: Memories of Ishmael Alunik* (Inuvik: Kolausok Ublaaq Enterprises, 1998), 11; Pierre's Creek on the Mackenzie River served as a boundary between the Gwich'in and the Inuvialuit about 200 to 300 years ago and was also a good place for blueberries and cranberries. I. Kritsch, *Gwich'in Territorial Park (Campbell Lake) Oral History Project Final Report: Prepared for Dept. of Economic Development and Tourism (GNWT)* (Tsiigehtchic: Gwich'in Social and Cultural Institute, 1994), 27.

[15] Heine et al., *Gwichya Gwich'in Googwandak*, 30; George Blondin, *Yamoria the Lawmaker: Stories of the Dene* (Edmonton, AB: NeWest Press, 1997), 101–3.

[16] Alunik, *Ishmael*, 66. [17] Georgette McLeod, pers. corr., 17 May 2022.

[18] Yukon, *Gazetteer of Yukon* (Yukon Geographical Names Program, 2022).

north-west to its junction with the Ch'oodèenjik or Porcupine River, and then at Fort Yukon abruptly south-westward across Alaska to its mouth in the Bering Sea. To the east of what became an international border, along the shores of the river, its tributaries, and out on the land, live Gwich'in, Tr'ondëk Hwëch'in, Tlingit, Northern Tutchone, Southern Tutchone, Upper Tanana, and Tagish people.

Euro-Americans travelled to the north-west interior from the late eighteenth century for exploration and trade, with more arriving and more frequently in the nineteenth century. Akaitcho, a nineteenth-century Tetsǫ́t'ıné leader, met with John Franklin in July 1820. Franklin was not the first newcomer to Akaitcho's land; by the 1820s, the North West Company had established several posts around the shores of what they called Great Slave Lake. Having brought meat to the posts in trade, Akaitcho agreed to guide and provision Franklin and his men on their journey northward. They set out together, but Akaitcho soon questioned his initial optimism about their journey. In mid-August, he informed Franklin that it would take a further forty days to descend the river 'and during the whole journey the party must experience great sufferings for want of food, as the reindeer had already left'. When pressed about why he had changed his timeline for their journey, Akaitcho replied that 'he had been unacquainted with our slow mode of travelling', and winter was coming. Franklin's response was painfully naïve given his ultimate arctic fate: 'We now informed [Akaitcho] that we were provided with instruments by which we could ascertain the state of the air and water, and that we did not imagine the winter to be so near as he supposed; however, we promised to return on discovering the first change in the season.' Akaitcho accepted their decision but emphasized that they would be going to their deaths. Akaitcho's persuasion, combined with some 'recent changes in the weather', finally led Franklin and his men to winter at a place they called Fort Enterprise on Winter Lake.[19]

Although newcomers, such as Franklin and the North West Company traders, came as colonizers, at their outset their power and significance was limited. Akaitcho's importance to Dene history lies not in his role guiding Franklin, but foremost in his leadership in negotiating a lasting peace with Tłı̨chǫ leader Edzo in the mid-nineteenth century at Nǫhdlatì/Gots'ǫkàtì/Mesa Lake.[20] Akaitcho's critique of Franklin's 'slow mode of travelling' exposed European weakness: explorers were encumbered by their instrumentation – the burdens of European society that they insisted on carrying with them – and by their ignorance of northern environments. Although they emphasized their

[19] John Franklin and John Richardson, *Narrative of a Journey to the Shores of the Polar Sea in the Years 1819, 20, 21 & 22* (Philadelphia: H. C. Carey & I. Lea, 1824), 200–2, 226.

[20] This story is told by Dene. For two written accounts see George Blondin, 'Edzo Overpowers the Great Enemy', in *Yamoria*, 93–100; Yellowknives Dene First Nation, *Proposed Dinàgà Wek'èhodì Protected Area YKDFN Traditional Knowledge Report* (31 Mar. 2018), 12–15.

work of exploration and discovery, people like Franklin and Alexander Mackenzie followed in the footsteps of northerners, led by guides and visiting well-known places, such as fish camps in use for hundreds of years, on their journeys down Nagwichoonjik.[21] Traders followed northerners for furs and missionaries followed them to their camps to proselytize, only later establishing missions for Dene, Gwich'in, and Inuvialuit to discover.

From 1795 until 1821, the North West Company dominated the trade in the Mackenzie River District. From 1821 until 1895–1900, the Hudson's Bay Company (HBC) monopolized trade with posts along the Mackenzie River from Great Slave Lake to Peel River Post, along the tributary Liard River, with Fort Simpson the district headquarters, at the junction of the two rivers (hence its original name, the Fort of the Forks). Peel River Post was renamed Fort McPherson and, here, Gwich'in acted initially as intermediaries to Inuvialuit, although after 1853 Inuvialuit traded directly at the fort, as well as at Fort Anderson on the Anderson River.

The upper Yukon River and its watershed was the last part of the Mackenzie and Yukon region where fur traders established posts. There were existing Indigenous trade networks reaching into this region and contacts with Russian traders to the east. Then the HBC erected five posts in the 1840s. In 1842, Robert Campbell established Fort Frances on Frances Lake and shortly thereafter Pelly Banks on the upper Pelly River. In 1846, to the north, LaPierre's House was built as a satellite post – just across the mountains – to Peel River Post. Both fell under the responsibility of a single officer. In 1847, Alexander Murray established Fort Yukon at the junction of the Porcupine and Yukon rivers and well within what was then Russian and would become American territory. Campbell erected the most significant central Yukon post, Fort Selkirk, at the confluence of the Yukon and Pelly rivers, one year later.[22] Fort Selkirk was abandoned in 1852, after a raid by Chilkat Tlingit, who felt their trade position threatened by the HBC. The Russian American Company had been trading in Alaska since the end of the eighteenth century and focused their attention on the sea otter pelt trade along the coast. Even after over-harvesting otters led to declining returns, the Russians only came as far inland as Nulato, establishing a post there in the early 1840s. Russian and HBC traders travelled from their respective posts at Nulato and Fort Yukon to the junction of the Yukon and Tanana rivers.[23] Of all these posts, Fort Yukon flourished until the

[21] Heine et al., *Gwichya Gwich'in Googwandak*, 169; See also Alexis Arrowmaker, Madeline Judas, Pierre Judas, et al., *We Know and Love Tłı̨chǫ Ndè: Comments and Concerns From the Dechı̨laot'ı Elders to the Environmental Assessment Review Panel, February 1996* ([Yellowknife]: Dene Cultural Institute, 1996), 10.

[22] Greg Hare and Ruth Gotthardt, *A Look Back in Time: The Archaeology of Fort Selkirk* ([Yukon: Selkirk First Nation], 1996), 24.

[23] Thomas J. Turck and Diane L. Lehman Turck, 'Trading Posts along the Yukon River: Noochuloghoyet Trading Post in Historical Context', *Arctic* 45, no. 1 (1992): 51–61 (p. 51).

sale of Alaska to the United States forced the HBC across the border. The closing of Fort Yukon in 1869 led to the decline of LaPierre's House. The HBC withdrew up the Porcupine River to Rampart House, which moved several times until the boundary was settled.[24] Chapter 4 picks up this historical thread.

Christian missionaries arrived in the 1840s. The Methodist Wesleyans reached Fort Chipewyan ahead of the Roman Catholic Oblates of Mary Immaculate (OMI), but the Roman Catholic and Anglican presence would be the most consequential.[25] The Oblate Alexandre Taché visited Fort Chipewyan in 1847 and returned the following year as well. He was succeeded by Henri Faraud, who spent much of 1849–50 at the post. The rapid expansion of missionary activity along the Mackenzie River began in 1858. By this time, the Roman Catholic Oblates had secured permission from George Simpson and the HBC to proceed with establishing northern missions. This permission ensured that the HBC would provide free transportation and accommodation to missionaries. The Anglican church at Red River was, in historian Kerry Abel's words, 'suddenly roused'.[26] Much has been made of the competition between Anglicans and Roman Catholics along the Mackenzie River and the Arctic Coast, although both groups benefited from larger institutions that enabled northern missions to draw on personnel and financial resources from outside.[27] The Roman Catholic Oblate missions relied on the support of lay brothers and Grey Nun sisters in furthering the work of priests. The Grey Nuns took responsibility for schools and did much of the work in the hospitals. In effect, the Roman Catholic mission families had brothers, sisters, mothers, and fathers labouring together. Anglicans, by contrast, could bring their immediate family to share the work, encouraging what Myra Rutherdale referred to as 'last minute' marriages.[28] By the end of the 1880s, there were twelve Oblate priests, seven Grey Nuns, and thirteen lay brothers operating fifteen missions from Fort Chipewyan to Arctic Red River (Tsiigehtchic) and two residential schools at Fort Providence (1867) and Fort Chipewyan (1874). At this time, the Anglican Mackenzie River Diocese included eight clergy and four school-masters and catechists, operating ten missions in the Mackenzie district and Yukon Territory combined, in addition to a mission post at Fort Chipewyan.

[24] Vuntut Gwitchin First Nation and Smith, *People of the Lakes*, 118.

[25] Morris Zaslow, *The Opening of the Canadian North, 1870–1914* (Toronto: McClelland and Stewart, 1971), 64.

[26] Kerry Abel, *Drum Songs: Glimpses of Dene History* (Montreal: McGill-Queen's University Press, 1993), 115–16.

[27] Martha McCarthy, *From the Great River to the Ends of the Earth: Oblate Missions to the Dene, 1847–1921* (Edmonton: University of Alberta Press, 1995), ch. 4; Zaslow, Opening, 63–76; Abel, *Drum Songs*, ch. 6.

[28] Myra Rutherdale, *Women and the White Man's God: Gender and Race in the Canadian Mission Field* (Vancouver: UBC Press, 2002), xiii, 50–1.

From this diversity of lands, cultures, languages, history, and relations, the Dominion of Canada delineated an international border with the United States of America, carved out two territories, the Yukon and the Northwest Territories, and would sign Treaties 8 and 11 with some of the Indigenous people of these lands. The Northwest Territories were soon subdivided into three districts, the Mackenzie, Keewatin, and Franklin. The District of Mackenzie corresponded to the fur trade's Mackenzie River District and includes the lands that along with the Yukon, and with some spilling over boundaries, are considered in this book. Collapsing northern Indigenous historical diversity into the geographic categories of the Yukon and the Mackenzie district is a simplification deployed in this book only to better examine the structures imposed and sustained at the moving edges of Canada's settler colonial state.

Disease, Medicine, and Colonialism

The most powerful narrative about the arrival of Europeans in the Americas hinges on the role of epidemic diseases in shaping this encounter. That story goes like this: Europeans who crossed the Atlantic brought with them infectious diseases, with which they had co-evolved in crowded urban centres and through close proximity to domestic animals. This relationship ensured greater immunity among first-generation European settlers and sojourners. By contrast, Indigenous peoples in the Americas had not acquired immunity to the most common European childhood diseases – smallpox, measles, scarlet fever, to name a few. When these pathogens arrived, they encountered populations of Indigenous Americans who had no immunity and who, in consequence, died en masse. The catastrophic impact of these diseases was reinforced by traditional healing practices such as sweating that could aggravate respiratory illnesses, for example, and by ignorance of effective quarantine measures. The diseases spread like wildfire, carried by the infected-but-unaware, who fled their villages and travelled to other communities bringing the diseases with them. So powerful was this disease tsunami that it cleared the land of Indigenous people, in many instances in advance of the arrival of explorers or colonists, creating the impression of an emptied land. The effects of these 'virgin soil epidemics', which killed large numbers of adults of reproductive age, were such that they led to catastrophic depopulation, conceivably as great as 90 per cent in parts of the Americas.[29]

This story has been told time and again since the 1970s and 1980s when it was articulated by Alfred Crosby and William McNeill, then popularized by writers like Jared Diamond, in a fashion that found wide resonance among

[29] Crosby, 'Virgin Soil Epidemics', 289–99.

scholars and the reading public.[30] The power of this narrative arises in several ways. The story has hemispheric reach: it offers a single narrative thread to the history of European colonialism that is accessible in a way that complex, multifaceted, localized stories rarely are. Authors, especially popularizers, of this story rely heavily on quantification and biological explanations. In particular, those who emphasize the role of 'virgin soil epidemics' harness the authority of dispassionate science and hard numbers of population sizes in reconstructing the causal mechanisms at work. They turn a language of childhood disease and 'virgin soil' that simultaneously infantilizes, naturalizes, and genders Indigenous populations to render them submissive and vulnerable, into a biological inevitability.[31] Lastly, the narrative conveys the horrific drama of colonization, while displacing the responsibility for its worst effects onto nature – onto viruses and pathogens that lack intentionality – and by extension away from the colonizers and settlers who profited from this catastrophe.

There is a well-established revisionist interpretation of 'virgin soil epidemics' that disputes their value in understanding the experience of disease as part of the history of European colonization in the Americas. This historiographical position, clearly articulated in 2003 with the publication of 'Virgin Soils Revisited' by David S. Jones, does not deny that infectious diseases, introduced by European colonizers, had catastrophic effects on Indigenous communities and populations. However, in works covering many different locales in the Americas, historians have undermined the singularity of this narrative and the simplistic resort to immunological explanations.[32] Suzanne Alchon situated sixteenth- and seventeenth-century contact-era epidemics in global disease context, demonstrating that high mortality in epidemics was not unique to Indigenous peoples in the Americas at this time.[33] What was exceptional about the colonial context, Alchon shows, was the role of European colonial policy in disrupting Indigenous societies and the effects of the arrival of multiple overlapping pathogens.

The colonizing work done by the idea of 'virgin soil epidemics' was the subject of David Jones's *Rationalizing Epidemics: Meanings and Uses of*

[30] Alfred W. Crosby, *Ecological Imperialism: The Biological Expansion of Europe, 900–1900* (Cambridge: Cambridge University Press, 1986); William McNeill, *Plagues and Peoples* (Garden City: Anchor Press, 1976); Henry F. Dobyns, *Their Number Become Thinned: Native American Population Dynamics in Eastern North America* (Knoxville: University of Tennessee Press, 1983).

[31] Jocelyn Thorpe, *Temagami's Tangled Wild: Race, Gender, and the Making of Canadian Nature* (Vancouver: UBC Press, 2012), 45, 64–5; David S. Jones, 'Virgin Soils Revisited', *The William and Mary Quarterly* 60, no. 4 (2003): 703–42 (p. 714).

[32] For a summary of this literature, see David S. Jones, 'Death, Uncertainty, and Rhetoric', in *Beyond Germs: Native Depopulation in North America*, ed. C. M. Cameron, Paul Kelton, and A. C. Swedlund, 16–49 (Tucson: University of Arizona Press, 2015).

[33] Suzanne Austin Alchon, *A Pest in the Land: New World Epidemics in a Global Perspective* (Albuquerque: University of New Mexico Press, 2003).

American Indian Mortality since 1600 (2004). Jones attended to sickness and mortality among Indigenous peoples, but the cultural construction of the 'Vanishing Indian', which shaped ideas about Indigenous mortality and depopulation, has long shaped American and Canadian colonial policies.[34] 'Virgin soil' interpretations have a long history in understandings of tuberculosis, in particular as part of early efforts to explain the apparent greater susceptibility of Indigenous peoples to TB. Christian McMillen shows how 'virgin soil' explanations were overly simplistic in the context of tuberculosis and were ultimately supplanted.[35] Jones and Paul Kelton, in advancing our understanding of Indigenous mortality as part of colonization, distinguished between the idea of 'virgin soils' and what Jones termed 'the social contingency of depopulation'.[36] Kelton argued in *Epidemics and Enslavement* (2007) that, along with the novel pathogens that arrived with colonizers and the epidemics that ensued, 'the nonbiological aspects of colonialism mediated the spread and impact of those diseases'.[37] In a subsequent work, Kelton showed how the Cherokee responded creatively and effectively to the new dangers of smallpox, including by implementing their own culturally specific quarantines.[38]

In the historiography of Indigenous peoples whose lands became Canada, there have been key works that have traced colonial epidemics, their course and consequences. Some of the earliest work was done by Arthur Ray in the 1970s and by Jody Decker in the 1980s and 1990s.[39] Regional explorations have been most sophisticated. Paul Hackett, Ann Carlos, and Frank Lewis describe epidemics around Hudson Bay and the Petit Nord. Robert Boyd's work on the Pacific Northwest and Ted Binnema on the western plains detail the impacts of major epidemics upon diverse Indigenous societies and economies.[40] These works all acknowledge the importance of historical

[34] Brian W. Dippie, *The Vanishing American: White Attitudes and U.S. Indian Policy* (Middletown: Wesleyan University Press, 1982).

[35] Christian W. McMillen, *Discovering Tuberculosis: A Global History, 1900 to the Present* (New Haven: Yale University Press, 2016), 25–7.

[36] David S. Jones, *Rationalizing Epidemics: Meanings and Uses of American Indian Mortality since 1600* (Cambridge: Harvard University Press, 2004), 57.

[37] Paul Kelton, *Epidemics and Enslavement: Biological Catastrophe in the Native Southeast, 1492–1715* (Lincoln: University of Nebraska Press, 2007), 161–3.

[38] Paul Kelton, *Cherokee Medicine, Colonial Germs: An Indigenous Nation's Fight Against Smallpox, 1518–1824* (Norman: University of Oklahoma Press, 2015).

[39] Arthur J. Ray, *Indians in the Fur Trade: Their Role as Trappers, Hunters, and Middlemen in the Lands Southwest of Hudson Bay, 1660–1870* (Toronto: University of Toronto Press, 1974); Jody F. Decker, 'Depopulation of the Northern Plains Natives', *Social Science & Medicine* 33, no. 4 (1991): 381–93; Jody F. Decker, 'Tracing Historical Diffusion Patterns: The Case of the 1780–82 Smallpox Epidemic Among the Indians of Western Canada', *Native Studies Review* 4, nos. 1 & 2 (1988): 1–24.

[40] Paul Hackett, *'A Very Remarkable Sickness': Epidemics in the Petit Nord, 1670–1846* (Winnipeg: University of Manitoba Press, 2002); Ann M. Carlos and Frank Lewis, 'Smallpox and Native

circumstance, colonial objectives and responses, and environmental context in shaping mortality and the spread of disease. None of these works, however, go much farther north than the 60th parallel or much later than 1850. Within the northern historiography that considers the lands that became the Yukon and the Northwest Territories, less attention has been paid to the history of epidemic disease. The only comprehensive works on northern health are Robert Fortuine's books on Alaska.[41] Epidemics discussed in the chapters to come appear also in works by Kerry Abel, Martha McCarthy, Patricia McCormack, and others.[42] The general assumption has been that colonial epidemics operated in these lands much as the wider literature showed they operated elsewhere.

Within Canadian historiography, the significance of novel pathogens and immunities is secondary to the role of colonialism and racism in shaping persistent and significant health disparities. Mary-Ellen Kelm, Maureen Lux, James Daschuk, Lisa Stevenson, Mary Jane McCallum, Adele Perry, and others have emphasized that it was, in McCallum's words, the 'colonial policies and practices of the Canadian government' that created ill health, as much as, if not more so than, pathogens.[43] These works draw on the international literature on imperialism, colonialism, and medicine to show how public health and sanitation became tools to control and manage 'problem' populations – including

American Mortality: The 1780s Epidemic in the Hudson Bay Region', *Explorations in Economic History* 49, no. 3 (2012), https://doi.org/10.1016/j.eeh.2012.04.003; Robert Boyd, *The Coming of the Spirit of Pestilence: Introduced Infectious Diseases and Population Decline among Northwest Coast Indians, 1774–1874* (Vancouver: UBC Press, 1999); Theodore Binnema, *Common and Contested Ground: A Human and Environmental History of the Northwestern Plains* (Toronto: University of Toronto Press, 2004); Ted Binnema, '"With Tears, Shrieks, and Howlings of Despair": The Smallpox Epidemic of 1781–82', in *Alberta Formed, Alberta Transformed*, vol. 1, ed. Michael Payne, Donald Wetherell, and Catherine Cavanaugh, 110–31 (Edmonton: University of Alberta Press, 2006).

41 Robert Fortuine, *Chills and Fever: Health and Disease in the Early History of Alaska* (Fairbanks: University of Alaska Press, 1992); Robert Fortuine, *'Must We All Die?': Alaska's Enduring Struggle with Tuberculosis* (Fairbanks: University of Alaska Press, 2005).

42 Abel, *Drum Songs*; Kenneth Coates, *Best Left As Indians: Native–White Relations In the Yukon Territory, 1840–1973* (Montreal: McGill-Queen's University Press, 1993); McCarthy, *Great River*; Patricia McCormack, 'The Athabasca Influenza Epidemic of 1835', *Issues in the North* 1 (1996): 33–42; Patricia McCormack, *Fort Chipewyan and the Shaping of Canadian History, 1788–1920s: 'We Like to Be Free in This Country'* (Vancouver: UBC Press, 2010).

43 Quotation in Mary Jane Logan McCallum, 'Starvation, Experimentation, Segregation, and Trauma: Words for Reading Indigenous Health History', *Canadian Historical Review* 98, no. 1 (2017): 96–113 (p. 100); Mary-Ellen Kelm, *Colonizing Bodies: Aboriginal Health and Healing in British Columbia, 1900–50* (Vancouver: UBC Press, 1998); Maureen K. Lux, *Medicine That Walks: Disease, Medicine and Canadian Plains Native People, 1880–1940* (Toronto: University of Toronto Press, 2012); Maureen K. Lux, *Separate Beds: A History of Indian Hospitals in Canada, 1920s–1980s* (Toronto: University of Toronto Press, 2016); James Daschuk, *Clearing the Plains: Disease, Politics of Starvation, and the Loss of Aboriginal Life* (Regina: University of Regina Press, 2013); Frank James Tester and Paule McNicoll, 'Why Don't They Get It? Talk of Medicine as Science. St Luke's Hospital, Panniqtuuq, Baffin Island', *Social History of Medicine* 19 (2006): 87–106.

Indigenous populations as viewed by settler states.[44] In *Rationalizing Epidemics*, Jones described the importance of moral communities to understanding why Europeans and Americans acted opportunistically when confronted with Indigenous sickness and mortality. For many early colonizers, notes Jones, Indigenous Americans lay outside their moral community, 'the limits of its empathy and concern', and they therefore did not 'feel an obligation to intervene and provide assistance'.[45] In the late nineteenth- and early twentieth-century North, moral communities were not drawn exclusively around categories of what we now term 'Indigenous' people and 'settlers'. Local circumstances, family relations, and individual personalities held greater sway in shaping relations of care. The creation and reinforcement of categories of racial difference between those designated as 'half-breeds', 'Eskimos', 'Indians', and 'whites', part of the governing colonial bureaucracy that emerged after 1900 especially, contributed to growing indifference towards the health and well-being of northern Indigenous peoples. If, as David Goldberg writes, race is one of the 'central conceptual inventions of modernity', in the construction of the modern North it contributed directly to the creation of the 'structures of indifference', detailed by McCallum and Perry, that constitute health care as produced by settler colonialism.[46] In her work on Inuit health in the Canadian Arctic in the 1940s and after, Lisa Stevenson writes of the 'murderous' indifference of the bureaucratic state, 'always couched in terms of benevolence and care'.[47]

Ideas and experiences of isolation shaped northern health history in critical ways. Spatial isolation was, according to Alison Bashford and Carolyn Strange, a 'persistent strategy for the management of problem populations in liberal and non-liberal nations, in colonial and post-colonial states'.[48] Public health figured importantly in the reproduction of liberal democratic values as part of the rise of local settler governance in Canada's territorial north. Quarantine became a tool for epidemic management, and spatial control – including isolation and exclusion – was one way that racial constructions shaped infrastructures of care in the North, as we will see in Chapters 5 and 6. McCallum emphasizes that

[44] See Warwick Anderson, *Colonial Pathologies: American Tropical Medicine, Race, and Hygiene in the Philippines* (Durham, NC: Duke University Press, 2006); Alison Bashford and Carolyn Strange, 'Isolation and Exclusion in the Modern World: An Introductory Essay', in *Isolation: Places and Practices of Exclusion*, ed. C. Strange and A. Bashford, 1–18 (London: Routledge, 2003); David Arnold, *Colonizing the Body: State Medicine and Epidemic Disease in Nineteenth-Century India* (Berkeley: University of California Press, 1993).

[45] Jones, *Rationalizing Epidemics*, 13.

[46] As cited in Bashford and Strange, 'Isolation and Exclusion', 4–5; Mary Jane Logan McCallum and Adele Perry, *Structures of Indifference: An Indigenous Life and Death in a Canadian City* (Winnipeg: University of Manitoba Press, 2018).

[47] Lisa Stevenson, *Life beside Itself: Imagining Care in the Canadian Arctic* (Oakland: University of California Press, 2014), 73.

[48] Bashford and Strange, 'Isolation and Exclusion', 1.

segregation was a defining feature of Indigenous health, whether on reserves, in schools, or in hospitals, including the post-war Indian Hospital system erected to house tuberculosis patients and which served as an extension of the residential school system.

Isolation also worked in other ways in the history of northern epidemics. Geographic isolation was an essential part of how northern Indigenous populations were imagined in the mid-twentieth century as 'virgin soil'. By thus defining isolated populations, medical researchers and later historians articulated that these populations were *endangered* – as also understood by liberal democratic states that deemed it necessary to isolate people 'considered a danger to themselves or to others'.[49] In a 2005 article, McCallum deftly charted how ideas of Indigenous bodies as 'isolated' were constructed first through geographic location – at a distance and remote from – then through the ways that the idea of isolation was part of larger constructions of civilization and primitivism.[50] Indigenous peoples were 'isolated from' civilization, and this produced a set of paradoxes, namely that isolation had meant both greater health and greater susceptibility to disease. McCallum observes that this 'did not translate into a policy of non-interference . . . [or] a desire to recognize and protect the integrity of Native and Inuit cultures, resources, and territories'; instead, it served to justify greater, more intrusive colonial medical interventions that included segregation and isolation.[51] The language and construction of 'isolation' was most powerful in the North, where it resonated with and reinforced colonial ideas of northern environments as a frontier and wilderness that persist into the present.[52]

Dene, Gwich'in, Inuvialuit, Métis, and other northern Indigenous populations were *not* isolated, remote, or disconnected. People were profoundly connected with one another, forming rich, diverse, historic socio-ecological worlds, travelling long distances, and holding and sharing expertise across territories the Canadian state – with far, far less knowledge – would come to claim. In the latter half of the twentieth century, the conceptual isolation of northern populations served to disconnect Indigenous people in the service of

[49] Bashford and Strange, 'Isolation and Exclusion', 3; Lux, *Separate Beds*, 7–8.

[50] See Paige Raibmon, *Authentic Indians: Episodes of Encounter from the Late-Nineteenth-Century Northwest Coast* (Durham: Duke University Press, 2005), 7–9; Gail Bederman, *Manliness and Civilization: A Cultural History of Gender and Race in the United States, 1880–1917* (Chicago: University of Chicago Press, 1995); Bruce Mazlish, *Civilization and Its Contents* (Stanford: Stanford University Press, 2004).

[51] Mary Jane McCallum, 'This Last Frontier: "Isolation" and Aboriginal Health', *CBMH/BCHM* 22, no. 1 (2005): 103–20 (p. 108).

[52] Daniel Chester Forest Sims, 'Balloon Bombs, the Alaska Highway, and Influenza: Tsek'ehne Perspectives on the 1943 Flu Epidemic', *BC Studies* 203 (2019): 111–30 (p. 126); Shelagh D. Grant, 'Arctic Wilderness – And Other Mythologies', *Journal of Canadian Studies* 33, no. 2 (1998): 27–42; Sherrill Grace, *Canada and the Idea of North* (Montreal: McGill-Queen's University Press, 2001).

a model of 'island evolution' that provided an easy-to-understand interpretation of the effects of novel pathogens as part of colonization.[53] To say that this interpretation was 'easy to understand' presupposes a system of knowledge in which this model of disease made sense. This system of knowledge was the inheritance of settler colonialism in the Americas that witnessed the collapse and 'extinction' of Indigenous peoples, purported inhabitants of a virgin wilderness, while colonizers stood by helpless – refusing to help. These were stories that, although reformulated in the 1970s, had been told for over a century in northern North America, a narrative trajectory traced in the chapters to come.

This work builds on ecological approaches to disease, exemplified by Linda Nash, that consider pathogens and people as situated in place, in time, in seasons, in relations with other people, and in relations with other-than-human nature.[54] Chapter 2 opens in the 1860s with a scarlet fever pandemic. Tracing scarlet fever and influenza down river and out on to the land reveals emerging colonial ecologies in the late nineteenth century. Chapter 3 considers stories told about good and ill health, epidemics and mortality, in the late nineteenth century. These stories, told at the time and since, articulate colonial motifs and fictions. This chapter also addresses the early history of smallpox and vaccination in the North. Chapter 4 opens at the turn of the twentieth century in the midst of the gold rush, an event that brought tens of thousands of people to the confluence of the Klondike and Yukon rivers. These men, women, and children carried with them countless pathogens, creating outbreaks and epidemics from Alaska to the Arctic Coast to Lake Athabasca. Beginning in 1898, the Canadian state's desire to access northern resources led it to seek title through treaties to northern lands. In return, treaty commissioners made promises to provide for the health of northern Indigenous peoples. Chapter 5 considers these promises, made to enable an infrastructure of extraction, which produced anaemic infrastructures of care. Chapter 6 extends the spatial analysis illuminated by these infrastructures to the public health measures introduced in the Yukon and the Mackenzie district, primarily in response to smallpox. Colonial authorities used health tools to disproportionately control the movement of Indigenous people, part of the gravitational forces asserted by settler colonialism in the North. Chapters 7 and 8 examine the 1928 influenza epidemic in detail. First, the course of the epidemic is traced. This serves to better understand its relationship to previous influenza outbreaks and pandemics, as

[53] Radin, 'Latent Life', 494.

[54] Linda Nash, *Inescapable Ecologies: A History of Environment, Disease, and Knowledge* (Berkeley: University of California Press, 2006); J. D. Mathews, J. M. Chesson, J. M. McCaw, J. Mc Vernon, 'Understanding Influenza Transmission, Immunity and Pandemic Threats', *Influenza and Other Respiratory Viruses* 3, no. 4 (2009): 143–9. https://doi.org/10.1111/j.1750-2659.2009.00089.x.

well as to demonstrate the profound impact of this epidemic. Chapter 8 examines the growing significance of racial constructions in this period and how colonial racism shaped critical decisions and the transformative outcomes of the 1928 influenza. This chapter also assesses the importance to any interpretation of its effects of situating epidemic disease in time and place. Finally, while the narrative arc in this book moves from scarlet fever in 1860 to influenza in 1928, throughout this period tuberculosis was spreading, with greatest intensity in the 1920s and 1930s. The impacts of tuberculosis in changing relationships with the land and as part of the history of residential schooling are examined in detail in Chapter 9. The book closes with the 1940s influenza epidemics that were used in the construction of 'virgin soil epidemics', returning us to where we started.

Oral Histories and Archives

This research relies on oral histories conducted with past generations of Elders in northern Indigenous communities. Beginning in the 1970s, systematic efforts were made to record, transcribe, and disseminate the stories, expertise, and knowledge of Elders and communities across the North. These efforts took many different forms and were closely connected to political organizing around land claims through, for instance, the work of the Committee for the Original People's Entitlement (COPE), the first Inuvialuit political organization, and the Dene Mapping Project of the National Indian Brotherhood. In the past fifty years, northern Indigenous heritage organizations, including the Gwich'in Social and Cultural Institute – now the Gwich'in Tribal Council's Department of Culture and Heritage, the Dene Cultural Institute – now the Yamozha K'ue Society, and the Tr'ondëk Hwëch'in Heritage Department, among others, have become important repositories for oral histories and interviews recorded with several generations of Elders. There have also been countless smaller oral history projects conducted through schools and colleges, others funded by Parks Canada or the Yukon Heritage Branch, others in conjunction with environmental impact assessments for major development projects, that have recorded interviews with Elders and community members, chronicling memories and life experiences going back to the nineteenth century and before. The transcripts of the Mackenzie Valley Pipeline Inquiry represent a distinct contribution to the archive of lived experience and northern Indigenous history, expertise, and politics.

These existing oral histories are found in many different places and forms. Some of the transcripts used in this research were accessed through agreements with northern heritage organizations, specifically the Gwich'in Tribal Council's Department of Culture and Heritage, the Tr'ondëk Hwëch'in Heritage Department, and the Inuvialuit Cultural Centre. I also relied on historiographical interpretations, set forth in published works such as Dene Elder George Blondin's three books, and in the interviews themselves, that share clear interpretations about not only what happened but also its historical significance.[55] Other oral histories are held in archives, such as the Salt River Oral History collection and the Metis Heritage Association interviews in the Northwest Territories Archives in Yellowknife. Archives also hold individual interviews. Some transcripts were printed and bound or published and have found their way into library collections. Others have been used as the foundation for major published works, including the Vuntut Gwitchin First Nation's *People of the Lakes* and the Gwichya Gwich'in's *Gwichya Gwich'in Googwandak*.[56]

From these collected oral histories, I have been able to learn much more about northern history over the last 150 years than would otherwise have been possible. Interviews conducted beginning in the 1970s included the life experiences of men and women born in the last decades of the nineteenth century as well as those who came after. Some of these Elders, like Inuvialuk Felix Nuyaviak, were known for their stories about historical epidemics (Figure 1.1).[57] Moreover, as was described in the *People of the Lakes* collection, 'Elders knew stories from before their time'.[58] Sarah Abel, a Gwich'in Elder, emphasized, 'Even me, I never saw it but it was spoken about in front of me. That is what I talk about. This is how I know, but really it happened before them.'[59] When interviewed, Elders would often explicitly state how they knew about events that had happened before they were born or when they were very small, identifying who they had heard the story from. Elders thus established their authority to share a particular story. When Gwich'in Elder Hannah Netro shared a story about the smallpox epidemic at Rampart House in 1911, she noted that 'I heard a story that was passed down from my dad'. Netro also specified that she remembered the year it happened because that was when 'my sister Ellen Bruce was born in 1911'.[60]

[55] On George Blondin as a storyteller, see Richard Van Camp, foreword to *Trail of the Spirit: The Mysteries of Medicine Power Revealed*, by George Blondin (Edmonton: NeWest Press, 2006).

[56] To ensure proper attribution, I identified in the footnotes where I am quoting or referencing the words of an interviewee or Elder, whether the quotation appears in a published volume, interview transcript, or elsewhere. For example, in abbreviated form: Name of Interviewee in *Title of Published Collection*, page number. This is distinguished from where I am quoting the ideas or otherwise referencing the editors or compilers of a collection that includes extended oral histories or transcriptions. For example, Editors of Volume, *Title* etc. Likewise, I have not changed the original language or used [*sic*] when quoting from oral histories or interviews.

[57] Felix Nuyaviak (1892–1981): for his expertise on stories about disease, see Willie Gruben, interview with Florence Nasogaluak and Cathy Cockney, 26 Jul. 1996, Kitigaaryuit, tape 16B, transcript, in Cathy Cockney, *Kitigaaryuit Oral Traditions Research Project 1996* (Inuvik: Inuvialuit Social Development Program, 1997), 244.

[58] Vuntut Gwitchin First Nation and Smith, *People of the Lakes*, 65.

[59] Sarah Abel in *People of the Lakes*, 65.

[60] Hannah Netro interviewed by Shelagh Beairsto, in *Rampart House: Stories Told By Our Elders* (Old Crow: Te'sek Gehtr'oonatun Zzeh College, 1993), 14.

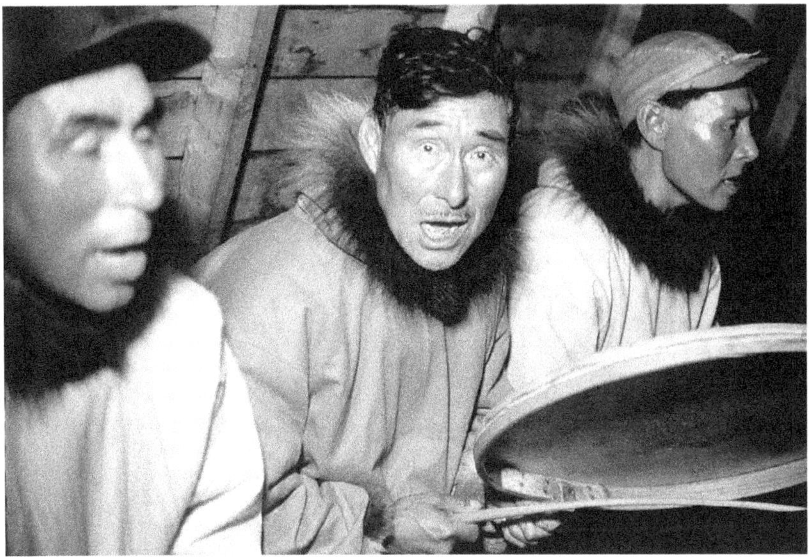

Figure 1.1 Felix Nuyaviak (1892–1981), in centre, drumming at Tuktoyaktuk. ©NWT Archives/Terrance Hunt fonds/N-1979–062: 0064.

Using oral histories collected in such diverse ways required constant attention to the contexts of production.[61] Stories and experiences, ways of framing expertise, as shared before the Berger Inquiry or in the context of environmental impact assessments, were very different from how stories and experiences were shared in community collections intended to teach young people about their heritage. There was anger apparent in the Berger transcripts, as witnesses gave testimony and challenged colonial authorities to take responsibility for their actions.[62] There was also, at times, language like that found in the opening quotation from Dene Elder Philip Simba, where he qualifies what he is saying by observing, 'because he is all alone now and no old person here to say that he is telling you the truth' (Figure 1.2). Simba was asserting the importance of collectively held knowledge and acknowledging that in colonial settings like the Inquiry, Indigenous expertise was not given its proper weight. The breadth of oral histories that have been collected over

[61] Malin Thor Tureby, 'To Hear with the Collection: The Contextualisation and Recontextualisation of Archived Interviews', *Oral History* 41, no. 2 (2013): 63–74.

[62] See also Sarah A. Nickel, *Assembling Unity: Indigenous Politics, Gender, and the Union of BC Indian Chiefs* (Vancouver: UBC Press, 2019), 39–41; Sara Ahmed, *Complaint!* (Durham, NC: Duke University Press, 2021), 13.

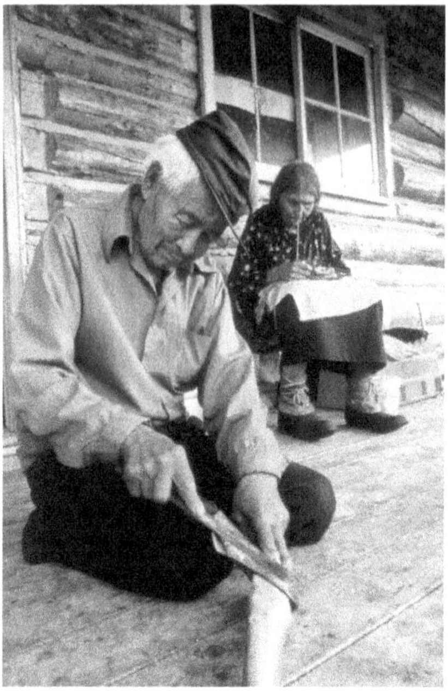

Figure 1.2 Philip Simba and Madelaine Simba, 1984. Photograph by Tessa Macintosh. NWT Archives/©GNWT. Dept. of Public Works and Services/ G-1995–001–5544.

the years meant that health and disease came up specifically in many transcripts. Major epidemics were the subject of focused attention.[63] Likewise, as interviews were often collected in conjunction with archaeological and heritage projects, this could involve visiting gravesites, which in turn prompted people to tell stories about sickness and epidemics.[64] That said, the experience of sickness itself can be a challenge to access through interviews and oral histories. As Gwich'in Elder Julienne Andre pointed out, 'I was sick many times and those parts I don't remember' (Figure 1.3).[65]

This book is foremost a history of colonialism, not a community-based history of epidemics. For those interested in the latter, these can be found in many of the sources I have referenced here, especially the larger comprehensive collections.

[63] For example, 'Influenza Epidemic, July 1928', in *That's the Way We Lived. An Oral History of the Fort Resolution Elders* (Yellowknife: Northwest Territories Culture and Communications, 1987), 75–8.

[64] For example, Yukon Territory, Heritage Branch, *Fort Selkirk Elders Oral History Project* (Whitehorse: Yukon Heritage Branch, 1987).

[65] Julienne Andre in *Gwichya Gwich'in Googwandak*, 282.

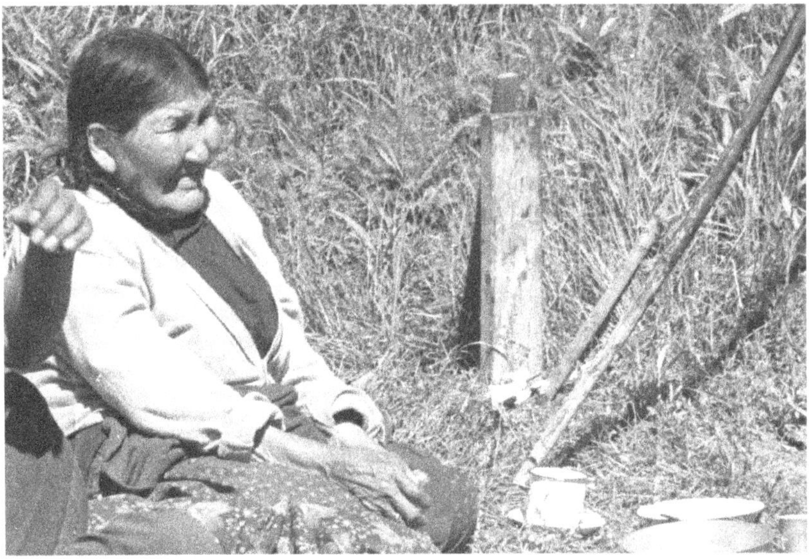

Figure 1.3 Julienne Andre at fish camp at Tree River, July 1978. Photograph by James Jerome. ©NWT Archives/James Jerome/N-1987–017: 0864.

This book relies as well on government, missionary, and fur-trade archival records used to understand both what happened and how different people, especially those with power, responded to epidemic disease. Access to some archival records was contingent on research agreements that required me to ensure the anonymity of those whose personal health information was revealed. These restrictions informed my use of pseudonyms or the omission of names altogether in places throughout this book. The few instances where I used pseudonyms, I have used only first names (e.g. 'Alex', 'Catherine'), and these are clearly identified.

Access restrictions applied most significantly to the burial registers used to construct a cause of death database, which provided quantitative evidence supporting the arguments laid out here. This database and its interpretation are discussed in the Appendix. The database includes over 7,000 records of death from 1860 to 1970 and was used to trace the regional extent of outbreaks, to assess the scale and impacts of epidemics, to understand the broad contours of health, sickness, and medicine, and to identify smaller outbreaks that were not always apparent in other materials. That said, while this database turns lives into statistics, I have throughout this book subordinated data to story, using numbers to better understand the dynamics of disease but not to obscure experience. The records in the database are all anonymized. Each was entered by me, usually in an archive, as for most of the registers I was not permitted to make copies that could be removed from the premises.[66] In this process, I encountered thousands of men, women, and children in the context of their passing. I found this experience deeply moving. In the course of working on this book, I gave birth to two premature babies, both of whom spent their first weeks of life in neonatal intensive care units, likely surviving only because of medical interventions that our family was fortunate to be able to access. It was impossible for me to read and record the deaths of premature infants from the burial registers with detachment, and more than once I found myself in tears. I would like those reading this book to know that I have treated all these records, and the lives they represent, with the utmost respect and care throughout the process of research and interpretation.

This also speaks to one last methodological issue in weighing the significance of northern history. Northern populations are small. Collectively, present-day populations of the Northwest Territories and the Yukon are less than 100,000 people. In the period studied in this book, the total population was in the tens of thousands, at most. In some ways, these small numbers work against circumpolar peoples from the perspective of global historical significance. Throughout this book, the numbers who died in epidemics, even the largest epidemics, are relatively small – much, much less than, say, the 40,000 deaths from COVID-19 in Canada in its first two years. Noted Inuit leader and activist Siila Watt-Cloutier wrote about the issue of numbers, drawing from her experiences working to limit persistent organic pollutants and their toxic effects at high latitudes:

> I remember quite clearly a person from The Malaria Project suggesting, in his presentation, that if we continued with the goal of eliminating POPs, including DDT, we would be bringing death to many thousands and perhaps millions of people. He used images of jumbo jets filled with people to show the numbers that would die each year if DDT were not available to help fight malaria. As I was listening to this presentation I started to question how 150,000 Inuit could compete with these stark figures of potential deaths. Our team, which included Shirley Adamson of the Yukon First Nations, had to develop a strategy to circumvent seeing this solely in terms of numbers; if numbers were going to be part of the equation the Inuit and Aboriginal peoples of the circumpolar world would surely lose.[67]

Watt-Cloutier was speaking to the larger moral issue in our contemporary world of what is happening to small communities and small societies, not

[66] A small number of records were drawn from publicly accessible registers, for example the Dawson City Mortuary Records 1898–1938, www.alaskaweb.org/dawmort/c_d.html.

[67] Sheila [Siila] Watt-Cloutier, 'The Inuit Journey towards a POPs-Free World', in *Northern Lights Against POPs: Combatting Threats in the Arctic*, ed. Terry Fenge, Inuit Circumpolar Conference, David Leonard Downie (Montreal: McGill-Queen's University Press, 2003), 259–60.

just in the northern villages destabilized by melting permafrost and generations of colonial trauma, but also island nations facing the deluges and hurricanes of a heating earth. This book offers an exploration of how history is made, not just at the centres of population and power, but in the countless small communities, in the hamlets and villages, and among families and camps out on the land, through the mountains, along the coast, and on the banks of rivers.

2 When Scarlet Fever Came to This Country

> And after that, through Archdeacon McDonald, we know when what they call scarlet fever came to [this] country. Moses Tizya, 11 August 1977[1]

In 1985, Effie Linklater and Lee Sax recorded the story of Ttssietla, a Gwich'in man who converted to Christianity in the 1860s.[2] Ttssietla met Robert McDonald, an Anglican missionary and Linklater's grandfather, on the banks of Teetł'it Gwinjik (the Peel River) and was moved by the interaction; Ttssietla returned and spent two months with McDonald before going home to his people. That winter, Ttssietla and his wife Bitsikotrig travelled upriver to their camps in the mountains. Soon after, their daughter was born. 'Ttssietla was so happy. He got out his drum and spent all night chanting his spirit song', the story went. Time passed, spring came, and there was plenty of meat and goose eggs.

> Then it came, like a black cloud of evil spreading over the land. People suddenly became ill, seized by something that no one had seen before, and within a few days were dead. Ttssietla spent day after day with his drum, singing, entreating the spirits to come to the aid of his people, but all to no avail. He heard stories of the same thing happening in other camps. Then the deadly thing came upon his child. Ttssietla watched in agony as the deep cough wracked her small body. The child looked entreatingly at her father, even as the light faded from her eyes. His child was dead.[3]

Ttssietla's infant daughter died that year of scarlet fever, part of a mid-nineteenth-century pandemic that brought sickness and death to families in Western Europe, the United States, and across the lands that were becoming Canada. The same year that the fever descended upon the Peel River, an article appeared in *The Lancet* describing this disease as it appeared in cities and towns: 'The deadliest of fevers ... often pestilential in its progress, sparing neither the young nor the old, but chiefly infecting the very young, and not unfrequently [*sic*] sweeping off the whole of the children of a family – its

[1] Moses Tizya in Vuntut Gwitchin First Nation and Smith, *People of the Lakes*, 91.
[2] Lee Sax and Effie Linklater, *Gikhyi: One Who Speaks the Word of God* (Whitehorse: Diocese of Yukon, 1990), v–vi.
[3] Sax and Linklater, *Gikhyi*, 7–8.

irruption into a household is regarded with dismay.'[4] Scarlet fever was called a disease of childhood, one in a gauntlet of infections run by children born in crowded cities. As a disease of childhood, scarlet fever was particularly deadly in the mid-nineteenth century. In these years, scarlet fever significantly 'outweighed diphtheria, measles, and whooping cough as causes of mortality for those under 15 years of age'.[5] Scarlet fever tied metropolitan centres – London, Montreal, Saint Petersburg – to the lands that bordered the Mackenzie and Yukon rivers and their tributaries. There were shared experiences of sickness and sorrow that spanned the geographical and cultural divides that made this space.

Colonialism created an axis along which the experiences and effects of scarlet fever in the mid-nineteenth century diverged. The colonial context shaped where scarlet fever travelled in 1865–6 and how people dealt with what was for many of them a new disease, amid larger economic, social, and cultural upheaval. In Linklater and Sax's telling, the death of his daughter shaped Ttssietla's path to religious conversion. In his grief, Ttssietla confronted McDonald, rejecting the solace and comfort the missionary offered. But after a year had passed, Ttssietla and Bitsikotrig went again to see McDonald, now to be baptized John and Alice. Thereafter, John Ttssietla became an important Anglican leader among the Gwich'in.[6]

At the time, the 1865–6 scarlet fever was perceived as the most significant nineteenth-century epidemic, with effects from Fort Chipewyan on Lake Athabasca to Peel River Post in the delta, east to Fort Anderson and west to Fort Yukon. Such a momentous event figured prominently in fur-trade and missionary records. Linklater and Sax's story about Ttssietla, written down and published in 1990, was rooted in the oral history of the Gwich'in. While there are older stories about 'epidemics' or 'sickness', the scarlet fever is the first major epidemic from which unambiguous oral histories have endured into the present. The years from 1865 to 1868 also saw seasonal influenza outbreaks. One trailed after scarlet fever in the autumn of 1865 and into the winter of 1866. The other arrived in the region with the boat crews in 1867, causing sickness and deaths into 1868. It is possible with this syndemic to trace scarlet fever with its distinctive rash separately from influenza, particularly from the second influenza, which returned on its own. However, in considering the historical impacts of ill health in the latter half of the 1860s, the interaction of these two diseases had devastating consequences, and this chapter addresses both. We will follow scarlet fever and influenza as they moved down rivers, through trade posts, and into camps, to illuminate how local relations with people and

4 'The Limitation of Scarlet Fever', *The Lancet* (4 Feb. 1865), 129.

5 Andrew Cliff, Peter Haggett, and Matthew Smallman-Raynor, *World Atlas of Epidemic Diseases* (London: Arnold, 2004), 75–7.

6 Sax and Linklater, *Gikhyi*, vi.

the land shaped this pandemic. This chapter conveys the scale of this sickness through estimates of deaths and the geographic extent of disease spread. The chapter then assesses the effects of ill health and mortality and the loss of adults and children on the larger processes of colonial change underway in the nineteenth century.

Sickness before 1860

Traders, explorers, and missionaries carried many different pathogens along Nagwichoonjik, Chu kon' dëk, and their tributaries in the early nineteenth century. Details of outbreaks and epidemics are more accessible after 1840, when missionaries began writing letters and sharing their experiences with audiences in Canada, Europe, and beyond. Between 1800 and 1860, several outbreaks of introduced infectious disease were linked to epidemics in more distant regions. Fur traders and John Franklin described an outbreak of measles and whooping cough in 1819–20 that was widespread across the Athabasca District.[7] In 1827 and 1828, whooping cough, which had been prevalent in the northern plains, was also reported in Fort Chipewyan and at Fort Simpson on Dehcho.[8] Influenza was a problem from the Canadas to the Petit Nord from 1835 to 1838.[9] Richard King, surgeon and naturalist with George Back's expedition to the Great Fish River from 1833 to 1835, reported on the influenza at Rapid River Fort and in the Athabasca District.[10] Patricia McCormack detailed its impacts in Fort Chipewyan in 1835–6.[11] Fur-trade records further indicated a 'fatal disease that rages' that reached along the Mackenzie River as far north as the Dene on Great Bear Lake.[12] Then in 1846, measles was reported from Fort Chipewyan and around Great Slave Lake, as well as a sickness along the Peel River in 1846–7.[13] Other places in the North experienced similar

7 Decker, 'Depopulation', 390; Hackett, *Remarkable Sickness*, ch. 7.

8 Abel, *Drum Songs*, 110; Shepherd Krech III, 'The Influence of Disease and the Fur Trade on Arctic Drainage Lowlands Dene, 1800–1850', *Journal of Anthropological Research* 39, no. 1 (1983): 123–46 (p. 128); Decker, 'Depopulation', 391.

9 Arthur J. Ray, 'Diffusion of Diseases in the Western Interior of Canada, 1830–1850', *Geographical Review* 66, no. 2 (1976), 139–57 (p. 144); Hackett, *Remarkable Sickness*, 196. Influenza pandemic in Canada more broadly, J. J. Heagerty, 'Influenza Epidemic of 1918', in RG 29, vol. 1192, file 311-J2-2, part 1, LAC.

10 Richard King, *Narrative of a Journey to the Shores of the Arctic Ocean in 1833, 1834 and 1835, under the Command of Capt. Back, R.N.* (London: R. Bentley, 1836), 219–20. For more on King, see Efram Sera-Shiar, 'Civilizing the Natives: Richard King and His Ethnographic Writings on Indigenous Northerners', in *Made Modern: Science and Technology in Canadian History*, ed. E. Jones-Imhotep and T. Adcock, 39–59 (Vancouver: UBC Press, 2018).

11 McCormack, 'Influenza Epidemic', 33–42.

12 Quotation from Krech, 'Influence of Disease', 128.

13 Abel, *Drum Songs*, 110; Krech, 'Influence of Disease', 129; Shepard Krech, III, 'Disease, Starvation, and Northern Athapaskan Social Organization', *American Ethnologist* 5 (1978): 710–32 (p. 714).

epidemics this same year, including influenza, measles, and dysentery in the Petit Nord and influenza or possibly measles along the north-west coast of Hudson Bay.[14] Epidemics bound people across the north together, connected by the river systems that were the highways of the fur trade.

There were also outbreaks that were locally significant, as they spread between communities and camps, but which cannot be connected to regional epidemics or wider pandemics. Between 1805 and 1807, a sickness was recorded by traders on the Liard River and at the Fort of the Forks.[15] In this same period a 'sickness in the Animal species' was reported by Willard Ferdinand Wentzel at the Forks, and he thought that it spread to people who consumed the flesh of dead animals.[16] In 1825, reports of sickness appeared at Fort Resolution, Tulita, and Fort Good Hope. Two years later, K'áhshó Got'ı̨nę stayed away from Fort Good Hope as they 'did not want to go close to an area where "so many" of their relatives had died'.[17] There was a significant outbreak of influenza that spread along Dehcho to the Peel River in the early 1850s.[18] Émile Petitot, in writings published after the fact, described 'a strange epidemic sickness' that became known as the *Mal du Fort Rae*, and which by 1862 had left 788 survivors from a population of 1,200 Tłı̨chǫ.[19] From other Oblate records, illness and many deaths prevailed not only at Fort Rae but also at Fond du Lac and as far north as Fort Good Hope.[20] While Petitot had his own reasons for highlighting this epidemic, his decision to identify it as a northern epidemic and to link it to Nishì or Old Fort Rae, with a name that endures in local memory, highlights the local and regional impact of those outbreaks that did not have wide geographic repercussions.

It is possible that *Streptococcus pyogenes* spread north before 1860: there are reports of sore throats and general 'sickness' in records and oral histories, the cause of which remains unknown, but no specific reports of scarlet fever. Along Nagwichoonjik, the Porcupine River, and the Peel River, traders, missionaries, and Indigenous peoples were all vulnerable to infection – particularly those children and adults who had no previous experience with the disease. We see then the significance in Moses Tizya's observation that it was at this time that scarlet fever 'came to this country'.

14 Hackett, *Remarkable Sickness*, ch. 9; Renée Fossett, *In Order to Live Untroubled: Inuit of the Central Arctic 1550–1940* (Winnipeg: University of Manitoba Press, 2001), 159.

15 Lloyd Keith, ed., *North of Athabasca: Slave Lake and Mackenzie River Documents of the North West Company, 1800–1821* (Montreal: McGill-Queen's University Press, 2001), 274, 297–8, 321.

16 Keith, *North of Athabasca*, 302.

17 Krech, 'Influence of Disease', 128; Krech, 'Disease, Starvation', 713.

18 Abel, *Drum Songs*, 110; Krech, 'Disease, Starvation', 714.

19 Émile Petitot, *Autour du Grand Lac des Esclaves* (Paris: Albert Savine, 1891), 189. All references to the *Mal du Fort Rae* that I located refer back to the Petitot volume. All translations from French sources by author.

20 McCarthy, *Great River*, 197.

Although scarlet fever may have been a novel pathogen, by the mid-nineteenth century Indigenous northerners had enough experience with outbreaks and epidemics to have arrived at their own measures to mitigate the spread of infectious diseases. Most effective and commonly used were when families and bands disrupted their seasonal rounds to avoid the trade posts and mission stations from which diseases spread.[21] People with medicine powers advised their kin and communities against shaking hands with missionaries. This advice was reported by missionaries to illustrate the backwardness of 'medicine men' but, when followed, would have helped to disrupt disease transmission.[22] Yet these measures and the therapies offered by Indigenous healers, as well as new medicines brought by fur traders and missionaries, would not have sufficed to control scarlet fever in the 1860s.

Scarlet Fever

In June of 1862, two men took their first trip with the Hudson's Bay Company boats from Red River to Fort Chipewyan. They travelled with a shared purpose: both were missionaries en route to the Mackenzie district. That common ground aside, two men could hardly be more different. One was the Roman Catholic Oblate Father Émile Petitot. He would be based in the Mackenzie district for sixteen years, until 1878, when he was transferred south to the diocese of St Albert. By 1884, Petitot had returned permanently to France. The other, Anglican Reverend Robert McDonald, would remain in the region for forty-three years. Their encounter on the barge was cordial. Petitot described McDonald as a gentleman and an 'excellent travelling companion'.[23] At Great Slave Lake, the missionaries parted ways. Petitot proceeded to Fort Providence, while McDonald continued down the Mackenzie.[24]

Petitot was twenty-four years old. Born and educated in Marseilles, France, where his father was a clockmaker, Émile joined the Oblates in 1860. In the North, Petitot was stationed at Fort Providence, Fort Resolution, and Fort Good Hope, staying longest at the last place, where he helped to construct and decorate the chapel. From this posting, Petitot travelled several times eastwards to K'áhbamį̀túé (Colville Lake) and the Sahtú (Great Bear Lake) region, and north to Fort Anderson. Petitot is best remembered for his artistic contribution at Fort Good Hope, as well as for his voluminous and detailed writings on

[21] Diary [hereafter McDonald Diary], 5 Jun. 1866, Robert McDonald Fonds, MSS 195–MSS 196 (85/97), YA; also Abel, *Drum Songs*, 110; McCormack, 'Influenza Epidemic', 41.

[22] 'The Youcon Mission', *The Church Missionary Intelligencer* 4 (London: Church Missionary Society, 1868): 100–10 (p. 106).

[23] Robert Choquette, *The Oblate Assault on Canada's Northwest* (Ottawa: University of Ottawa Press, 1995), 60.

[24] McDonald Diary, 17 Jul. and 2 Aug. 1862.

Dene, Gwich'in, and Inuvialuit. He authored books and manuscripts and published letters that have been mined by historians, anthropologists, and researchers from northern communities interested in the nineteenth-century North. And yet Petitot's superiors moved him back and forth between these posts because of repeated sexual relationships with young Indigenous men and episodes of violence.[25] Robert Choquette has addressed Petitot's career in detail, describing the father as a 'nightmare' for his Oblate colleagues.[26] In letters to his superiors, Petitot detailed how many days he spent on snowshoes, alongside the number of people he baptized and whose marriages he solemnized, demonstrating that, for him at least, travel was as important as proselytizing (Figure 2.1).[27] The extreme elements of his personality, including how Petitot projected his internal torment over his desires onto the Indigenous people among whom he lived and worked, his mental illness, and the fact that his most detailed writings have survived only in published form, while his

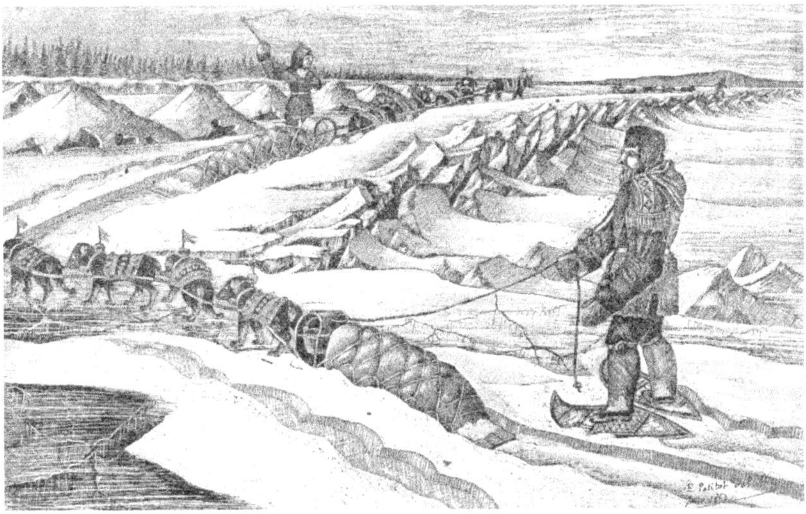

Figure 2.1 Émile Petitot's preferred mode of self-presentation. Missionaries travelling on Great Slave Lake. Petitot, *Autour*, plate 2.

[25] See Choquette, *Oblate Assault*, 59–66; John S. Moir, 'Petitot, Émile', *Dictionary of Canadian Biography* (1998), www.biographi.ca/en/bio/petitot_emile_14E.html.

[26] Choquette, *Oblate Assault*, 59.

[27] Émile Petitot to T. R. P. Supérieur Général, Good Hope, 15 Jan. 1866, *Missions de la Congrégation des Missionnaires Oblats de Marie Immaculée*, vol. 7 (Paris: Hennuyer, 1868), 291.

original diaries have not endured, complicate the contribution of his perspective to northern history.

Robert McDonald continued on down the Mackenzie River in August of 1862, past Fort Providence, Fort Simpson, and Fort Good Hope, and then moving to the Peel and Yukon rivers onwards to his posting at Fort Yukon, which he reached on 23 September. At thirty-three years of age, McDonald was a little older than Petitot (Figure 2.2). Born in the Red River settlement, his father, Neil, was a retired HBC employee and his mother, Anne, the daughter of a Scots-born North West Company employee and an Anishinaabe woman. McDonald was fluent in Anishinaabemowin and French but had been educated 'to identify himself with the white, English-speaking, Protestant element of the Red River establishment'.[28] While we might describe McDonald as Métis, he

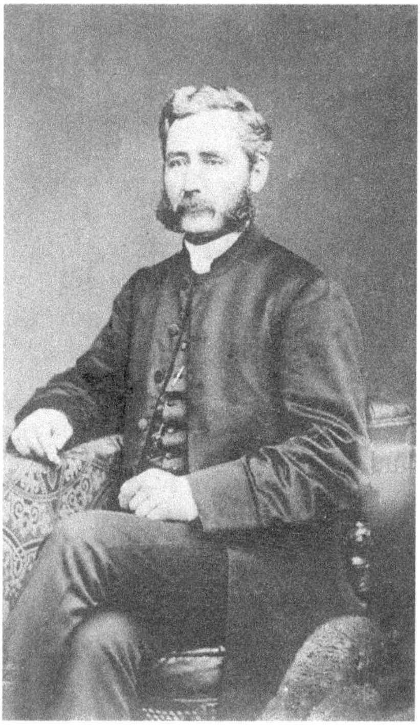

Figure 2.2 Robert McDonald as a young man. The General Synod Archives, Anglican Church of Canada.

[28] Frank A. Peake, 'Robert McDonald (1829–1913): The Great Unknown Missionary of the Northwest', *Journal of the Canadian Church Historical Society* 17, no. 3 (1975): 54–72 (p. 56).

was silent about his own identity. However, he was perceived, according to historian Frank Peake, as 'a curious mixture' by the Church Missionary Society. Letters from colleagues and superiors refer at times to 'European missionaries and Archdeacon McDonald'. McDonald was passed over for promotion to bishop, notwithstanding his successes as a missionary in the North, on account of his mixed heritage.[29] Historian Myra Rutherdale argued that his Métis heritage gave McDonald more faith in Indigenous believers as potential recruits to the ministry than some of his superiors.[30] Equally if not more important was McDonald's marriage to Julia Kutug (Gepik or Ooghaii in her own language), a Teetł'it Gwich'in woman.[31] Together, they translated the Bible, prayer and hymn books, and other religious writings into Dagoo and raised nine children.[32] Marriage with local peoples, while relatively common in the fur trade, was rare amongst missionaries in this period – Anglicans often came north with their wives, and the Oblates were celibate. McDonald was based at Fort Yukon until 1872. When the boundary with the United States was enforced, he moved to Rampart House and then Fort McPherson. McDonald lived in McPherson for another thirty years, always travelling widely throughout the Peel River watershed and along the Yukon River. After spending half of his long life in the North, McDonald left his family behind when he returned to Winnipeg in 1905 to live out his final years.

Petitot troubled his superiors with his volatile behaviour and because he valued exploration as much as, if not more than, proselytizing. McDonald was a steady, hard-working, well-respected man who left a long legacy for the Anglican Church in the northern Yukon and Mackenzie delta. Their role in the colonial project saw both men engage in scientific work, although Petitot was by far the more enthusiastic. Yet McDonald, like Petitot and many fur traders, gathered fossils and sent biological samples and Gwich'in cultural objects to the Smithsonian.[33] Their principal goal was to convert northern Indigenous peoples, to persuade them to abandon their pre-existing beliefs and practices that were incompatible with Christianity, and to minister to their bodies as well as their souls. Attention to Indigenous bodies made both Petitot and McDonald important recorders of health and significant participants in the nineteenth-century history of disease.

29 Cited in Peake, 'McDonald', 56. 30 Rutherdale, *Women and the White Man's God*, 144.

31 Leslie McCartney and Gwich'in Tribal Council, *Our Whole Gwich'in Way of Life Has Changed = Gwich'in K'yuu Gwiidandài Tthak Ejuk Gòonlih: Stories from the People of the Land* (Edmonton: Polynya Press, 2020), xxxix.

32 See Craig Mishler, 'Missionaries in Collision: Anglicans and Oblates among the Gwich'in, 1861–65', *Arctic* 43, no. 2 (1990): 121–6 (p. 125); Patrick Moore, 'Archdeacon Robert McDonald and Gwich'in Literacy', *Anthropological Linguistics* 49, no. 1 (2007): 27–53.

33 McDonald Diary, 20 Jul. 1863 and 17 Jul. 1865. See also Ted Binnema, *Enlightened Zeal: The Hudson's Bay Company and Scientific Networks, 1670–1870* (Toronto: University of Toronto Press, 2014).

McDonald and Petitot crossed paths more than once. Three years after their shared journey, McDonald arrived at Fort Good Hope in early September in a party of four boats. Petitot was based at the mission but made no mention of his Anglican counterpart. Petitot was most interested in the arrival of his bishop, Henri Faraud. Petitot also described twenty Dene men lying in the boats, sick with scarlet fever.[34]

Scarlet fever or scarlatina is an acute infectious disease caused by Group A *Streptococcus pyogenes* bacteria. Infection by *S. pyogenes* produces toxins to which the body responds in different ways: as strep throat, impetigo, erysipelas, puerperal sepsis, tonsillitis, and middle ear infections and, more severely, necrotizing fasciitis and rheumatic fever, all in addition to scarlet fever. The condition of scarlet fever refers to a red rash with the texture of sandpaper that appears across the body – on the neck, chest, elbow, groin, and inner thighs – and which is accompanied by a swollen and bumpy 'strawberry' or 'raspberry' tongue. Before the rash appears, people develop a sore throat, high fever, and swollen glands. The rash can last for several days, and infection with scarlet fever can lead to severe complications and death. The many different serotypes of *S. pyogenes* bacteria (over 150) mean that, while infection with one strain confers immunity against the toxins produced by future infection from that same strain, it does not confer immunity against future infection by different strains.[35] Not as infectious as measles, scarlet fever caused disproportionate mortality among those aged two to fifteen and was particularly frightful for how it could tear through the children in a family. While a childhood disease in the sense that children were more vulnerable to death, even those who survived were not necessarily well protected as adults against future infection. Adults could also suffer serious consequences from the infection, even death, although unlike polio or measles they were not at higher risk of severe or fatal outcomes. The severity of the infection and the likelihood of death reflected the virulence of the bacteria in a given outbreak, the synergistic effects of *S. pyogenes* bacteria with another viral or bacterial infection, and the body's ability to mount an effective immune response.[36]

Along with plague and cholera, scarlet fever is an 'epidemic-prone bacterial infection', in contrast to viral infections (smallpox, influenza, and measles) or bacterial infections that rarely lead to outbreaks.[37] We can infer a long-standing

[34] Émile Petitot, *Quinze ans sous le Cercle Polaire: Mackenzie, Anderson, Youkon* (Paris: E. Dentu, 1889), 158.

[35] Manisha Pandey, Victoria Ozberk, Ainslie Calcutt, et al., 'Streptococcal Immunity Is Constrained by Lack of Immunological Memory Following a Single Episode of Pyoderma', *PLOS Pathogens* 12, no. 12 (Dec. 2016), http://doi.org/10.1371/journal.ppat.1006122.

[36] On scarlet fever and influenza, see Elizabeth M. Perks and Richard T. Mayon-White, 'The Incidence of Scarlet Fever', *Journal of Hygiene* 91 (1983): 203–9.

[37] Samson S. Y. Wong and Kwok-Yung Yuen, '*Streptococcus pyogenes* and Re-emergence of Scarlet Fever as a Public Health Problem', *Emerging Microbes and Infections* 1, no. 7 (Jul. 2012), http://doi.org/10.1038/emi.2012.9.

relationship between *S. pyogenes* and human beings given the high number of different infectious serotypes – a product of long co-evolution. However, accurate diagnoses of scarlet fever in the historical record are complicated by the challenge of distinguishing one rash-causing disease from another.[38] The first recorded epidemic dates only to 1553 in Palermo, Italy, with major, irregular outbreaks appearing more frequently in Europe and the Americas in the seventeenth and eighteenth centuries. There were long intervals between epidemics, and by the late eighteenth century, the disease appeared to have declined in virulence. This milder phase did not last. After 1840, outbreaks of scarlet fever reappeared with such a vengeance that the period from 1825 to 1885 was characterized by a global pandemic of scarlet fever, with its peak in the 1860s. In 1843, a severe epidemic of scarlet fever spread through Rupert's Land. Arthur Ray described this as the first occurrence 'for at least a generation', which caused significant loss of life among both Indigenous people and Europeans, with the highest mortality among children.[39] Since the late nineteenth century, scarlet fever has declined significantly in virulence, and its treatment with antibiotics for several decades has shaped its later evolutionary history.

Historians connected the northern scarlet fever epidemic in the 1860s with epidemics elsewhere.[40] But when Petitot reflected on the cause of the disease, he believed that a 'slow and rainy autumn' had encouraged its spread. The cold, dry winter, which would have destroyed 'the putrid microbes', was delayed that year.[41] Petitot was summarizing prevailing nineteenth-century ideas about the relationships between environment, climate, and germs in causing sickness.[42] Contrary to Petitot's speculation, the *S. pyogenes* bacteria – like the influenza virus – thrives in colder weather. Historically, scarlet fever has caused more deaths in winter, which represents a combination of more cases of the disease and greater susceptibility to its effects on the body in those months.[43] In nineteenth-century Europe, dry conditions even more so than

[38] Alan R. Katz and David M. Morens, 'Severe Streptococcal Infections in Historical Perspective', *Clinical Infectious Diseases* 14 (1992): 298–307 (p. 299).

[39] Ray, 'Diffusion', 150–1.

[40] Abel, *Drum Songs*, 149–50; Linea Sundstrom, 'Smallpox Used Them Up: References to Epidemic Disease in Northern Plains Winter Counts, 1714–1920', *Ethnohistory* 44, no. 2 (1997): 305–43 (table 1, p. 309).

[41] Petitot, *Quinze ans*, 165.

[42] Conevery Bolton Valenčius, *The Health of the Country: How Americans Understood Themselves and Their Land* (New York: Basic Books, 2002); Gregg Mitman, 'In Search of Health: Landscape and Disease in American Environmental History', *Environmental History* 10, no. 2 (2005): 184–210.

[43] Peter R. Martin and E. Arne Høiby, 'Streptococcal Serogroup A Epidemic in Norway 1987–1988', *Scandinavian Journal of Infectious Diseases* 22 (1990): 421–9; Joseph MacLean Parish, 'An Analysis of the 1875–1877 Scarlet Fever Epidemic of Cape Breton Island, Nova Scotia', PhD diss., University of Missouri–Columbia, 2004, 75.

cold temperatures correlated with scarlet fever mortality.[44] This connection, in light of the warmer, wetter conditions in 1865, suggests that the role of climate in this epidemic was secondary. Most important was the virulence of the *S. pyogenes* strain that arrived in the 1860s; this strain had caused higher mortality even in those places where the bacteria was long established.

Beyond the virulence of the scarlet fever that year, there were also the synergistic effects of other pathogens circulating at that time. William Hardisty, Chief Trader for the Mackenzie River District, wrote to Strachan Jones, the clerk at Fort Rae, to advise additional caution against the spread of scarlet fever with that autumn's boats. Hardisty observed that 'the Indians of Fort Rae being already infected with disease, the fever is more likely to be communicated to them than to those who are comparatively healthy'.[45] Hardisty here was referring to the *Mal du Fort Rae*, the disease that had caused hundreds of deaths among the Tłı̨chǫ in the preceding five years. He recognized the danger of synergistic effects that arose when the body confronted more than one pathogen at a time. Beyond Nishì, seasonal influenza contributed to mortality in 1865–6. Influenza was a relatively common visitor along the Mackenzie, Yukon, and tributary rivers and the coast. Petitot had described influenza at Fort McPherson and among the Inuvialuit in the delta as recently as 1864.[46] The majority of the crews and some of the passengers on the boats that arrived in Fort Good Hope in September were reported sick with scarlet fever *and* influenza.[47] People fell sick with influenza in the autumn and winter of 1865–6, even as the scarlet fever subsided.

The Course of the Epidemic

At Fort Simpson in early September 1865, Robert McDonald and Henri Faraud prepared to board the HBC boats while William Hardisty lay in bed, 'quite prostrated' by scarlet fever.[48] Within a month, thirty people died at Fort Simpson.[49] Scarlet fever arrived in Fort Good Hope with the boats and, attesting to the contagiousness of the outbreak, within two days 'at least half' of those in the community had fallen ill, including the HBC servants.[50] Jean Séguin, the other Oblate missionary stationed at Good Hope, omitted any mention of his own illness at this time, an omission Hardisty made as well.

[44] Susan Scott and Christopher J. Duncan, *Human Demography and Disease* (Cambridge: Cambridge University Press, 1998), 311.

[45] William Hardisty to Strachan Jones, 28 Nov. 1865, B.200/b/35, fo. 62b–62c, HBCA.

[46] R. P. Petitot to J. Fabre, Notre-Dame de Bonne-Espérance, 11 Nov. 1864, *Missions de la Congrégation*, vol. 6, 476; McCarthy, *Great River*, 120.

[47] Sax and Linklater, *Gikhyi*, 60; McDonald Diary, 2 Sept. 1865.

[48] McDonald Diary, 2 Sept. 1865.

[49] W. L. Hardisty to W. J. McLean, 29 Sept. 1865, B.200/b/35, fo.61a, HBCA.

[50] Jean Séguin to mother and sister, 1 Jun. 1866, 71.220 / 7343, OMI, PAA.

That 'whites' fell ill was observed by Petitot, who suggested their sickness spread fear among the community as a whole.[51] By the next spring, almost 100 people had died at Fort Good Hope, predominantly Dene, but also Gwich'in and Nahanni.[52] The epidemic spread eastwards, killing as many as sixty Sahtu Dene.

S. pyogenes travelled rapidly and over long distances with the HBC boats (Map 2.1). Dënesųłıné, Gwich'in, Métis, and Dene men who made up the boat crews were among the first to fall ill; it was 'the men in the brigade' who unintentionally brought the disease from Portage La Loche home to families in Fort Chipewyan in August 1865, from whence it departed and moved down-river. McDonald spent the winter at Fort Yukon, travelling to LaPierre's House, Peel River Post, as well as to smaller camps out on the land. Illness among his companions disrupted his travels. McDonald had difficulty finding men 'to carry packages over to LaPierre's House for me'. One man turned back when he fell ill.[53] More than once, McDonald noted they had to camp after only a few hours on account of illness among the boat crews.[54] Crews, passengers, and even trade goods carried the bacteria.[55] But the impact on the crews, because of the effects on trade, raised serious concerns. Hardisty wondered whether the boats might not reach Fort Yukon before freeze-up, keeping scarlet fever from that place. He was mistaken.[56] However, the disruption that the scarlet fever introduced to the HBC's normal operations kept the disease from Fort Halkett, near the confluence of the Smith and Liard rivers. Sickness at Fort aux Liards meant that a crew could not be raised to carry the annual outfit to Fort Halkett. With no boat sent, scarlet fever never reached Fort Halkett and the families who traded there. With the exception of two men who were at Fort aux Liards when the scarlet fever passed through that place, the forty-three families that made up 'the Halkett branch of the [Tsek'ehne] tribe' escaped the epidemic.[57]

In the weeks that followed the first appearance of scarlet fever, McDonald spent much of his time visiting with the sick, offering prayers and medicine. This was along with the regular coming and going of hunters and families. In September and early October 1865, McDonald travelled to Fort Good Hope, Tsiigehtchic, Fort McPherson, and then back across the mountains, with visits

51 R. P. Petitot to T.-R.P. Supérieur Général, Fort Anderson, 18 Nov. 1865, *Missions de la Congrégation*, vol. 7, 183.

52 Codex Historicus, Fort Good Hope, Acc. 97.109/Box 90 (7) Item 1988, OMI, PAA; Petitot to Supérieur Général, 15 Jan. 1866, p. 292; Séguin to mother and sister, 1 Jun. 1866.

53 McDonald Diary, 13 and 17 Sept. 1865.

54 McDonald Diary, 21 and 26 Sept. 1865.

55 As cited in Parish, 'An Analysis', 35.

56 As cited in Katherine Louise Arndt, 'Dynamics of the Fur Trade on the Middle Yukon River, Alaska, 1839–1868' (PhD diss., University of Alaska, 1996), 161.

57 W. L. Hardisty to Governor, Chief Factors, Chief Traders, Northern Department, 30 Jul. 1866, B.200/b/36, fo. 93b, HBCA; see also Allen A. Wright, *Prelude to Bonanza: The Discovery and Exploration of the Yukon* (Sidney, BC: Gray's Publishing, 1976), 88–9.

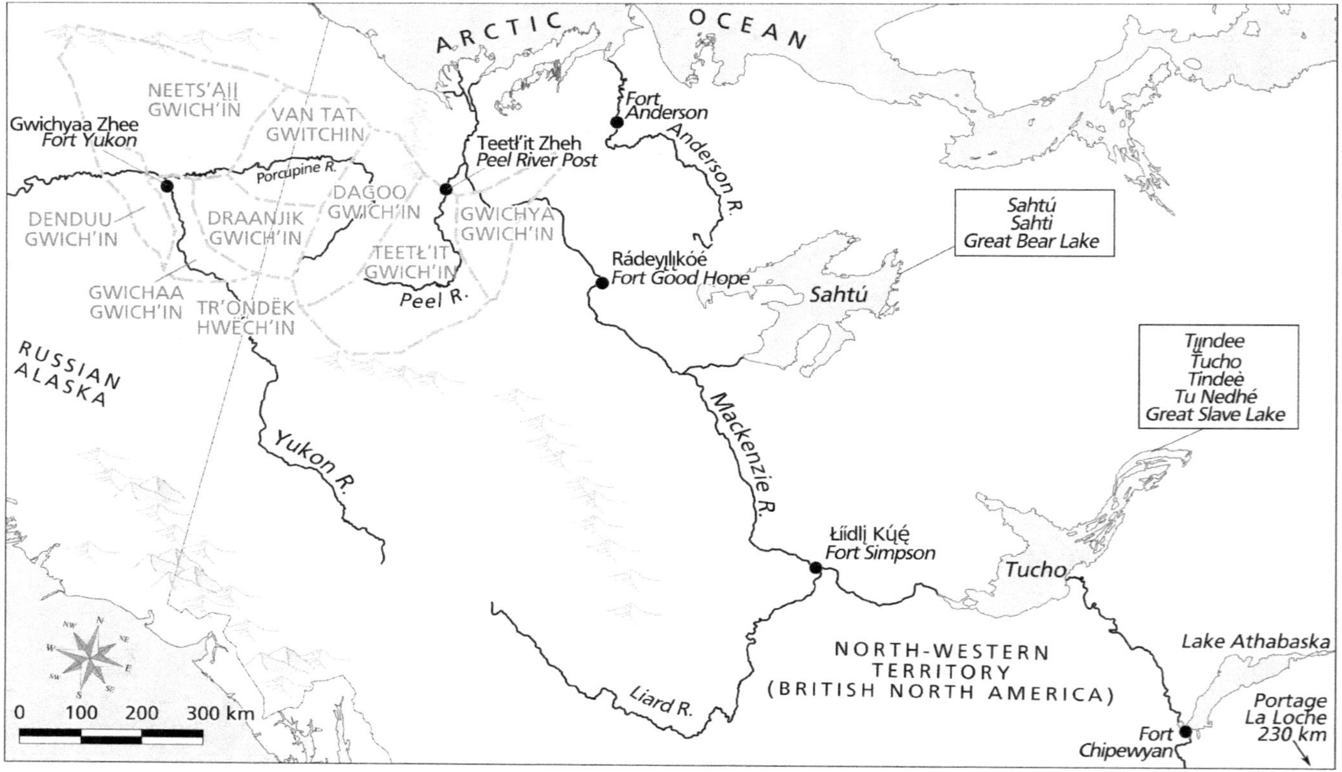

Map 2.1 Map of scarlet fever epidemic, 1865–6.

to camps on the smaller rivers en route. At Fort Yukon he described visits from Tr'ondëk Hwëch'in, Draanjik Gwich'in, Gwichaa Gwich'in, Neets'ąįį Gwich'in, and others – evidence of dense nineteenth-century social networks.[58] Many of those who came and left from Fort Yukon were in good health. 'Two young men arrive from Netsi-kutchin [*sic*] country. They brought news of all being well, and of having collected large quantities of provisions.'[59] Sadly, when McDonald travelled to them two months later, he reported that twenty-seven had died in the epidemic, almost a third of the band.[60] Katherine Arndt argued that epidemic did not spread much farther west than Fort Yukon, with timing and rumours (which kept people away from the trade post) playing a role in checking the disease.[61]

Many who survived scarlet fever and influenza struggled in the months to come as the epidemic disrupted not only trade but also the seasonal round of subsistence. Some of the Dagoo Gwich'in were reported to have died from scarlet fever and starvation. For although climate did not amplify the epidemic, the seasonality of the scarlet fever – its arrival at an important time in the annual harvesting cycle – deepened its impact.[62] In December 1865, the *Gens du large* told McDonald that 'they incurred great losses of provisions this fall, owing to their not having had time to secure them before they were seized by scarlet fever'.[63] K'áhshó Got'ı̨nę living near Fort Good Hope were so sick they could not fish.[64] Autumn fisheries and meat hunts provided food for families and provisioned trade posts along the Mackenzie, the Yukon, and their tributaries. At Peel River Post, fishermen fell ill or died during the autumn. Postmaster Andrew Flett reported he had 'none to replace them with till the best season was over'.[65] Then, the two fort hunters fell ill only days after they had embarked on their autumn hunt. Nagwichoonjik Gwich'in found them and brought them back to the fort 'in a most pitiful condition', but for three months they could not walk, possibly suffering from the effects of exposure. As a result, Flett wrote in February, 'we have had no fresh meat this winter as yet'. At Peel River Post, the problem of provisioning was deepened by the disproportionate number of deaths among hunters. Flett noted that 'with respect to hunters the best are all dead'.[66] Gwich'in who traded out of LaPierre's House had their provisions 'eaten by the Bears during their illness'.[67] Deaths came not just from infection with *S. pyogenes* but also from the ways the severe infection left otherwise healthy adults vulnerable to exposure and starvation. Thankfully, the epidemic

[58] McDonald Diary, 29 and 30 Sept. 1865. [59] McDonald Diary, 8 Oct. 1865.
[60] 'The Youcon Mission', 103. [61] Arndt, 'Dynamics', 163–4.
[62] Scott and Duncan, *Human Demography and Disease*, 311–14.
[63] 'The Youcon Mission', 103.
[64] Petitot, *Quinze ans*, 163, refers to them as the Batard-Loucheux.
[65] Andrew Flett to W. L. Hardisty, 1 Feb. 1866, B.200/b/36, fo. 40, HBCA.
[66] Flett to Hardisty, 1 Feb. 1866.
[67] James Flett to William Hardisty, Jan. 1866, B.200/b/36, fo. 42, HBCA.

and its disruptions aside, 1865–6 was not a bad year for meat or fish. When the main hunts failed, there were rabbits and smaller game. The epidemic came after earlier summer fisheries and hunts that had been generally successful, leaving stores that kept families, traders, and missionaries through the duration and aftermath of the epidemic.

The scarlet fever pandemic passed, and there was a brief period of respite. In the spring of 1867, Dene from Fort Good Hope were hired to crew the boats carrying the returns south to Portage La Loche; they were to come back, as always, in late summer with the new year's outfit. While in Portage La Loche, the crew again fell sick. The men from Fort Good Hope caught influenza, possibly brought west by their counterparts from Red River. Nine men died within days, creating immediate problems for the brigade. Hardisty observed, 'several others are at the point of death and those who are well are so dispirited that they cannot or will not work'.[68] The crews tarried so long their provisions ran out, and they had to slaughter oxen for meat. Twelve men died at Portage La Loche, at least ten from Fort Good Hope alone, 'while many of those who recovered continued so weak that they were unfit for work during the remainder of the voyage'.[69] Hardisty hired replacement men from Jack Fiddler's crew, but the delay was such that those in the posts down Dehcho began to worry that something had happened. Hardisty also recognized the possibility that the boat crews would carry the disease into the district, and, given the dramatic impact on the tripmen, he feared the consequences would be more dire than the recent scarlet fever.[70] In spite of Hardisty's foresight, when the brigade returned with five boats at the end of August 1867, they carried the virus into the Mackenzie district. They arrived just before the autumn freeze-up, when people congregated at posts and then left for their winter hunting grounds. Within two weeks of the brigade's arrival, Robert McDonald reported from Fort Youcon that 'nearly all the Dagoo [are] ill of cold'.[71] The cold and catarrh that McDonald described soon turned into reports of influenza and eventually deaths. That autumn, the weather was 'dreadful', with incessant snow and rain.[72] Across the region, people fell sick, disrupting autumn hunts at forts Nelson and Liard. When the river reopened the following spring of 1868, there were more accounts of sickness and deaths. The 1867–8 influenza was not as deadly as the 1865–6 scarlet fever; the influenza killed less than a third of the number whose deaths were attributed to *S. pyogenes*. Nevertheless, it was a dangerous

[68] William Hardisty to J. W. Wilson, 7 Aug. 1867, B.200/b/35, fo. 114a, HBCA.

[69] William Hardisty to The Governor, Chief Factors, Chief Traders, Northern Department, 2 Dec. 1867, B. 200/6/37, fo. 1, HBCA; R. MacFarlane to J. W. Wilson, 1 Aug. 1868, B.200/6/37, fo. 45, HBCA.

[70] William Hardisty to Governor Mactavish, 16 Aug. 1867, B.200/b/35, fo. 120b, HBCA.

[71] McDonald Diary, 31 Aug. and 11–13 Sept. 1867.

[72] Hardisty to The Governor etc., 2 Dec. 1867.

epidemic, and delirium was a hallmark of that year's virus.[73] The number of deaths in the winter of 1867–8 may have been greater because of difficulties in securing food, when sickness disrupted autumn hunts and then snowshoe hare and lynx populations went through a cyclical crash, a coincidence that people had been spared in the winter of 1865–6.[74] Passing through the region so soon after the scarlet fever, the 1867–8 influenza deepened the emotional, social, demographic, and economic effects of the previous epidemic.

Mortality and Effects

Ttssietla's loss and grief were repeated hundreds of times over. Although many recovered from their sickness, and some camps were spared altogether, reports of deaths began circulating in the autumn of 1865. Petitot wrote in 1866 of Néyollé, the head of a family that evaded the epidemic in their camp at K'áhbamį̨túé. On learning of the deaths of his younger brother, his two sisters, and many cousins and nephews, 'he sat, with his head in his hands, and stayed in this position for a long while saying nothing. He then sat up, shed countless tears and sobbed so hard as to rent his soul.'[75] Young people, described as the only survivors of large families, and others who did not die joined new camps and kin groups.[76] Many adults who died were important hunters and leaders, and some had strong medicine powers. When McDonald arrived at Birch River in November 1865, he learned of the death of Chutsugvihti, a well-known medicine man and leader of the camp.[77] In January, reports reached Fort Yukon of the deaths of many Van Tat Gwich'in, including Mary Flett, the wife of James Flett the post officer at LaPierre's House. Their daughter Jane's earliest memory was her father sobbing over her mother's death bed.[78] The chief of the Teetł'it Gwich'in, Atechyo, died in the epidemic, as did the chief of the Nagwichoonjik Gwich'in.[79]

Deaths in the scarlet fever epidemic may have amounted to 20 or 25 per cent of the population along Nagwichoonjik and among the Gwich'in who traded at

[73] Andrew Flett to William Hardisty, 7 Jan. 1868, B.200/b/36, fo. 131, HBCA.

[74] Hardisty to The Governor etc., 2 Dec. 1867.

[75] Petitot to Supérieur Général, 15 Jan. 1866, p. 285.

[76] Petitot to Supérieur Général, 15 Jan. 1866, p. 283; see also Émile Petitot, *Les Grands Esquimaux* (Paris: E. Plon, Nourrit et Cie., 1887), 278.

[77] McDonald Diary, 8 Nov. 1865.

[78] Robert Lampard, 'William Morrison MacKay, MD 1836–1917', in *Alberta's Medical History* (Red Deer: R. Lampard, 2008), 35 n. 13; Jane Flett was William MacKay's wife, see Chapter 3. Mary Flett appears only as Mrs James Flett in Anglican, HBC, and other textual sources. In biographies of Jane Flett, her mother is named Mary. See 'Jane Flett MacKay, 1857–1947', *Alberta Medical Association*, www.albertadoctors.org/about/medical-history/pioneering-alberta-doctors/flett-mackay. Mary was a common name for northern Indigenous women who converted to Christianity. Andrew Flett's Indigenous wife was also Mary Flett, and their daughter was also Jane.

[79] McDonald Diary, 17 Jan. 1866; Flett to Hardisty, 1 Feb. 1866.

Teetł'it Zheh (Fort McPherson), Zheh Gwitsal (LaPierre's House), and Fort Yukon.[80] The most commonly cited figure was that given by William Hardisty, who reported over 1,000 deaths, noting that this was more than in any previous epidemic. Direct reports (Table 2.1) tallied between 690 and 790 deaths, although these include reports shared before the epidemic had ended and do not include every camp or trade post. After the second influenza epidemic, when Chief Trader Roderick MacFarlane sat down at Portage La Loche in August 1868 to write his annual report, he recorded that a further '250 Men, Women and children perished – 3 engaged Servants also died'. The influenza, like the scarlet fever two years previously, had reached right across the district, although there were more deaths at some posts than others. Fort Good Hope, from where the boatmen had originally left, was one of the hardest hit, with thirty-eight deaths attributed to influenza. Forty people died at Fort Resolution on the south shore of Great Slave Lake. In spring 1868, McDonald reported ten deaths among the Van Tat Gwich'in, 'since last autumn'.[81] In the first part of winter, 'there was no sickness' at Great Bear Lake, but then in February, 'Fever and Influenza broke out among them and did much injury'. 'Many Deaths' were also reported from Fort Simpson, 'several Indians died' at Fort Nelson, and families at Nishì and Big Island also suffered losses.[82]

The language used in the descriptions of deaths in these years is best understood as communicating the depth of impact but cannot be readily translated into numbers. The Van Tat Gwich'in, or 'people of the lakes', had eighty men in 1848. In January 1866, McDonald notes that they suffered a 'large number of deaths', although what this meant depended on the number of people in the band and their role in their community.[83] Greater nuance can be found in the description of losses among the 'Mountain Indians' or Dagoo Gwich'in. In April 1866, McDonald described 'fearful mortality' among the Dagoo Gwich'in. From HBC postmaster Andrew Flett's account from Peel River, we learn that this was 'a party of 38 men' from whom 'only 6 are now living'.[84] The loss of thirty-two from thirty-eight hunters would be devastating, significantly affecting the future health of a band. In remarking upon these deaths, Flett expressed concern for the future of the trade. 'Peels River', he wrote, 'is now a poor place with respect to hunters the best are all dead . . . this number are now so reduced that I don't see how we are to get along in future.'[85]

[80] See Petitot to Supérieur Général, 18 Nov. 1865, p. 184; W. L. Hardisty to Governor Mactavish, 27 Nov. 1866, B.200/b/35, fo. 100b, HBCA; James McDougall to W. L. Hardisty, 5 Jul. 1866, B.200/b/36, fo. 58b, HBCA; 'The Youcon Mission', 109; McCarthy, *Great River*, 122; Abel, *Drum Songs*, 150.

[81] McDonald Diary, 14 Jun. 1867

[82] All quotations from R. MacFarlane to The Governor, Chief Factors and Chief Traders, Northern Department, 3 Aug. 1868, B.200/b/37, fo. 55–9, HBCA.

[83] McDonald Diary, 17 Jan. 1866. [84] Flett to Hardisty, 1 Feb. 1866.

[85] Flett to Hardisty, 1 Feb. 1866.

Table 2.1 *Descriptions and counts of mortality and sickness in 1865–6 scarlet fever*

Place or people	Deaths (low)	Deaths (high)	Description	Source	Date
Fort Chipewyan / Athabasca	120	–	Two-thirds of population ill; whole families died	Oblates	Aug. 1865–May 1866
Slave Lake	60	–	–	Oblates	May 1866
Fort Simpson	44	60	More than sixty having died at and near Fort Simpson alone	HBC	Sept.–Nov. 1865
Fort Good Hope	69	100	Within two days 'at least half' of the community was ill	Oblates	Autumn 1865, Spring 1866
Great Bear Lake	60	–	–	Oblates	Spring 1866
Fort Anderson and Anderson River / Kuukugmiut	43	69	'Large numbers of Eskimos died of this disease'	Oblates	Nov. 1865
Peel's River Post	100	–	–	Oblates	May 1866
Fort Yukon	4	–	'Those at the post'	HBC	Jul. 1866
Gwichaa Gwich'in / 'Youcon Indians'	48	64	Includes Shahnuuti''s camp, the majority of whom fell ill in late October	HBC and McDonald	Nov. 1865–Jul. 1866
Tr'ondëk Hwëch'in / Gens de fous	22	–	–	HBC	Jul. 1866
Neets'ąįį Gwich'in	27	33	Sixty men, women, and children survived	HBC and McDonald	Dec. 1865
Denduu Gwich'in / Gens de milieu	15	22	Eight men and several women and children died. Eighteen survivors	McDonald	Jun. 1866
Draanjik Gwich'in	19	–	–	HBC and McDonald	Jul. 1866
Van Tat Gwich'in	–	–	'Large number' of deaths	McDonald	Jan. 1866

Table 2.1 (*cont.*)

Place or people	Deaths (low)	Deaths (high)	Description	Source	Date
'Rat Indians' (Either Dagoo or Van Tat Gwich'in)	26	–	–	HBC	Jul. 1866
Dagoo Gwich'in	32	–	'Fearful mortality'	HBC and McDonald	Feb. 1866
Boat crews	–	–	Twenty men lying sick in the boats, and others perished at Portage La Loche and en route	Oblates	–

Commerce and provisioning took precedence for traders with the HBC in interpreting the significance of the loss of life. In McDonald's account, at times his observations reflected not only the number who died, but also how they died. At least three of the 'Mountain Indians' committed suicide, which McDonald found deeply troubling.[86] In McDonald's attention to these self-inflicted deaths, we are reminded about his core preoccupation: he was a missionary who aimed to convert people to Christianity, not a dispassionate witness. McDonald's record of the outbreak is most evocative when he writes about sickness or deaths of people in the context of their faith.

Also clear from descriptions of the impact of the epidemic, and the limited demographic data which has survived, was the impact on adult men and the repercussions that flowed from these deaths. There were the scarlet fever deaths of the chiefs of the Teetł'it Gwich'in and the Nagwichoonjik Gwich'in, and of Chutsugvihti, the head of his band. Then, with the influenza, came the death of the chief of the Van Tat Gwich'in, 'Peter Taylor', in the winter of 1867–8.[87] Antoine Houle (sometimes also Hoole), the Métis interpreter at Fort Yukon, died in the fall of 1868, after the main epidemic had moved through the region, when there was still 'much sickness' about.[88] Houle's father, François, was an HBC interpreter born in Red River and stationed at Fort Halkett, Fort Simpson, and Fort Liard between 1829 and 1885. At the age of fourteen, François sent his

[86] McDonald Diary, 13 Apr. 1866.
[87] McDonald did not offer an Indigenous name for Peter Taylor. McDonald Diary, 17 Mar. 1868.
[88] McDonald Diary, 2 Mar. 1869.

son to live with the Gwich'in who traded at Peel River Post to learn their language and follow in his father's footsteps. Antoine went on to have two Gwich'in wives and was a key figure in the trade at Fort Yukon, a post he helped to found in 1847. It was from Fort Yukon in 1848 that Houle ordered two coils of violin strings. This represented, according to anthropologist Craig Mishler, the arrival of fiddle music among the Gwich'in, a momentous event in northern cultural history which was shared in Gwich'in historical memory as the story of the Grasshopper and the Ants.[89] In October 1868, the forty-one-year-old Houle fell dangerously ill. Within two days he had fallen delirious 'and at sunset he departed this life', wrote McDonald, who attended Houle's death.[90]

Two HBC censuses (Table 2.2) conducted in 1858 and 1871 show the demographic effects of these epidemics. Over thirteen years, the Mackenzie district population declined from 4,609 to 3,963 men, women, and children.[91] The evidence of effects by age and gender is striking. Between the two censuses, the population of adult men in the district declined steeply, with 343 fewer men in 1871 as compared to 1858. The loss of children in the scarlet fever epidemic is under-accounted for by these censuses, as it is in this age group where deaths in the epidemic would have been offset by children born after 1866. The significant loss in the number of adult men resonates

Table 2.2 *Hudson's Bay Company censuses, 1858 and 1871*

	1858	1871	1858	1871	1858	1871	1858	1871
HBC POST	Men		Women		Boys		Girls	
Fort Simpson and Big Isl.	268	90	163	108	171	110	143	75
Fort Rae	214	123	156	105	145	168	142	112
Peel's River & LaP. House	102	83	99	71	83	116	53	87
Fort Yukon	256	142	231	114	218	113	137	76
Fort Liard	113	67	86	65	111	91	87	63
Fort Resolution	98	104	149	104	119	63	103	49
Fort Good Hope	189	160	130	212	97	84	51	63
Fort Norman	120	56	88	47	93	30	62	26
Fort Halkett / Fort Nelson	106	54	96	77	71	72	59	50
Bear Lake	–	52	–	48	–	27	–	17
Fort Providence	–	144	–	151	–	87	–	58
Hay River	–	48	–	44	–	34	–	23
Totals	*1,466*	*1,123*	*1,198*	*1,146*	*1,108*	*995*	*837*	*699*

89 See Craig Mishler, *The Crooked Stovepipe: Athapaskan Fiddle Music and Square Dancing in Northeast Alaska and Northwest Canada* (Urbana: University of Illinois Press, 1993), ch. 1.

90 McDonald Diary, 22 Oct. 1868.

91 See copies of 1858 and 1871 censuses, File 2 – Ross MSS, and File Hardisty census respectively, N-2002–012 box 1, June Helm fonds, NWTA.

Table 2.2 (*cont.*)

	Change between censuses			
HBC POST	Men	Women	Boys	Girls
Fort Simpson and Big Island	−178	−55	−61	−68
Fort Rae	−91	−51	23	−30
Peel's River & LaP House	−19	−28	33	34
Fort Yukon	−114	−117	−105	−61
Fort Liard	−46	−21	−20	−24
Fort Resolution	6	−45	−56	−54
Fort Good Hope	−29	82	−13	12
Fort Norman	−64	−41	−63	−36
Fort Halkett / Fort Nelson	−52	−19	1	−9
Bear Lake	–	–	–	–
Fort Providence	–	–	–	–
Hay River	–	–	–	–
Totals	*−343*	*−52*	*−113*	*−138*

Note: Fort Halkett in 1858 census, Fort Nelson in 1871.

with the reports that circulated during the epidemic about the deaths of many of the district's leaders and best hunters. These reports came from the Dagoo and Teetł'it Gwich'in, as well as the 'Liard Thikannies'.[92] Although the Halkett Tsek'ehne avoided the scarlet fever, Hardisty reported that only seven men (and unknown numbers of women and children) survived from the Tsek'ehne who traded out of Fort Liard, this from a population of nineteen adult men and seventy-eight people total in 1858, meaning more than half the men perished.[93] In 1869, Roderick MacFarlane reported that 'the fearful epidemics of 1865 and 1867 carried off nearly a fourth of our best fur traders'.[94]

The deaths of adult men may reflect, in small measure, a bias in the colonial record, apparent also in the Cause of Death database. We see from Flett and Hardisty much greater concern within the HBC for the health and loss of men, which translated into more accurate record keeping. Why men were at greater risk may have had something to do with the nature of scarlet fever or the combined effects of scarlet fever and influenza on adult male bodies although the precise effects are unknown. We do know that men were more vulnerable to deaths from starvation. The global historical record shows lower female mortality during famines, attributed primarily to proportionately greater stores of

92 Daniel Sims, pers. comm., suggests that this group likely refers to the Fort Nelson Tsek'ehne or Tseloni.

93 Hardisty to Governor etc., 30 Jul. 1866.

94 R. MacFarlane to The Governor, Chief Factors and Chief Traders, 24 Jul. 1869, B.200/6/37, fo. 177, HBCA.

fat on female bodies.[95] Starvation played a role in the deaths of the Dagoo Gwich'in and others as well and may have amplified deaths among men at this time, particularly during the influenza epidemic in 1867–8, which saw more widespread hunger. Local context also offers insights: men were more involved in the trade and therefore more likely to be exposed to scarlet fever at the posts and as part of the boat crews. Some never made it home and died, as Petitot wrote, 'far, very far from the steppes where they were born'.[96] In this way, they may have spared their families from sickness. Only men among the Dagoo Gwich'in were reported to have committed suicide, suggesting other ways that men were vulnerable during these epidemics.

The loss of hunters had many repercussions. Such losses led the HBC to close Fort Anderson. Established in 1860, following repeated requests from the Inuvialuit to open a post in their region, Fort Anderson was located at a site chosen for strategic purposes and because of a diversity of available resources (fish, moose, caribou, and trees for construction and heating).[97] The Inuvialuit traded with the Russians to the west or at Peel River Post, which was largely controlled by their Gwich'in competitors. In general, Inuvialuit traded more frequently on the coast, and the decision to erect the post inland in the space between Awaq (Cape Bathurst) and the Coppermine River meant that Fort Anderson was poorly sited, given the HBC's strategic goals. Fort Anderson was supplied from Fort Good Hope, and it was most likely from that place that the scarlet fever arrived in the autumn of 1865. On his arrival at Fort Anderson in November that year, Petitot saw fifteen fresh graves. He gave medicine to the Kuukugmiut chief 'who was sick at the fort'.[98] When the chief died a few days later, this prompted rumours of vengeance against Petitot and other whites for the chief's death and for their responsibility in bringing disease among the people. There were at least another twenty-eight deaths among the Kuukugmiut, and Petitot speculated that more Inuvialuit perished on the coast. By 1870, survivors of the Kuukugmiut were now wintering with Kuukpangmiut and Kitigaaryungmiut (Mackenzie River Inuvialuit).[99] Among those buried at Fort Anderson, and those who died in the larger epidemic, were most if not all of the K'áhshó Got'ı̨nę hunters who had supplied Fort Anderson 'with the means of

[95] Cormac Ó Gráda, 'Making Famine History', *Journal of Economic Literature* 45, no. 1 (2007): 5–38 (p. 22).

[96] Petitot, *Quinze ans*, 158.

[97] Andrew Stuhl, *Unfreezing the Arctic: Science, Colonialism, and the Transformation of Inuit Lands* (Chicago: University of Chicago Press, 2016), 22–4; John K. Stager, 'Fort Anderson: The First Post for Trade in the Western Arctic', *Geographical Bulletin* 9, no. 1 (1967): 45–56 (p. 49).

[98] Jean Séguin to mother and sister, 5 Aug. 1866, 71.220 / 7343, OMI, PAA; Charles Arnold, Wendy Stephenson, Bob Simpson, and Zoe Ho, eds. *Taimani: At That Time* (Inuvik: Inuvialuit Regional Corporation, 2011), 26–7.

[99] Ishmael Alunik, Eddie D. Kolausok, and David Morrison, *Across Time and Tundra: The Inuvialuit of the Western Arctic* (Vancouver: Raincoast Books, 2003), 64–8; Stager, 'Fort Anderson', 56.

living'.[100] Trade at the post was already marginal, and there had been a recent crisis in 1864 when sixty-four dogs died of distemper. The HBC saw little reason to continue a failing enterprise, and the fort closed.

Most disruptive to the trade were the deaths of the Dene men at Portage La Loche in 1867. In November, Hardisty worried about securing a crew for the coming season, writing 'there may be a difficulty in getting Indians to go to the Portage next summer … [men] who have usually remained inland, will be required for the Portage'.[101] When the epidemic lasted through the winter months and reached many families along the river, Hardisty's concerns were realized. In the summer of 1868, MacFarlane described that season's 'Weak Crews', who lacked experience. Eight of fourteen men deserted, which meant that they could not 'travel as hard as usual'.[102] In 1870, Hardisty reported that the crews were 'mostly made up of mere boys, who are really unfit for the duty required of them: but as they were the only ones we could get to undertake the voyages'.[103] The difficulties securing crews created such considerable anxiety that both Hardisty and MacFarlane suggested to William Mactavish, then governor of Rupert's Land, that the best and 'perhaps cheapest means of communication with this District' was no longer by rivers but rather through the Bering Strait to the delta by sea.[104]

The danger that sickness posed for the men who made up the boat crews cannot be exaggerated. Even in 1868, what MacFarlane characterized as a 'comparatively healthy' year, two men – one from Big Island (near Fort Providence) and the other from Great Slave Lake – died from influenza.[105] Much of the resistance to working on the boat crews stemmed directly from concern about sickness, which even if it did not kill could still be brought into the district and spread to families. Crewing the boats was arduous: men suffered lung haemorrhages and other physical effects. Hunting, trapping, and fishing allowed much greater independence of movement in the midst of kin and community, rather than the manual labour of moving hundreds of pieces of goods along a fixed route in the direct employ of the HBC. Lucy Vaneltsi, born in 1901, told stories about the HBC's York boats and the people who 'worked very hard all summer long'. Vaneltsi said that the HBC paid them for the summer's work, but 'they didn't eat properly and they worked hard. When they got back to Arctic Red River or Fort McPherson, they were just half starving.'[106] The work fell to

[100] Hardisty to Governor etc., 30 Jul. 1866, refers to them as the 'Batard Loucheux'.
[101] William Hardisty to William King, 27 Nov. 1867, B.200/b/37, fo. 17, HBCA.
[102] MacFarlane to The Governor etc., 3 Aug. 1868, fo. 55.
[103] William Hardisty to The Governor, Chief Factor and Chief Traders, 2 Aug. 1870, B.200/b/37, fo. 255, HBCA.
[104] Hardisty to Mactavish, 16 Aug. 1867, fo. 121; R. MacFarlane to William Mactavish, 3 Aug. 1868, B.200/b/37, fo. 60, HBCA.
[105] R. MacFarlane to William Mactavish, 23 Nov. 1868, B.200/b/37, fo. 82, HBCA.
[106] Lucy Vaneltsi, 'Traditional Life #2', in 'Gwich'in COPE stories' (Fort McPherson, NT: Gwich'in Social and Cultural Institute, 2010), 719–20.

Indigenous men because of the racialized division of labour within the fur trade and belies characterizations of the fur trade as an 'economic partnership'.[107] Men hired to work on the boat crews were not paid at set or promised rates, in contrast to fishermen, labourers, or interpreters, but were given assurances that they would be treated fairly, 'like the other voyageurs'.[108] This was not sought-after or well-remunerated labour, and European servants aimed to find better positions within the company. In December of 1867, Hardisty reported that a great number of European servants were leaving the district because the additional work they had to perform when the influenza broke out, including the transhipment of goods, 'has quite disgusted them with the service, and they will not be persuaded to renew their Engagements on any terms'.[109] It was for these reasons that being 'kept inland' and off the boat crews was 'considered the greatest privilege a man can receive in McKenzie River'.[110]

Resistance to the HBC and to work on the boat crews peaked in 1870. Malingering and desertion had been a concern in years previous, and Séguin, writing in June 1869, described fear of an uprising at Fort Good Hope.[111] But it was in the summer of 1870 that the Portage brigade turned back just above 'the Grand Rapids' on the north-west corner of Lake Winnipeg and only a fraction of the distance the outfit had to travel, meaning that 300 pieces never made it to Portage La Loche. The failure of the annual transhipment left the Mackenzie district without goods (ammunition, clothes, tools, foodstuffs, tobacco) required or desired by the company's servants, as well as those with whom the HBC traded.[112] Immediately to the south, the Athabasca District received its full outfit that year, and Hardisty, back in charge after a furlough, hoped that William McMurray, chief factor in Fort Chipewyan, could help make up some of the difference.[113] Other goods from Norway House made their way slowly west, but Hardisty could not persuade his crews to go further than the Portage, and so the work fell to crews from the east.[114] This disruption to the trade was tied to the formation of the Provisional Government in Red River and deep-rooted discontent with the HBC at the moment of their transfer of Rupert's Land to the Dominion of Canada. Hardisty reserved his harshest criticism for the 'rascally Red River tripmen' who had abandoned the goods at Grand Rapids, although his own crews from the Mackenzie

[107] Binnema, *Enlightened Zeal*, 31.
[108] R. MacFarlane to William King, 29 Mar. 1869, B.200/b/37, fo. 167, HBCA.
[109] William Hardisty to James Stewart, 3 Dec. 1867, B.200/b/37, fo. 10, HBCA.
[110] William Hardisty to Samuel Parson, 30 Jul. 1871, B.200/b/38 fo. 96, HBCA.
[111] Jean Séguin to mother and sister, 1 Jun. 1869, 71.220 / 7344, OMI, PAA.
[112] Hardisty to The Governor etc., 2 Aug. 1870, fo. 255.
[113] John Rae to G. Simpson, 23 Apr. 1851, E.15/8, HBCA.
[114] The problems continued into the following year; see Robert Hamilton to W. L. Hardisty, 19 Jun. 1871, B.200/b/38, fo. 120, HBCA.

district also worked to rule that year.[115] This episode must be understood not only within the context of the assertion of Indigenous and Métis rights in what became Manitoba; it was also a direct product of the epidemics of 1865–6 and 1867–8 in the North. Certainly, Hardisty's anxiety about the Mackenzie district trade reached its peak that summer. While Hardisty conveyed confidence to his superiors that even in the absence of goods the trade would still proceed and that there was sufficient ammunition and other necessities to make it through winter, he nevertheless wrote that if the provisions trade should fail, 'we may not be able to bring up all the boats that will be required to fetch down the supplies next summer, which we must have or give up the business altogether – for as we shall be bare of Everything and probably *naked* by that time'.[116]

The loss of life, sickness, and fear that attended scarlet fever and influenza in the late 1860s wreaked havoc on the fur trade. A marginal post (Fort Anderson) closed, but it was in the labour of transportation and the dangers posed by work to the brigades and at transhipment points that ill health became a critical concern and part of broader opposition to the role of the HBC. Epidemics contributed directly to changes in fur-trade operations in the latter part of the nineteenth century. The experiences of scarlet fever and influenza shaped social relations in the North, as sickness and grief created new dependencies and opportunities for missionaries and traders in their relations with Indigenous northerners.

Care, Compassion, and Cruelty

There was no cure for scarlet fever in the 1860s. The best chances for survival and future good health came with attentive care from those who were well. Shared Dene, Gwich'in, Tr'ondëk Hwëch'in, and Inuvialuit values of generosity and helping the weak meant that people would have done what they could to help those who suffered. Indigenous medicine was the main source of healing for northerners at this time. Even though many Indigenous northerners caught scarlet fever in the trade and mission posts, as soon as they could they moved on to their wintering grounds where, in Séguin's words, they 'could breathe a little'. Out on the land their families cared for them, 'so long as the one who was sick could light a fire'.[117] Hardisty complained that 'the Indians . . . will not hunt when death occurs in their families'.[118] And it was not just families who cared for one another, as we saw with the Nagwichoonjik Gwich'in who rescued the Teetł'it Gwich'in hunters in the autumn of 1865.

[115] Hardisty to The Governor etc., 2 Aug. 1870, fo. 257.
[116] Hardisty to The Governor etc., 2 Aug. 1870, fo. 258. Emphasis in original.
[117] Séguin to mother and sister, 1 Jun. 1866. [118] Hardisty to Governor etc., 30 Jul. 1866.

Missionaries such as McDonald also spent much time visiting the sick, bringing medicines, and offering care not just at the trade posts but also at the camps out on the land. This was part of a missionary's responsibilities to minister to bodies and souls.

Some HBC employees cared for people at the trade posts, although this appears to have been the exception rather than the rule. HBC correspondence was preoccupied with the business and provisioning implications of the scarlet fever epidemic. Hardisty, for instance, spilled much ink persuading his superiors that the falling off in returns was a direct consequence of the epidemic, not a product of his decision to end the debt system that had underpinned the Mackenzie district trade up to that point.[119] Hardisty called for 'a Medical Officer attached to this District'. He wanted a doctor to provide care to those who were ill in the district, to 'prevent our Men and Indians from pretending to be sick on the voyage', and to save the company money in keeping experienced men who fell ill in the district, rather than forcing them to retire so they could leave.[120] Hardisty was nothing if not a man preoccupied with the company's bottom line.

Some of his men emulated Hardisty's single-mindedness. James McDougall, then apprentice clerk at Fort Yukon, wrote to his superior in November of 1865 reporting on the spread of the scarlet fever. He directed attention to François Boucher, a Métis employee of the HBC, who with his eldest son had re-engaged at Fort Yukon. McDougall criticized Boucher as 'a discontented fellow' at best, who was 'at the bottom of many of the quarrels that took place between the Whites and Indians within the last few years'. McDougall complained that Boucher, when hired to fish, 'spends the time hunting and otherwise amusing him self in the woods'.[121] Robert McDonald also wrote about Boucher and his family in his diary, although never disparaging him but rather describing Boucher's successes at hunting and how he 'received a hearty welcome' from Boucher at his camp 'in a deep valley surrounded by mountains whose peaks tower up to the height of about 1500 feet or more. The view around grand.'[122] When McDonald solemnized François's marriage to 'Eliza Ross a Tukudh woman' in October 1866, François was forty-one years old and Eliza twenty-eight. François, Eliza, and their son François Jr. participated in the 1885 Northwest Resistance.[123] Boucher's conflicts with the HBC evidently arose not simply from a desire to 'amuse him self in the woods' but were rooted more deeply in Indigenous opposition to Euro-Canadian colonial domination.

[119] Hardisty to Mactavish, 27 Nov. 1866; Abel, *Drum Songs*, 147, 206.

[120] Hardisty to Mactavish, 27 Nov. 1866.

[121] J. McDougall to W. L. Hardisty, 25 Nov. 1865, B.200/b/36, fo. 43, HBCA.

[122] McDonald Diary, 24 Mar. 1863.

[123] Lawrence J. Barkwell, *Veterans and Families of the 1885 Northwest Resistance* (Saskatoon: Gabriel Dumont Institute, 2011), 54.

McDougall gave Boucher reason to oppose the HBC. Boucher and his family – his wife and three sons – all fell ill with scarlet fever while travelling down the Mackenzie River. McDonald visited them at Tsiigehtchic.[124] McDougall asked Andrew Flett to take advantage of the Bouchers' sickness and to keep them at Peel River Post 'until the return of the Packet from Fort Simpson' carrying the mail. McDougall then called on Hardisty to use the opportunity to revoke the engagement of father and son.

But it was Andrew Flett's empathy and care for people at Peel River during the scarlet fever outbreak that Hardisty cited in promoting him to Clerk. 'When all his people and family were ill', Hardisty wrote, Flett

> attended almost day and night to the Sick, and besides to the usual duties of his post, laced nets and personally prosecuted the principal fishery, which undoubtedly saved the establishment during Winter – for the Sickness continued most of the Winter among the Indians of the Lower Posts, who could not have otherwise supplied a sufficiency of provisions to the Fort.[125]

Flett's family included his wife, Mary, the daughter of Robert Campbell (the HBC chief factor at Fort Selkirk in the 1850s) and a Northern Tutchone woman.[126] Flett also had at least two children from a previous wife Cachoza (or Jane Gaucher/Boucher), a Dene woman from Echaot'ı̨e Kų́ę́ (Fort Liard) who died around 1854. The younger of the two children, also Jane, was eleven years old when the scarlet fever arrived at Peel River. That Flett's family lived at Peel River Post goes some way to explain his greater concern for the well-being of the community. Colonialism in Northern North America created overlapping moral communities delineated along the lines of race, family, and religion. These were the limits that explain why epidemics brought out compassion in some and ruthlessness in others.

Christian missionaries too could lack compassion, and their work in medicine and healing was inseparable from their colonial objectives. This was acutely apparent in stories told by Séguin and Petitot of the death of Nitchontchèlè and five of his family in 1867.[127] These deaths were part of the epidemic's toll among K'áhshó Got'ı̨nę and Sahtu Dene who visited and

[124] McDonald Diary, 10 Sept. 1865; McDougall to Hardisty, 25 Nov. 1865.

[125] Hardisty to Mactavish, 27 Nov. 1866.

[126] Nora Lande (descendant of Andrew Flett), pers. corr., 23 Jan. 2019; Victoria Castillo, 'Fort Selkirk: Early Contact Period Interaction Between the Northern Tutchone and the Hudson's Bay Company in Yukon' (PhD diss., University of Alberta, 2012), 85, 88, which describes Campbell referring to a Northern Tutchone woman as 'Beloved'. Campbell was hostile to the idea of 'country wives', and his only legal marriage was to Eleanora Stirling of Scotland. There was also a second Andrew Flett, who married Maria at Fort McPherson, 20 Dec. 1867. Most commonly known as Andrew Bonnetplume, he was sometimes also called Andrew Flett. The Orkney-born Andrew Flett and his wife Mary served as witnesses to Bonnetplume's marriage.

[127] Jean Séguin to mother and sister, 30 May 1868, 71.220 / 7344, OMI, PAA; also Petitot, *Quinze ans*, 123.

traded at Fort Good Hope. Nitchontchèlè was a powerful medicine man and a large physical presence. Also known as Kochon/Cochon, he was, in Sahtu Dene Elder George Blondin's telling, 'a medicine man to fear'.[128] 'He helped people, but he was a cruel warrior too', according to Blondin. Petitot and Séguin referred to him as a 'sorcerer' or a 'conjuror', belittling his skills and medicine powers as wizardry and demonic possession.[129] Petitot, Séguin, and McDonald were interested in Indigenous men and women with significant medicine powers. Séguin and Petitot described conflicts with powerful medicine men, including instances where they blamed missionaries for bringing diseases.[130] Powerful spiritual leaders were not only perceived as key opponents but also presented opportunities for broader success in converting their kin and communities. In the minds of missionaries, the deaths of powerful spiritual leaders, or at least the death of their beliefs, created space for Christianity.

Petitot called Nitchontchèlè 'Le Petit Cochon' or 'the Little Pig', and his family members were likewise named. There was an older esteemed hunter known as 'Big Pig', Nitchontchèlè's wife was 'Big Sow', and his brother was 'Middle Pig'. Séguin and Petitot made much of these names, ridiculing the family for not knowing the significance of pigs in European culture. This ridicule aimed to expose Nitchontchèlè's ignorance and was a device used by Petitot and Séguin to highlight the righteousness of their proselytizing. Petitot devoted a section of his book, *Quinze ans*, to 'The Family of Pigs', where he writes that the name arose from the family's participation in the fur trade. Three or four of the family members ate bacon and ham while at Portage La Loche, presumably working on the boat crews. According to Petitot, they were so taken by these 'tastiest' of meats that they wanted to distinguish themselves with the name of the animals from which they came. Similarly the children of 'Middle Pig' were named for more traditional foods: Little Beaver Belly and Fattened Hare.[131]

After the arrival of the Oblates in Fort Good Hope, Nitchontchèlè initially kept his distance. For five years, he refused to set foot in the mission house. Petitot appears to have had a better relationship with Nitchontchèlè than Séguin, who described quarrelling with him. Before his death, Nitchontchèlè drew a map for Petitot of territory lying to the east of Dehcho between Fort Good Hope and Tulita that the missionary wished to explore.[132] After his death, Nitchontchèlè's surviving male kin, Tatékoyé and Dzan-you, refused to guide Petitot into this area, describing the land as haunted by evil spirits. Eventually,

[128] George Blondin, 'Kochon: Strong Warrior and Medicine Man', in *When the World Was New: Stories of the Sahtu Dene* (Yellowknife: Outcrop, 1990), 87–93.
[129] Petitot, *Quinze ans*, 120.
[130] Petitot to Supérieur Général, 15 Jan. 1866,p. 289; Séguin to mother and sister, 30 May 1868.
[131] Séguin to mother and sister, 30 May 1868; Petitot, *Quinze ans*, 119–23.
[132] Émile Petitot, *Exploration de la région du Grand Lac des Ours* (Paris: Téqui, 1893), 285.

when there was a scarcity of caribou and fish in January 1870, they relented.[133] Nitchontchèlè and his family were clearly conflicted in their relationships with the Oblates. Nitchontchèlè wished on some level to share his knowledge and expertise with the missionaries – or at least with Petitot – but in other respects, Nitchontchèlè and his family remained adamantly situated within their own culture.

With this in mind, the Oblate reactions to Nitchontchèlè appear grotesque. Nitchontchèlè fell ill in the winter of 1865, in the midst of the scarlet fever epidemic, and came to Petitot and Séguin for help. Petitot describes Nitchontchèlè's sickness not as an infectious disease, but as something more akin to a possession. Nitchontchèlè acted out with gestures and expressions how in his sickness he felt physically possessed, a 'pantomime', which prompted Séguin to laugh out loud. In Petitot's words, Séguin's was 'un rire homérique' – a Homeric laugh, or 'a loud and long-continued burst of merriment'.[134] Petitot uses this story to describe how he, unlike his colleague, took care not to laugh but rather to convey to this 'frank soul' and 'candid man' – Nitchontchèlè – that Petitot took him seriously. Describing this episode served to portray Petitot as a man with great empathy for Indigenous people. Petitot also aimed to demonstrate his own skill at securing conversion to Christianity through empathy in contrast to Séguin's combative and 'rational' approach.[135] In Petitot's account, Nitchontchèlè then asks to be baptized, and Petitot tells him that if he does so, Nitchontchèlè will have to renounce his spirits and his 'occult practices', and that going forward Jesus Christ 'alone will be your medicine'. To this, Nitchontchèlè agrees. He and his wife are baptized that Christmas, and he is given a third name, Noël. In Séguin's recounting of his death two years later, Nitchontchèlè never truly converted but went through with the baptism only to please his wife. When dying of influenza and delirious, Nitchontchèlè reportedly cried out that if he was to die, it was his own fault as he had continued to 'fait l'inkanzé' (practise his own medicine) and so God was making him die.[136]

The didactic and rhetorical aims of these accounts are obvious: Petitot and Séguin were arguing over the most effective means of conversion. They made efforts to diminish the strength and value of Indigenous spiritual beliefs, and they

[133] 'Travelling in the land of the devil', chapter 8 in Petitot, *Exploration*. See also Séguin to mother and sister, 30 May 1868.

[134] Petitot, *Quinze ans*, 122; Joseph William Hewitt, 'Homeric Laughter', *The Classical Journal* 23, no. 6 (1928): 436–47 (p. 436).

[135] I use the word rational here not to suggest that Séguin's approach made more sense, but because he aimed to contradict Indigenous beliefs with European logic and reason. See D. Tricoire, 'The Enlightenment and the Politics of Civilization: Self-Colonization, Catholicism, and Assimilationism in Eighteenth-Century France', in *Enlightened Colonialism: Civilization Narratives and Imperial Politics in the Age of Reason*, ed. D. Tricoire, 25–45 (Cham: Palgrave Macmillan, 2017).

[136] Séguin to mother and sister, 30 May 1868.

highlighted the significance of their work in the North. The truths amid these accounts are more difficult to discern. These are only the missionary perspectives. We see how Séguin and Petitot disagreed about the significance of Nitchontchèlè's life, beliefs, and death. Sickness and the fear generated by epidemics, combined with the presence of missionaries, created opportunities for the deepening inter-penetration of colonial and Indigenous ways of life. Men and women turned to religion as medicine, whether Indigenous spiritual medicine or Christian medicine, and the missionaries represented the value of conversion to Christianity in these ways as well. Petitot and Séguin's stories of Nitchontchèlè show clearly how conversion in the context of epidemics was not a moment of change or transformation, but a negotiation and a process that was incomplete, partial, and opportunistic for all parties. Most strikingly, though, these stories show the violence of colonization even when enrobed in the mantle of Christian love: Séguin's Homeric laughter at a sick man, echoing in his and Petitot's ridicule of the Cochon name, reveals the harshness and 'hideous grimaces' that accompanied the accounts of care and concern from missionaries in the north-west.[137]

The Opening of Residential Schools

Adult deaths disrupted subsistence and trade and left orphaned children. As part of the values of care held by Gwich'in, Dene, Inuvialuit, and others, orphaned children were adopted by other families, often but not exclusively kin. As Myra Moses, a Van Tat Gwich'in Elder born in Alaska in 1884 said about the time when she was a child, 'orphans, too, we took them in and took care of them. This is what we did. People took care of each other at that time.'[138] Sarah Abel spoke of Shahnuuti', whose leadership was evident in his care for orphans.[139] George Blondin told a story about adoption as a means of establishing peace between Dene in conflict.[140] Among fur traders, however, orphans were perceived as a problem. In the wake of the epidemic, when Flett wrote to Hardisty about the deaths of the Peel River hunters, he added, 'those now remaining are so incumbered [*sic*] with Orphan children'.[141] By November, HBC employees were asked to contribute 'in aid of MacKenzie River Orphan Asylum', with the funds used to build a schoolhouse at Tulita.[142] Soon thereafter, according to historian Robert Choquette, schoolmaster Murdo

137 Jean Séguin to mother and sister, 14 Jan. 1868, 71.220 / 7344, OMI, PAA.

138 Myra Moses in *People of the Lakes*, 85. 139 Sarah Abel in *People of the Lakes*, 113.

140 Blondin, *When the World Was New*, 46; Helene Rabesca in June Helm, *The People of Denendeh* (Montreal: McGill-Queen's University Press, 2000), 347.

141 Flett to Hardisty, 1 Feb. 1866.

142 J. McDougall to W. L. Hardisty, 2 Nov. 1866, B.200/b/36, fo. 73, HBCA; H. A. Cody, *An Apostle of the North: Memoirs of the Right Reverend William Carpenter Bompas, D.D.* (London: Seeley and Co., 1908), 57–8.

McLeod was charged with assaulting two female students. The school closed abruptly in 1868.[143] Another school opened at Fort Providence in 1867, staffed by Grey Nuns recently arrived from Red River. Grey Nuns opened a second school at Fort Chipewyan in 1874. The Anglicans established their first permanent boarding school in the North in 1895 at Hay River.[144] Children orphaned in the 1860s and thereafter were essential to what religious and state authorities perceived as the 'success' of these schools. Inseparable from the larger Canadian system of residential schooling, the opening of residential schools in the North arose directly from the impact of scarlet fever.

The founding of residential schools in the late nineteenth century served multiple purposes: they provided for the education of children of HBC employees, as well as other children whose parents sought additional education at this time; they enabled the fuller conversion of northern Indigenous peoples to Christianity; and they provided a place where the HBC could send orphaned children so that they would not disrupt trade. Yet even as these schools were a colonial response to the impacts of epidemic disease, they became almost immediately new sites of ill health in the North. We close this chapter, then, by looking at one example of the ways in which residential schools came to amplify infectious disease in the wake of the scarlet fever.

Whooping Cough

Whooping cough, or pertussis, is a highly contagious infectious disease which, like scarlet fever, is caused by bacteria rather than a virus. In the case of whooping cough, the bacterium in question is *Bordatella pertussis*, which spreads when someone infected with the disease sneezes or coughs, although it does not survive long outside of human hosts. Typical infection with *B. pertussis* leads to an incubation period that lasts from a week to ten days, followed by an initial stage (one to two weeks) of the disease when it is 'indistinguishable from the common cold'.[145] The second stage of the disease is when distinctive symptoms appear including vomiting and paroxysms of coughing, as many as forty times a day. The common name – whooping cough – comes from a 'characteristic inspiratory "whoop"' that follows on the coughing fits.[146]

143 Choquette, *Oblate Assault*, 158; Journal de R. P. Petitot, 30 May 1868, *Missions de la Congrégation des Missionnaires Oblats de Marie Immaculée*, vol. 9 (Paris: Hennuyer, 1870), 61–2.

144 TRC, *Canada's Residential Schools: The Inuit and Northern Experience*, vol. 2 (Montreal: McGill-Queen's University Press, 2015), 14–15.

145 Anne Hardy, *The Epidemic Streets: Infectious Disease and the Rise of Preventive Medicine, 1856–1900* (Oxford: Clarendon Press, 1993), 13.

146 Alan R. Hinman and Walter A. Orenstein, 'A Shot at Protection: Immunizations Against Infectious Disease', in *Silent Victories: The History and Practice of Public Health in*

The second stage can last up to six weeks, and the third stage is when the cough eases and the infected person recovers. Sickness with whooping cough can last up to three months, although it is in the first relatively asymptomatic period that someone is highly infectious. Deaths from whooping cough are most common in young children and typically result from secondary infection, with pneumonia especially.[147] Whether vaccinated or infected by *B. pertussis*, a person can be infected later in life, although infected (or re-infected) adolescents and adults may not exhibit the characteristic paroxysms in the second stage but rather sickness more akin to a common cold.

As Kerry Abel describes, whooping cough travelled through the Athabasca and Mackenzie districts repeatedly in the nineteenth century. In 1819, a severe epidemic of measles and whooping cough reached as far north as Great Slave Lake. As with scarlet fever, children, whether along Dehcho or in London, England, were most vulnerable to deaths from whooping cough, and this was evidenced in outbreaks in 1827–8 and thirty years later in 1857–8.[148] From then until the end of the century, there were no further major whooping cough outbreaks when the pathogen acted alone or in concert to cause large numbers of deaths. Nevertheless, where the disease did appear in the late nineteenth century illuminates important new aspects of colonial disease ecologies.

After 1860, whooping cough broke out twice along the Mackenzie and into the Yukon. In the autumn of 1874, whooping cough appeared among the children at the Fort Providence residential school, and several died. At Fort Liard, the sickness interfered with the autumn hunt on account of 'the distress which it occasioned', although no deaths were reported.[149] Pertussis broke out in Fort Good Hope that winter and contributed to some of the twenty-five deaths reported in 1874.[150] It was not by random chance that the disease had appeared first and with greater severity at the Fort Providence school. Rather, this reflected not only the vulnerability of children to whooping cough, but also the role of overcrowded living accommodations in mortality from the disease. Nineteenth-century urban observers commented that 'the more whooping-cough patients there were in one apartment, the more violent were their symptoms and the more difficult their relief'.[151] The Fort Providence school was one of the few places in the North that approached the kind of crowded conditions found in Victorian cities. A two-storey building, fourteen by fifteen metres in size, served as 'orphanage, boarding school, classrooms, hospital and sisters' residence', which in 1874 housed at least six Grey Nuns and thirty

Twentieth-Century America, ed. J. W. Ward and Christian Warren (Oxford: Oxford University Press, 2007), 72.

147 Hardy, *Epidemic Streets*, 13. 148 Abel, *Drum Songs*, 109–10.

149 W. L. Hardisty to James Grahame, 1 Jul. 1875, B.200/e/14, HBCA.

150 McCarthy, *Great River*, 200. 151 Hardy, *Epidemic Streets*, 17.

children, if not more.[152] While not as crowded as some of the subsequent schools opened in the region, from 1867 until 1899 the children 'slept in berths, like the shelves of a bookcase, ranged one above the other from the floor to the ceiling . . . In this children's dormitory, of which we speak, the one free corner was occupied by the Sisters' beds, laid side by side.'[153] Living space for the children would therefore have been far more crowded at the Providence 'orphelinat-hôpital' than in any other interior space in the nineteenth-century North, producing the kinds of conditions that contributed directly to greater mortality from whooping cough.[154]

Pertussis was endemic in southern urban areas, with outbreaks every two or three years causing significant mortality among young children before the introduction of an effective vaccine in the late 1930s. In the North, whooping cough was never endemic but travelled into the region with traders, colonizers, and visitors. The second appearance in this period was in 1886–8, first in the autumn at Fort Chipewyan (where there were no deaths) then by March 1887 again at the Fort Providence residential school. The sister superior wrote to Séguin telling him that all forty children had fallen ill. Séguin anticipated that the disease would spread to Good Hope: 'It will probably arrive in summer and ravage the little children.'[155] This was what he recalled happening a decade before. Sure enough, in the autumn of 1887, two newborn infants died at Fort Good Hope after the disease arrived in that community, while others died 'in the woods' and over the winter.[156] The Fort Providence residential school served as a site of whooping cough infection and deaths within its own walls and spread the disease elsewhere along Dehcho. The school exemplified the unhealthy environments produced by colonialism. We will return to northern residential schools later in the book, in the discussion of tuberculosis in Chapter 9 most significantly.

As a syndemic in 1865–6, followed so closely thereafter by a further, serious wave of influenza in 1867–8, this pandemic experience of scarlet fever and influenza had dire consequences for the people of the North. There was grief and loss; economic instability and disruption tied to political unrest; and new

[152] Thérèse Castonguay, *A Leap in Faith: The Grey Nuns Ministries in Western and Northern Canada*, vol. 2 (Edmonton: Grey Nuns of Alberta, 1999), 161–6, quotation p. 165.

[153] R. P. Duchaussois, *The Grey Nuns in the Far North* (Toronto: McClelland and Stewart, 1919), 129.

[154] R. P. Duchaussois, *Aux Glaces Polaires, Indiens et Esquimaux* (Lyons, France: Oeuvre Apostolique de Marie Immaculée; Ville La Salle, PQ: Noviciat des Oblats, 1921), 92. Vol. 2 of the TRC attributes a description of crowding to Providence, where it in fact describes the early years of the school at Fort Resolution (St Joseph's Hospice). See TRC, *Inuit and Northern Experience*, 14.

[155] Jean Séguin to sister, 5 Jun. 1887, 71.220 / 7346, OMI, PAA.

[156] Jean Séguin to sister, 6 Feb. 1888, 71.220 / 7346, OMI, PAA; Codex Historicus, Fort Good Hope, Oct. 1887–May 1888.

assertions of colonial power, not only through the introduction of residential schooling but also in missionary efforts to convert people to Christianity amid the fear and great mortality. By reconstructing the geographic scope, course, and effects of scarlet fever and influenza, we have to recognize that not all introduced pathogens produced this scale of devastation, nor did they all prompt the same depth of colonial intrusions and change. In our own times, we could compare this to the different effects of SARS CoV-1 in 2002–4 with SARS CoV-2 in 2020. The degree of disruption and transformation between the two events are on completely different levels, notwithstanding similarities in the pathogens and their novelty in global human populations. The degree of disruption produced by the scarlet fever pandemic in 1865 was transformative in the history of the lands along Nagwichoonjik, Chu kon' dëk, and their tributaries. While contemporary observers did not hide the severity of the scarlet fever, the impacts were nevertheless obscured at the time and since by other narratives: of constant epidemics and depopulation, of Indigenous ill health, hardship, and weakness, and even of 'extinction'. These stories will be familiar to many readers, and if they did not reflect the experience of 1865–8, where, then, did they come from?

3 Colonial Motifs and Medicine

In December 1867, William Hardisty ruminated whether 'MacKenzie's River ... [is] getting less healthy than it used to be, especially during the Summer months'. Hardisty mused, 'whether the change is in the Climate, or in the constitutions of the Indians themselves, I am not confident to determine'.[1] Hardisty neatly conveyed prevailing colonial interpretations about disease causation in the late nineteenth-century north-west. He expressed a sense of decline among Indigenous peoples in the region, one that fit with other contemporary ideas about Indigenous peoples and their 'constitutions' rooted in racist ideologies. Missionaries echoed traders' sentiments. Historian Martha McCarthy wrote that in the aftermath of the 1860s epidemics, 'a series of less-destructive ailments followed; they so weakened the people that any slight illness could cause their deaths'. Oblate bishop Henri Faraud 'compared his missionaries to the gleaners coming behind the harvesters, picking up the few who were left of disappearing tribes'.[2] McCarthy takes Faraud's assessment at face value. I do not.

Histories of the nineteenth century offered by Elders in the early and mid-twentieth century contradict the assertion that it was a period of rampant ill health. George Blondin, in telling the story of Karkeye born late in 1855, emphasized, 'people were healthier and stronger than they are today'.[3] For Julienne Andre, recalling life on the land at the end of the nineteenth century, 'there were no white men and nobody got sick. We travelled all year from spring through the fall and nobody got the flu or cold.'[4] Nauyavuik, one of Vilhjalmur Stefansson's Inuvialuit informants in the delta between 1908 and 1912, concurred: 'before the ships (whalers) came there were some epidemics, but between times few were ever sick'. According to Nauyavuik, there 'were no colds'.[5] In the early 1990s, Sarah Meyook shared stories with interviewers at Qargialuk (Ptarmigan Bay) along the Yukon coast. She spoke about her

1 William Hardisty to William Mactavish, 2 Dec. 1867, B.200/b/37, fo. 6, HBCA.
2 McCarthy, *Great River*, 123; see also Abel, *Drum Songs*, 158.
3 Blondin, *When the World Was New*, 116.
4 Julienne Andre in *Gwichya Gwich'in Googwandak*, 262, 269.
5 Vilhjalmur Stefansson, *The Stefánsson–Anderson Arctic Expedition of the American Museum: Preliminary Ethnological Report* (New York: Published by Order of the Trustees, 1914), 380.

grandmother's and mother's skills and knowledge, including making parkas from caribou skin and ground squirrels. Meyook's mother 'said people never get sick too in those days'.[6] Jean Séguin, the Oblate missionary, expressed a similar view about the health of the country. Writing in August of 1866, after the scarlet fever had passed:

> We all found ourselves still radiant with health. This country is not like others because except for some epidemics brought to us by the boats, there is no disease. The good Lord does all he does well, because if there was as much illness as in France, in less than a year we would have to depart for lack of inhabitants. Still a disease like last year's, and there would not be a savage left.[7]

Séguin distinguishes here between the good health of the land and the weakness of its Indigenous inhabitants, echoing Hardisty's ruminations on climate versus constitution.[8] If we see Blondin, Andre, Nauyavuik, and Meyook as offering evidence of good health as well as explaining why people were healthy, can we reconcile the competing reports of good and ill health in this time and place?

This chapter examines the stories told about early epidemic disease in the North by missionaries, traders, and eventually anthropologists. Stories from people at that time – Petitot, Hardisty, and others – were grounded in experience but embellished to better serve colonial objectives. Twentieth-century anthropologists did not embellish their stories so much as interpret from flawed evidence. Where these interpretations fell under the sway of the 'virgin soil' model, epidemics took on a different and more menacing character, more in keeping with that presented a century earlier by participants in the colonial enterprise. Here we consider the implications of how we interpret evidence of past epidemics in the North to understand how often disease arrived with Europeans and thereby strive for a better understanding of how northerners could respond to novel pathogens. From our most recent pandemic experience, we see how, with time and rest, communities can recover from devastating encounters with disease. But repeated waves of sickness – like with the scarlet fever followed by influenza – challenge that resilience. So the question of the frequency and intensity of outbreaks and epidemics is an important one. The severe epidemics in the 1860s led the HBC to hire a physician, William MacKay, who along with missionaries provided medical care to the Mackenzie district posts. Colonial biomedicine existed alongside, and was still secondary to, traditional healing practices. This chapter considers some of these practices and the introduction of new tools to deal with new pathogens.

6 Sarah Meyook, interview with Renie Arey and Murielle Nagy, 19 Jul. 1991, Qargialuk (Ptarmigan Bay), tape 28B, in Murielle Nagy, ed., *Yukon North Slope Cultural Resources Survey*, book 2 (Inuvik: Inuvialuit Social Development Program, 1994), 2.

7 Séguin to mother and sister, 5 Aug. 1866.

8 Europeans considered the North healthy, relative to tropical colonies. See Binnema, *Enlightened Zeal*, 8–9.

The Anthropologists Debate

Fur-trade scholarship flourished in the 1970s and 1980s, in the wake of the transfer of the Hudson's Bay Company (HBC) Archives from London, England to Winnipeg, Manitoba.[9] This included new ethnohistorical and anthropological research on the North that aimed to historicize the communities anthropologists worked with in the twentieth century. June Helm and Shepard Krech III both studied the Dene (whom they called northern Athapaskans). They each turned to HBC records for insight into population changes as a result of contact with Europeans beginning in the late eighteenth century, in the lands that became the Mackenzie district, Yukon Territory, and Alaska. From their overlapping archival forays, Helm and Krech drew competing conclusions about post-contact demographic change.

This debate was animated by wider scholarship on epidemics and depopulation in Indigenous America. There were two key lines of argumentation that pertained to Dene history. First, scholars sought to understand whether subarctic environments were inherently severe. Second, anthropologists were interested in the influence of nineteenth-century demographic changes on kinship and social organization. Underpinning both lines of inquiry was the role of epidemics in causing dramatic population declines in the nineteenth century.

Helm argued, as early as 1965 and drawing on work by Julian Steward, that the challenges of survival in an inherently harsh environment meant that Dene along the Mackenzie had both maternal and paternal kinship relations and that this social organization endured throughout the nineteenth century.[10] In 1980, Helm argued further that the practice of female infanticide, used to regulate population size, ended in order to dampen the demographic impacts of epidemic diseases.[11] Krech, by contrast, argued that the apparent environmental severity was in fact evidence of socio-ecological upheaval linked to introduced diseases and the fur trade.[12] Embracing the idea of 'virgin soil epidemics', Krech detailed epidemics beginning around 1820 and enduring for the rest of the century. He calculated that the population was reduced to one-fifth of its

[9] Adele Perry, *Colonial Relations: The Douglas-Connolly Family and the Nineteenth-Century Imperial World* (Cambridge: Cambridge University Press, 2015), 6; Ray, *Indians in the Fur Trade*; Sylvia Van Kirk, *Many Tender Ties: Women in Fur Trade Society in Western Canada, 1670–1870* (Norman: University of Oklahoma Press, 1983); Jennifer S. H. Brown, *Strangers in Blood: Fur Trade Company Families in Indian Country* (Vancouver: University of British Columbia Press, 1980); Robert R. Janes, 'The Athapaskan and the Fur Trade: Observations from Archaeology and Ethnohistory', *Western Canadian Journal of Anthropology* 5, nos. 3–4 (1975): 159–86; J. C. Yerbury, *The Subarctic Indians and the Fur Trade, 1680–1860* (Vancouver: University of British Columbia Press, 1986).

[10] June Helm, 'Bilaterality in the Socio-Territorial Organization of the Arctic Drainage Dene', *Ethnology* 4 (1965): 361–85.

[11] June Helm, 'Female Infanticide, European Diseases, and Population Levels among the Mackenzie Dene', *American Ethnologist* 7 (1980): 259–85.

[12] Krech, 'Disease, Starvation', 710–32; 'Influence of Disease', 123–46.

pre-contact size, where Helm used much the same archival material to argue for a less dramatic decline. In a 1978 article, Krech drew on works that argued 'post-contact shocks' led to changes in social organization and the rise of bilateral kinship in the nineteenth century. Krech argued against the historical significance of female infanticide. He did not link changed social organization solely to drastic depopulation, but rather to a range of demographic and environmental changes, all of which were tied to the fur trade. In 1983, for instance, he argued that caribou were killed unsustainably for their tongues because of new demands for meat created by traders. This last piece foreshadowed his comprehensive, influential, and problematic book *The Ecological Indian: Myth and History* (1999).[13]

Their debate makes for compelling reading, not least because of its gendered dynamics. Helm was a prominent anthropologist. She served as Chair of the American Association for the Advancement of Science in 1978, was a consultant to Justice Thomas Berger during the Mackenzie Valley Pipeline Inquiry, and was later President of the American Anthropological Association. She collaborated closely with other women, most notably Beryl C. Gillespie and Nancy Lurie. Helm clashed with a junior male scholar: Krech had completed his doctoral dissertation on Fort McPherson in 1974 and in the early 1980s was an associate professor at George Mason University.[14] They argued over – among other things – the relative importance of female infanticide and the significance of kinship organized patrilineally, matrilineally, or bilaterally. Krech advanced a complicated argument about the interrelationship of disease, environment, and social organization in the nineteenth century. Helm's contributions were more focused, and her research, which Krech critiqued as modelled rather than historical or contextual, was more systematic in its claims of the importance of social adaptations both to an inherently severe environment and to the new hazards of epidemic disease.[15] There were limitations to how both Krech and Helm used historical sources. Significantly, they placed greatest weight on documentary sources and drew very little on their own, late twentieth-century informants, a methodology at odds with twenty-first-century research norms in the North. They clearly saw archival research as a tool to assess the historical 'truth' of Dene stories.[16] Neither scholar anticipated Mary Black-Rogers's insights into the discourses of 'starving' in the fur trade, and

[13] Kimberly TallBear, 'Shepard Krech's *The Ecological Indian*: One Indian's Perspective', *IIIRM Publications* (Sept. 2000): 1–5; Lianne C. Leddy, 'Intersections of Indigenous and Environmental History in Canada', *Canadian Historical Review* 98, no. 1 (2017), 84–5.

[14] Krech thanked Helm in the acknowledgements of his 1976 article, 'The Eastern Kutchin and the Fur Trade, 1800–1860', *Ethnohistory* 23, no. 3 (1976): 213–35 (p. 232).

[15] Krech, 'Influence of Disease', 124.

[16] In addition to the works already cited by Krech and Helm, see also June Helm and Beryl C. Gillespie, 'Dogrib Oral Tradition as History: War and Peace in the 1820s', *Journal of Anthropological Research* 37, no. 1 (1981): 8–27; the Yellowknives Dene offered their critique

they always interpreted starvation and sickness literally.[17] Krech and Helm each subjected HBC census records to rigorous analysis. Krech, in particular, took all references in HBC materials to disease and famine, whether described by symptoms or named as whooping cough, smallpox, and the like, as signs of larger epidemics. In their assumption that references to infectious diseases in the documentary record were a minimum measure of epidemics among northern Dene, Helm and Krech were following on the main interpretations within anthropology and history in the late 1970s and 1980s.

Histories of the subarctic invariably cite Helm and Krech, although their profound disagreement is foregrounded only in works that address health and disease.[18] Martha McCarthy responded to both Helm and Krech by offering her own analysis of population changes along Dehcho. Drawing from Oblate sources, McCarthy asserted that notwithstanding 'the immediate effects of imported diseases', there was no evidence of permanent depopulation.[19] James Waldram, Ann Herring, and Kue Young's *Aboriginal Health in Canada* (1995) distinguished between Helm and Krech as offering gradualist versus catastrophist theories respectively for understanding the role of introduced diseases and ill health in post-contact change. Waldram, Herring, and Young offered a nuanced overview of the impact of introduced diseases, emphasizing that the intensity of epidemics and scale of depopulation had to be understood at the community level, rather than assuming regional, national, or continental continuities.[20]

In spite of these differences, neither Helm nor Krech fabricated epidemics. Krech used the idea of depopulating 'virgin soil' epidemics to infer catastrophe from accounts of sickness, applying what was a theory of epidemic disease and historical change to his interpretation of the evidence from HBC records. This is what historians and anthropologists do when looking at accounts of sickness and disease in the past: they draw on the available evidence and conceptual frameworks to try to understand the nature and impacts of an epidemic. Such work becomes more complicated when we realize that one of the most prolific nineteenth-century European writers on northern disease and Indigenous peoples, Oblate father Émile Petitot, exaggerated, embellished, and even made up, epidemics.

of Helm and Gillespie on their website, 'Our People', *Yellowknives Dene First Nation*, https://ykdene.com/about/our-people/, last accessed 28 Sept. 2022.

17 Mary Black-Rogers, 'Varieties of "Starving": Semantics and Survival in the Subarctic Fur Trade, 1750–1850', *Ethnohistory* 33, no. 4 (1986), 353–83.

18 For example, in Abel, *Drum Songs*, 95, 105; McCormack, *Fort Chipewyan*, *passim*.

19 McCarthy, *Great River*, 124.

20 James B. Waldram, D. Ann Herring, and T. Kue Young, *Aboriginal Health in Canada: Historical Cultural, and Epidemiological Perspectives* (Toronto: University of Toronto Press, 1995), 46; Cameron, Kelton, and Swedlund, eds., *Beyond Germs*, 5–6.

How Many Epidemics?

Missionaries and fur traders had different interests in disease. For missionaries, tending to the body was as important as tending to the soul. As Martha McCarthy observed, 'health and faith were closely linked for both Oblate and Dene, making medical care an integral part of evangelization'.[21] Narratives of northern missions, published by Oblates in the nineteenth century to raise funds for their work, not only present details about sickness and healing but also lingered on the pathos of epidemics. Missionaries Émile Petitot, in his published books and letters, and Robert McDonald, in his voluminous diaries excerpted for global Anglican audiences in *The Church Missionary Intelligencer*, emphasized the number of deaths in an outbreak to highlight the number of souls they had secured – marked by crosses on the landscape, baptisms performed, or prayers before death. While in general Petitot, McDonald, and others were reliable observers (indeed, burial registers created by missionaries are indispensable to this book), they had powerful motivation to err on the side of *more* sickness, as ill health was a measure of the great need for mission work.

Fur traders, on the other hand, at times under-reported sickness and death. From 1805, Willard Ferdinand Wentzel, an employee of the North West Company, managed the Fort of the Forks, where the Liard and Mackenzie rivers meet. According to historian Lloyd Keith, Wentzel dismissed reports of sickness and their severity among the Dene.[22] Shepherd Krech referred to Wentzel as 'skeptical' about illness.[23] Wentzel was far from the only one. In 1800–1, John Thomson, clerk at Rocky Mountain Fort, north of Fort of the Forks on the other side of the river, grumbled that Dene hunters were deceitful, refused to pay their debts when they arrived, and 'say that they would have come sooner were it not that two or three of their relations are sick'.[24] Traders may have under-reported sickness when they perceived it as an excuse rather than a statement of fact. That is not to say, though, that Indigenous hunters did not deploy 'sickness' for reasons other than simply reporting on their health. In her analysis of the fur-trade glossary of starvation, Black-Rogers distinguished meaning based on the source of information ('Rumor, Report, Observed by writer, Self-starving') and organized the language of starvation into three categories: literal, technical (or fur-trade jargon), and manipulative (including both deliberately false statements and ritual routines of speech that served overlapping purposes).[25] In the case of sickness, not all reports were equal,

[21] McCarthy, *Great River*, 119.
[22] Lloyd Keith, ed., *North of Athabasca: Slave Lake and Mackenzie River Documents of the North West Company, 1800–1821* (Montreal: McGill-Queen's University Press, 2001), 54.
[23] Krech, 'Influence of Disease', 142, n.7.
[24] Keith, *North of Athabasca*, 145.
[25] Black-Rogers, 'Varieties of "Starving"', table 1, 356.

not all signalled a major outbreak, and not all counts of deaths could be trusted; nor did any of these reports arise from some objective viewpoint.

In 1865, the earliest reports of a serious disease came from Fort Chipewyan in August. The Fort was the gateway for goods and people destined for the Mackenzie River District, and Oblate missionaries there initially described an 'epidemic cold or possibly measles'; by the end of the month, the diagnosis of measles (*la rougeole*) was set forth, with symptoms including 'dysentery, swollen throat, ear discharge, and weakness'.[26] Further north at Fort Good Hope, Oblate father Jean Séguin also characterized the disease as measles.[27] Meanwhile, the same outbreak was simultaneously described by Robert McDonald, HBC traders, and other Oblates as scarlet fever. Most observers chose one disease or the other – for most, it was scarlet fever but in some Catholic documents, measles.[28] Measles and scarlet fever could have both been involved in the 1865 epidemic. Nineteenth-century observers frequently confused the two diseases. Medical literature used illustrations of the characteristic rashes to clarify clinical distinctions. Urban dwellers welcomed a diagnosis of measles, which did not require quarantine, in place of a scarlet fever diagnosis that could lead to months of bored isolation.[29] There was no such motivation in the North where, prior to the creation of a public health infrastructure, quarantines were not enforced. Missionaries and traders had experience with scarlet fever and measles but little formal training in distinguishing the two diseases. As Oblates, Petitot and Séguin relied on a German system of homeopathic medicine to treat sickness.[30] Petitot wrote to his superior in the midst of the epidemic saying that he did not know whether it was measles, scarlet fever, or both at once.[31] The secondary symptoms described at Fort Chipewyan – diarrhoea, swollen throat, ear discharge, and weakness – could have accompanied either disease. In Chapter 2, the epidemic is described as scarlet fever because that is what the evidence points to. Influenza was involved as well, but the diagnosis of measles appears to be a different characterization of the same disease, rather than the involvement of a third pathogen.

In Petitot's writings, however, measles became a separate epidemic. This did not appear in his letters from the 1860s but crystallized in a book published thirty years later, *Exploration de la Région du Grand Lac des Ours* (1893). Here, Petitot distinguished between the 1865 scarlet fever epidemic and an 1867 measles outbreak that killed 1,000 out of 4,000 people residing along the

[26] Codex Historicus, Fort Chipewyan, 10 Aug. and 30 Aug. 1865, PR1991.0345/74, OMI, PAA.
[27] Séguin to mother and sister, 1 Jun. 1866, and 5 Aug. 1866.
[28] An example of both scarlet fever and measles can be found in Hardisty to Mactavish, 27 Nov. 1866, fo. 105a.
[29] Hardy, Epidemic Streets, 44; Clement Dukes, 'On the confusion of two different diseases under the name of rubella (rose-rash)', *The Lancet* 156, 4011 (14 July 1900), 89–94.
[30] Petitot, *Quinze ans*, 162; McCarthy, *Great River*, 124–5.
[31] Petitot to Supérieur Général, 18 Nov. 1865, 183.

Arctic Coast.[32] Secondary sources have reproduced Petitot's claim. But Séguin, writing home in 1867, did not differentiate between the sickness at Fort Good Hope and Fort Anderson in diagnosis; both were 'rougeole', and both were part of the same 1865 epidemic.[33] In 1867, on a trip to the Arctic Coast, Séguin observed no illness, contrary to what Petitot published after the fact. There were the influenza outbreaks that year, but that was not what Petitot described. In effect, he was claiming that there was a second measles epidemic that killed a quarter of the population on the coast two years after the scarlet fever. Petitot alone made this claim.

Then there are reports from 1867 to 1868 that describe the illness as typhus, not influenza. These references all trace back again to Petitot, who wrote in letters and in his larger narratives that 'the typhus or some nervous fever' had had dire effects on the K'áhshó Got'ı̨nę, the Inuvialuit, and the Gwich'in.[34] It is possible that people may have been infected with and died from typhus in 1867–8, but it is implausible to characterize this as epidemic typhus or to identify that disease as the principal cause of the deaths that winter.

Typhus is a vector-borne disease caused by *Rickettsia* organisms, a very small species of bacteria that live in small mammals and insects. Fleas and lice, including the human body louse, carry *Rickettsia*.[35] Lice have long co-evolved with human hosts and are recorded in most parts of the world. Northern ground squirrels (siksiks) had lice, and there are references in archival documents and oral histories to these, as well as to body lice and 'vermin'.[36] However, the species of small mammals found in the Yukon and Mackenzie district are poor reservoirs for *Rickettsia*. Typhus could have been brought by men working on the HBC boat crews who came from urban centres or off of crowded ships. At LaPierre's House in 1869, Robert McDonald noted that during the winter 'One of the Co's men had Typhus fever'.[37] But McDonald's account of a single man falling ill with typhus is persuasive precisely because it does not set off an epidemic. Whether typhus could have achieved epidemic form in the north in this period is highly unlikely. While conditions among boat crews plying northern rivers in the

32 Petitot, *Exploration*, 374, n. 1.

33 Jean Séguin to mother and sister, 1 Jul. 1867 and 3 Aug. 1867, 71.220 / 7344, OMI, PAA; An HBC reference to 'measles' among Inuit connects to Séguin ('a rumor had also reached Good Hope'), Hardisty to Governor etc., 30 Jul. 1866, fo. 94.

34 R. P. Petitot to J. Fabre, Good Hope, 29 Feb. 1868, *Missions de la Congrégation des Missionaires Oblats de Marie Immaculée*, vol. 8 (Paris: Hennuyer et fils, 1869), 296, 306.

35 Hans Zinsser, *Rats, Lice, and History* (New Brunswick: Transaction Publishers, 2008); Amina Boutellis, Laurent Abi-Rached, and Didier Raoult, 'The Origin and Distribution of Human Lice in the World', *Infection, Genetics, and Evolution* 23 (2014): 210–11.

36 Mary Evik Ruben interview with Cathy Cockney, 21 Mar. 2001, Paulatuuq, Parks Canada, *Paulatuuq Oral History Project: Inuvialuit Elders Share their Stories* (Inuvik: Parks Canada Western Arctic Field Unit, 2004), 215; Fortuine, *Chills and Fever*, 33, 36, 64–5.

37 McDonald Diary, 2 Mar. 1869. Fortuine, *Chills and Fever*, 207.

nineteenth century left men vulnerable to sickness, they were not crowded and unsanitary like those found among early modern armies or in jails or crowded slums, where epidemic typhus flourished.

In the HBC records and McDonald's diary, the 1867–8 epidemic is exclusively described as 'influenza', with delirium also reported. Typhus is characterized by a headache, chills, high fever, and a blotchy rash; delirium and confusion eventually set in, and it was these symptoms that gave the disease its name: Hippocratic writings used the Greek word, *typhos* meaning 'hazy' or 'smoky' to describe the confused state of the victim. The delirium experienced in this influenza outbreak may account for Petitot's diagnosis of 'typhus'. There were no reports of a rash. Hardisty observed that the influenza brought with it 'a low, bilious fever' (bilious refers to nausea or vomiting). Typhus was sometimes confused with typhoid, a disease with gastrointestinal symptoms. Yet the epidemic moved between communities, breaking out at different times in a manner consistent with influenza rather than with a contaminated food or water source (typhoid) or unsanitary, overcrowded conditions (typhus). Only Petitot described a typhus epidemic at this time.

Petitot was a prolific writer, and – more than many other colonial observers – he was attentive to Indigenous languages and cultural practices. We cannot discard his writings wholesale as the fictions of an unreliable observer. When it came to disease, however, he was neither an expert nor did he pay close attention to symptoms and effects. He repeatedly confused who died when and from what disease. Petitot would have had it that between 1865 and 1867 the Mackenzie district was ravaged by major epidemics of scarlet fever, measles, influenza, and typhus, diseases which struck with fury and left people paralysed with fear.[38] Separate outbreaks of different diseases enhanced the drama of Petitot's published writings. The distinction between scarlet fever inland in 1865 and measles along the coast in 1867 reinforced racialized distinctions between Gwich'in and Inuvialuit, which Petitot was instrumental in constructing. The differential diagnosis of disease served a rhetorical function for Petitot, even if it was not tethered to reality. Most historians to date have erred on the side of Petitot, including his and others' descriptions of multiple pathogens. But if some of these outbreaks are exaggerated or imagined, repeating these fictions as history does not represent a comprehensive accounting of the history of disease but instead alters how we understand the health of these places at this time and the capacity of communities to contend with novel pathogens.

[38] The language I use here draws directly from Petitot's writings, including Petitot to Fabre, 29 Feb. 1868, 306.

Extinction Fictions

The most dramatic distortion of the fate of northern peoples claimed that two Gwich'in tribes, the Tatsa Kutchin and the Tennuth Kutchin, disappeared altogether in the scarlet fever epidemic. Historical references to the loss of these tribes trace back to a single source, William H. Dall's *Alaska and Its Resources*, published in 1870. Dall was a naturalist with the Scientific Corps of the Western Union Telegraph Expedition, which travelled eastwards up the Yukon River from Nulato, reaching Fort Yukon in the spring of 1867, after the scarlet fever had passed. Dall wrote, 'There were formerly a few bands of Indians between the mouths of the Porcupine and Tananáh, on the Yukon, but they have been swept away by scarlet fever. They were the *Tennúth-Kutchín* or Birch Indians (*Gens de Bouleaux*) and the *Tatsáh-Kutchín*.'[39] In 1934, anthropologist Cornelius Osgood clarified that the people Dall had referred to as the Tatsa Kutchin belonged to a larger group of 'Lower Yukon Kutchin' that were only 'partially extinct'.[40] Osgood otherwise supported Dall's findings, writing, 'No complete study of the Kutchin nation can ever be made. Within twenty-five years of their first discovery, the Birch Creek Kutchin were annihilated by an epidemic of scarlet fever.'[41]

Osgood and others used the experience of the Birch Creek Gwich'in to emphasize the 'extinction' or 'annihilation' of northern Indigenous people in epidemics. The notion of an Indigenous band or tribe 'going extinct' is deeply problematic in its own right and is closely tied to the long-standing narratives regarding Indigenous peoples' historical experiences of contact-era diseases. The prevailing image of a disease tsunami wiping out Indigenous villages is enhanced by the disappearance of specific peoples. Extinction is defined as '[of a species, family, or other larger group] having no living members' or, more generally, 'a situation in which something no longer exists'.[42] 'Partial' extinction is little more than an oxymoron that served to reinforce Dall's original observation, even as Osgood gently corrected it. Beyond that, the language of extinction is more commonly applied to other-than-human nature for the obvious reason that humans, as a species, have yet to go extinct. Describing an Indigenous community in this fashion is dehumanizing; it served to underline the place of Indigenous peoples as part of nature and individual tribes as appropriate discrete subjects of scientific study rather than members of the larger human community, while the prospect of 'extinction' justified the need for anthropological study in the present. Finally, it was, in this instance, wrong

39 William H. Dall, *Alaska and Its Resources* (Boston: Lee and Shepherd, 1870), 431.

40 Cornelius Osgood, 'Kutchin Tribal Distribution and Synonymy', *American Anthropologist* 36, no. 2 (1934): 168–79 (p. 177).

41 Cornelius Osgood, *Contributions to the Ethnography of the Kutchin*, reprint ed. (New Haven: Human Relations Area Files Press, 1970), 14–15.

42 *Oxford English Dictionary* and *Cambridge English Dictionary* definitions, respectively.

insofar as it was used to refer to a human social group that has persisted. On the website of the Tanana Chiefs Conference, a tribal consortium in Alaska, the Birch Creek or Denduu Gwich'in correct those who 'believe that this band was annihilated by scarlet fever'.[43]

Dall did not conjure his tale from thin air. He travelled with an artist, Frederick Whymper, whose maps show the error of their ways. In June 1867, the expedition passed deserted villages on the Yukon River, 'formerly inhabited by some Indians of the Kutchin tribes, who all died five years ago of the scarlet fever'.[44] Who these houses belonged to was muddled by Dall and Whymper: the former assigned them to the Birch Creek Gwich'in, the latter noted on his map that they were homes of the *Gens de milieu*. These two were one and the same band, a small group that numbered around thirty people, including nine hunters led by Bikkuinechatti, when Robert McDonald visited them in November 1862.[45] By June 1866, McDonald reported that from this camp there was 'but a feeble remnant' after the scarlet fever: three men, two teenage boys, six women, and seven children.[46] McDonald observed that 'they will doubtless be not much longer as a separate tribe, but be merged into the others'.[47] Indeed, that same June, while visiting a camp that included one man and three women from the *Gens de milieu*, McDonald recorded 'Two of the women taken to wife by two of the Indians from Fort Youcon.'[48] The *Gens de milieu* and the *Gens de Bouleaux*, distinguished by traders and travellers who did not employ consistent ethnographic categories, were one and the same. The survivors of the scarlet fever joined other families and bands, without losing their own identity or their relations to the lands by Birch Creek.[49]

The accounts shared by Elders which open this chapter describe the good health that they remember and which they were told of by their families.

43 'Birch Creek', *Tanana Chiefs Conference*, www.tananachiefs.org/about/communities/birch-creek/.

44 Dall, *Alaska*, 100. Of course, the date is wrong too.

45 McDonald Diary, 22 Nov. 1862. The Birch Creek Gwich'in are also called, in different sources, the 'people on the other side' (Beaumont, Osgood), a name which is also given to the Tennuth Kutchin. Kennicott called the Tennuth Kutchin the 'middle people' (Slobodin), and Murray called them the 'people of this side', a distinction – between 'this' and 'the other' – which could be accounted for depending on which side and which river you are starting from. Susan Beaumont, *Jijuu: Who Are My Grandparents? Where Are They From?* (Fort McPherson: Gwich'in Enrolment Board, 1998), 33; Osgood, 'Kutchin Tribal Distribution', 172; Richard Slobodin, 'Kutchin', *Handbook of North American Indians*, vol. 6, *Subarctic*, ed. June Helm (Washington: Smithsonian Institution, 1981), 532; Alexander H. Murray, *Journal of the Yukon 1847–48*, ed. L. J. Burpee, Publications of the Canadian Archives no. 4 (Ottawa: Government Printing Bureau, 1910), 82.

46 McDonald Diary, 13 Mar. 1866; 'Youcon Mission', 106.

47 'Youcon Mission', 106.

48 McDonald Diary, 2 Jun. 1866; Beaumont, *Jijuu*, 33.

49 Michael Koskey and Kristin Mull, 'Traditional Ecological Knowledge and Biological Sampling of Nonsalmon Fish Species in the Yukon Flats Region, Alaska', Technical Paper no. 362, Alaska Department of Fish and Game (May 2011), 23.

The incommensurability of their accounts with the 'virgin soil' model and the idea of prevalent sickness in the nineteenth century must give us pause.[50] Following on the work of Waldram, Herring, and Young, in this book, diseases are traced from community to community where possible. Regional continuities are not assumed but instead only examined where there is evidence showing the wider spread of disease. This approach raises significant questions about the long-standing historiographical assumption that smallpox was among the earliest pathogens introduced by Europeans to people living along the shores of the great northern rivers and lakes.

Smallpox

Smallpox holds an exceptional place in the history of disease: it is the sole major infectious disease that survives now only in captivity. Since its eradication in 1980, smallpox has been relegated to our collective imagination where its image is drawn with three main features. Smallpox was the first virus against which an effective vaccine was developed, by Edward Jenner in 1796. Smallpox had an awful physical manifestation. Historian Michael Bliss evoked the horrors of the disease in nineteenth-century Montreal, where 'mirrors were not allowed in smallpox hospitals'.[51] Lastly, smallpox holds a place of singular importance among contact-era epidemic diseases. Given its distinctive appearance and the scarring left in its wake, smallpox was easily identifiable among the pathogens that crossed oceans in this period. Smallpox was responsible for some of the most devastating epidemics introduced by Europeans.

The role of smallpox in contact-era epidemics stemmed from variola's capacity, under the right circumstances, to diffuse widely; to travel, in Alfred Crosby's words, 'with seven-league boots'.[52] Smallpox can vary significantly in virulence, producing different experiences of the disease and patterns of transmission.[53] A more virulent outbreak could burn out more quickly, leaving few survivors. The frequency of epidemics shaped viral transmission. Survivors from a previous epidemic would be immune to the disease, blocking its spread. Rather than a wave of disease that overwhelmed villages and communities across vast regions, smallpox travelled erratic paths.[54] A Tlingit headman, Saigakakh, recounted a smallpox epidemic from his childhood that

[50] Eve Tuck and K. Wayne Yang, 'Decolonization is Not a Metaphor', *Decolonization: Indigeneity, Education & Society* 1, no. 1 (2012), 35–6.
[51] Michael Bliss, *Plague: A Story of Smallpox in Montreal* (Toronto: Harper Collins, 1991), 39–42.
[52] Crosby, *Ecological Imperialism*, 201.
[53] Ana T. Duggan, Maria F. Perdomo, Dario Piombino-Mascali, et al., '17th Century Variola Virus Reveals the Recent History of Smallpox', *Current Biology* 26 (Dec. 2016): 3407–12.
[54] Ray, *Indians in the Fur Trade*, 183–7; Boyd, *Spirit of Pestilence*, 40; Fortuine, *Chills and Fever*, 236.

spread north from the Stikine into Alaska.[55] Witness accounts and smallpox scarring traced the contours of a 1775 outbreak near Cape Edgecumbe on the Alaska Panhandle, but it was only the people from that area who were pock-marked, 'none from the westward'.[56] The spread of smallpox depended on virulence and how the virus arrived and travelled. The different forms of seasonal transportation that prevailed over land, water, ice, and snow shaped disease transmission.

The ships that sailed between England, Spain, Russia, and North America brought crewmen from urban disease pools and created ample opportunity for smallpox to reach communities along the coast and those with whom they traded. As historian Robert Boyd argued, 'the relatively dense and continuous precontact populations, and the extensive social and economic networks characteristic of the aboriginal Pacific Northwest all suggest that smallpox, when first introduced, must have spread to the limits of settlement'.[57] Beyond these coastal regions, the movement of smallpox over lands and waters is less obvious. The Orkneymen who made up the European labour force in the northwest interior came from islands where smallpox was endemic.[58] But they appear to have rarely – if ever – carried the disease far inland. As Binnema noted, 'if smallpox ever hit the northwestern plains before 1780, there is scant evidence of it'.[59]

Historians have asserted that the great smallpox pandemic of 1775–82 reached the Mackenzie River District. The 'Pox Americana', in Elizabeth Fenn's words, originated in Mexico City, travelled along the Atlantic seaboard (with significant implications for the American Revolution), through the western states, and into British North America. In her map illustrating the transmission of smallpox across North America, Fenn drew a solid arrow – not a dashed 'probable' arrow – showing the epidemic's northernmost reach: the southern shore of Great Slave Lake.[60] Samuel Hearne is the source of evidence that smallpox reached Great Slave Lake. In a note appended to his posthumously published *Journey to the Northern Ocean* (1795), Hearne observed, 'the Northern Indians [Dënesųłıné], by annually visiting their Southern friends, the Athapuscow Indians [Cree], have contracted the small-pox, which has

[55] Recounted to a Russian official Kyrill T. Khlebnikov, in Fortuine, *Chills and Fever*, 227.

[56] Fortuine, *Chills and Fever*, 228. [57] Boyd, *Spirit of Pestilence*, 32.

[58] C. Stuart Houston and Stan Houston, 'The First Smallpox Epidemic on the Canadian Plains: In the Fur-Traders' Words', *Canadian Journal of Infectious Diseases* 11, no. 2 (March/April 2000): 112–15 (p. 113); B. Smith, 'Camphor, Cabbage Leaves and Vaccination: The Career of Johnie "Notions" Williamson, of Hamnavoe, Eshaness, Shetland', *Proceedings of the Royal College of Physicians Edinburgh* 29 (1998): 395–406 (p. 399). Binnema, *Common and Contested Ground*, 123–4.

[59] Binnema, *Common and Contested Ground*, 120. See also Binnema, 'With Tears, Shrieks, and Howlings of Despair', 110–31.

[60] Elizabeth A. Fenn, *Pox Americana: The Great Smallpox Epidemic of 1775–82* (New York: Hill and Wang, 2001), 7.

carried off nine-tenths of them, and particularly those people who composed the trade at Churchill Factory'.[61] Hearne was HBC chief at Prince of Wales's Fort (Churchill) from 1776 to 1782, when the epidemic hit.[62] And smallpox did reach Churchill and elsewhere in the Petit Nord with estimates of mortality in the Hudson Bay region ranging from 20 to 50 per cent.[63] Aside from Hearne's comment, there is no documentary record nor any evidence in oral histories that smallpox travelled to the north-west. Patricia McCormack wrote that it 'appears unlikely' that the people living in the vicinity of Fort Chipewyan experienced the epidemic, although it did reach Portage La Loche, where the Churchill and Athabasca river systems meet.[64] Paul Hackett relied on Krech to suggest that the epidemic 'had only limited penetration among the Athapaskan tribes of the Arctic drainage lowlands, perhaps striking only the southern groups who traded with the English'.[65] If this were indeed the case, the epidemic would have reached Dene living between Great Slave and Great Bear lakes, and Fenn drew her arrow short.

But Krech's analysis demands closer attention. Aside from Hearne, the only other evidence Krech brought to bear was Alexander Mackenzie's observations from 1789 that people camped near Great Bear River had legs 'full of Scabs by their frequent roasting them to the Fire'.[66] Krech did not state explicitly that this was smallpox scarring (that is Hackett's inference) but wrote that 'epidemic diseases might have produced these symptoms'.[67] It is unlikely that Mackenzie observed smallpox scars on the legs of Sahtu Dene and failed to make this explicit. He was familiar with the disease and its characteristic scarring, most commonly visible on the hands and face. Most eighteenth-century observers would be far more able to identify smallpox and its after-effects (blindness, in addition to scarring) than those of us who have never encountered the virus. Moreover, Mackenzie was the one who reported on the presence of smallpox near Portage la Loche, telling of traders who turned back because here 'they found, in every direction, the ravages of the small pox'.[68] Elsewhere, Krech speculated that a major smallpox epidemic from 1835 to 1840 caused 'heavy' mortality among 'the Dihai, Chandalar River, and Birch Creek Kutchin [Gwich'in]

[61] Samuel Hearne, *A Journey from Prince of Wales's Fort in Hudson's Bay to the Northern Ocean* ... (London: A. Strahan and T. Cadell, 1795), 178.

[62] On Hearne's reliability, see Emilie Cameron, *Far Off Metal River: Inuit Lands, Settler Stories, and the Making of the Contemporary Arctic* (Vancouver: UBC Press, 2015), 44, *passim*; I. S. MacLaren, 'From Exploration to Publication: The Evolution of a 19th-Century Arctic Narrative', *Arctic* 47, no. 1 (1994): 43–53.

[63] Ann M. Carlos and Frank Lewis, 'Smallpox and Native American Mortality: The 1780s epidemic in the Hudson Bay Region', *Explorations in Economic History* 49, no. 3 (2012), http://doi.org/10.1016/j.eeh.2012.04.003.

[64] McCormack, *Fort Chipewyan*, 280, n.8.

[65] Hackett, *Remarkable Sickness*, 117.

[66] Krech, 'Disease, Starvation', 712.

[67] Krech, 'Disease, Starvation', 712; See also Yerbury, *Subarctic Indians*, 147–8.

[68] Mackenzie in Abel, *Drum Songs*, 72; Decker, 'Historical Diffusion Patterns', 7.

bands' even though 'direct evidence ... is lacking'.[69] Krech asserted that the smallpox had spread among these people because of their trade ties with the Russians, but there were no reports of smallpox at this time among the Gwich'in, no deaths attributed to this disease, nor scars reported by traders or missionaries in the following decades. When, in 1843, Russian naval officer and explorer Lavrenty Zagoskin travelled downriver from Nulato (the place closest to the Gwich'in where this epidemic certainly reached), he noted that the disease had struck villages with different intensity.[70] Given that eighteenth- and nineteenth-century smallpox outbreaks never travelled reliably and uniformly along trade routes, Krech's conclusion tells us more about his assumptions about the diffusion potential of smallpox than the history of the virus.

Why does it matter whether the smallpox epidemic of 1775–82 or 1835–40 reached the Dene in the Mackenzie district or the Gwich'in on the lands that later became the Yukon? After all, as we will see, smallpox did arrive in these places in 1870, 1900, and after. Tracing the presence or absence of smallpox before 1870 illuminates issues around evidence and its interpretive weight. The historiography that has assumed smallpox reached the Mackenzie district in the late eighteenth century demonstrates how paper-thin evidence can be stretched to carry a virus all the way to Great Bear Lake. More than that, scholars built larger interpretations about depopulation and socio-cultural change around significant disease outbreaks before the 1820s. The 1780s smallpox has long stood as the best contender for a major, depopulating episode, given that pandemic's scale and mortality levels in communities with no previous exposure. If smallpox never reached the Mackenzie district or the eastern reaches of the Yukon River and its tributaries until the late nineteenth century, then – as observers said at the time – the 1860s scarlet fever *was* the worst epidemic in the history of the fur trade to that date. It is no minor issue whether an epidemic reached an area or not. Witness accounts of the smallpox epidemics among Northwest Coast peoples led Boyd to argue for the enduring impacts of the earliest experiences of disease on Indigenous relations with white people.[71] As we will see throughout this book, epidemics and how they were handled shaped foundational relationships between Indigenous peoples and settlers. Understanding the significance of an epidemic's course and impacts goes much deeper than counting those who died.

Medicine

In 1866, William Lucas Hardisty was forty-four years old. Born in northern Quebec, he was the son of HBC trader Richard Hardisty and Margaret Sutherland, the daughter of a Scottish man and Cree woman. William's younger

[69] Others have characterized Krech's findings as speculation: see Keith, *North of Athabasca*, 303.
[70] Fortuine, *Chills and Fever*, 236. [71] Boyd, *Spirit of Pestilence*, 23–31, 45–6.

brothers, Richard Charles and Joseph Wordsworth, had long careers with the HBC in Edmonton, Honolulu, and beyond. William's younger sister, Isabella Sophia, married Donald A. Smith (Lord Strathcona). William's wife, Mary Ann Allen, was the granddaughter of a Chinook woman and a British man, and four of their five children claimed Métis scrip. (Scrip refers to documents redeemable for land or money issued to Métis people in the West and parts of the North in exchange for their land rights.[72]) The fifth child of William and Mary Ann, Isabella Clark, married James Alexander Lougheed, a prominent Alberta settler politician of Protestant Irish background.[73] One of William and Mary's three sons, Richard Thomas Hardisty, served the British on the Nile Expedition (1884–5). Shortly after his return to Canada, he died from a wound to the head in the Battle of Batoche (1885) while serving with Frederick Middleton's federal troops.[74] As Adele Perry has shown, intimate family life is essential to understanding race and power in colonial societies; Hardisty and his immediate family's sense of identity and place within Canada's emerging colonial society would make for a rich in-depth study.[75] In this book, however, Hardisty is an important but passing actor, and one whose contradictions, as a Métis man whose allegiance lay principally with the company that employed him, were by no means unique in the nineteenth-century North.

William Hardisty entered the HBC's service in 1842 as a postmaster sent to work in the Mackenzie River District. He had been the Chief Trader in charge of the district for almost a decade when the scarlet fever broke out. In July of 1866, after the epidemic ebbed, Hardisty's duties brought him down to Portage La Loche. Here was the height of land between the Hudson Bay and Arctic watersheds. From 1826 to 1886, this was the trading nexus in the HBC's brigade system, where goods that arrived from England, eastern Canada, and the United States – including clothes, tools, and household items, but also meat-mincing machines and goggles – were exchanged with the returns in fur, castorum, leather, and caribou tongues from the Mackenzie River District posts.[76] When Hardisty sat down to compose his annual report to the Governor, Chief Factors, and Chief Traders of the Northern Department, he reflected on the scarlet fever

[72] For the use of scrip applications in Métis history and genealogies, see Brenda Macdougall, *One of the Family: Metis Culture in Nineteenth-Century Northwestern Saskatchewan* (Vancouver: UBC Press, 2010); and chapter 7 in Gerhard J. Ens and Joe Sawchuk, *From New Peoples to New Nations: Aspects of Metis History and Identity from the Eighteenth to Twenty-First Centuries* (Toronto: University of Toronto Press, 2015).

[73] Their grandson, Peter Lougheed, would serve as the tenth premier of the province of Alberta.

[74] See Lawrence Barkwell, 'Richard Hardisty: Métis Soldier', Louis Riel Institute, 2010; Richard Hardisty's mother, Mary Allen, claimed scrip on her son's behalf after his death. See R190-44-1-E, vol. 1369, C-15006, LAC.

[75] Perry, *Colonial Relations*. Several family members, including William Lucas, are in the *Dictionary of Canadian Biography*. See also Donna McDonald's *Lord Strathcona: A Biography of Donald Alexander Smith* (Toronto: Dundurn Press, 1996).

[76] William Cowan to William Hardisty, 10 Jun. 1867, B.200/b/36, fo. 96, HBCA.

and its impact on the trade. It was here that Hardisty estimated the loss at 1,000 people across the district, a tally which, while higher than the cumulative reports from each post, appears realistic in context. Recall too, the discussion in Chapter 2 of the ways in which fur traders often under-counted sickness, in contrast to missionaries who exaggerated (Petitot being an extreme example).

In accounting for the serious toll among Indigenous northerners, Hardisty speculated that 'they were frightened out of their senses, and gave themselves up to despair'. He continued: '[they] Fancied the end of the World was come, and that they were all going to die, which prevented them from taking the necessary precautions during the Crisis of the Fever which, in ordinary cases would have insured recovery'.[77] From his post at Fort Simpson, Hardisty had witnessed the effects of the scarlet fever pandemic in the North. Yet none of his other correspondence during the outbreak, that either Hardisty wrote or received from the posts in his district, communicated these sentiments. This perspective – that the people had given up, and this kept them from doing what they could when confronted with a virulent pathogen, or in their ignorance had done precisely the wrong things – echoes many other descriptions from the nineteenth century and earlier of the effects of infectious diseases among Indigenous populations in the Americas.[78] The failure and ineptitude of Indigenous peoples was the other side of a colonial coin minted to describe inherent, constitutional weakness in the face of introduced infectious diseases. The frequency with which colonial observers used these two explanations to account for Indigenous deaths across diverse communities and encounters with widely varying pathogens hints at its true status. The fatalism described by Hardisty was not an accurate description of Tłı̨chǫ or Gwich'in or Sahtu Dene experiences with scarlet fever in 1865–6, but a colonial motif: a way in which colonial societies understood and interpreted the sickness they were confronted with and which they often did little to stop.[79] As a child of the fur trade, Hardisty learned this interpretation at a young age, and it shaped his worldview.

Hardisty was also acknowledging, though, that more could have been done. 'Necessary precautions' could have been taken. In reporting to his superiors, Hardisty laid the blame for this failure on those who had fallen ill, deflecting his own responsibility for so many deaths in his district and that the trade had

[77] William Hardisty to The Governor etc., 30 Jul. 1866, fo. 93a.

[78] See R. P. Petitot to T.-R. P. Supérieur Général, Fort Anderson, 18 Nov. 1865, *Missions*, vol. 7, 184; Ray, *Indians in the Fur Trade*, 105–6; J. B. Tyrrell, ed., *David Thompson's Narrative of His Explorations in Western America 1784–1812* (Toronto: The Champlain Society, 1916), 322–3.

[79] Jones, *Rationalizing Epidemics*, 13, 56. There are other deep-rooted colonial and colonizing narratives of disease in diverse contexts; see Nükhet Varlık's, '"Oriental Plague" or Epidemiological Orientalism? Revisiting the Plague Episteme of the Early Modern Mediterranean', in *Plague and Contagion in the Islamic Mediterranean*, ed. N. Varlık (Kalamazoo: Arc Humanities Press, 2017).

suffered as a result. But within six months, Hardisty made his first request for a medical officer to serve the Mackenzie River District, and his second a year later.

The MacKays

The deaths at Portage La Loche in 1867, their role in magnifying the challenges of transportation and crewing the boats at this time, and coming as they did in the wake of the scarlet fever epidemic, drove home the need for a physician. In December 1867, Hardisty wrote to Mactavish asking again for a permanent Medical Officer in the Mackenzie River District. Hardisty argued for the great need, 'even at the sacrifice of an additional £100 or so of Salary, to induce some one to come. It is doubtful whether we will be able in future to induce a sufficient number of Indians . . . to engage for the trip to Portage La Loche, unless a Doctor accompanies the Brigade.'[80] The doctor was needed to keep the crews healthy and to discourage malingering. The HBC had long played a significant role in the provision of medical care in western and northern Canada.[81] It was in the company's interest to ensure the good health of employees, Indigenous hunters, and their families. From the seventeenth century, the HBC recruited surgeons (physicians) for their posts on the shores of Hudson Bay. In the nineteenth century, full-time surgeons were stationed at the largest posts – Red River, Edmonton, and York Factory – while itinerant surgeons could attend to medical needs elsewhere in Rupert's Land.[82] William Todd worked at Fort Wedderburn on Lake Athabasca in 1819–20 and was a rare exception of a physician stationed at a farther-flung trade post in the nineteenth century. In 1864, the company recruited William Morrison MacKay, a Scottish-trained physician, to work in the North, first at York Factory and Norway House. In 1868, he was sent to the Mackenzie and was based at Simpson, Rae, and Resolution for over a decade, while also travelling to the other district posts. In the 1890s, he was Chief Trader at Fort Chipewyan before retiring to Edmonton in 1898.

Ideas about the causes of ill health common among residents of the northern interior were neither uniform nor rooted principally in biomedicine. Environmentalist ideas about disease prevailed among traders and missionaries in the 1860s. Petitot expressed these when he attributed the scarlet fever to the

80 Hardisty to Mactavish, 2 Dec. 1867, fo. 6.

81 Lux, *Medicine That Walks*; Hackett, *Remarkable Sickness*; Paul Hackett, 'Averting Disaster: The Hudson's Bay Company and Smallpox in Western Canada during the Late Eighteenth and Early Nineteenth Centuries', *Bulletin of the History of Medicine* 78, no. 3 (2004): 575–609; Jody F. Decker, 'The York Factory Medical Journals, 1846–52', *CBMH/BCHM* 14, no. 1 (1997): 107–31.

82 Decker, 'York Factory', 108–9.

'slow and rainy autumn' and Séguin when he described the country as healthier than France. Hardisty had similarly connected the apparent decline in the health of the Mackenzie district to a changing environment. In his December 1867 letter, Hardisty wrote that even though the influenza had been spreading through the district, 'I trust, however, that the pure air of winter will have restored them to their usual health and spirits'.[83] Unfortunately, as we know, 'the pure air of winter' did not suffice to check the passage of the virus that season. Echoes of humoral theory also appear, as when W. Cornwallis King, the HBC clerk at Fort Rae, wrote to Hardisty in March 1867 describing ill health among the families based at his post: 'I think their blood is turning into bile.'[84] King did not have formal medical training. Other HBC employees did, including the aforementioned Todd, and also John Rae, best known for his travels by snowshoe, and William MacKay.[85]

MacKay received advanced medical education at Edinburgh University. He studied under Joseph Lister, famous for his advances in antiseptic surgical practices developed in the 1860s. Bacteriological research by Louis Pasteur and Robert Koch, essential to the success of germ theory, remained very much in the laboratory before practical applications appeared in the 1870s, 1880s, and thereafter. And so the medicines sent in with the 1869 outfit to assist MacKay in his northern practice had exotic names but still relied heavily on herbal-derived remedies designed to act as laxatives or purgatives, or to otherwise bring about relief of symptoms without offering much by way of cures or specific therapies (Figure 3.1). Spirits of hartshorn were smelling salts, used to arouse people from unconsciousness; mixed with water, they were aromatic spirits of ammonia, also listed in MacKay's requisition. The purge of choice for English physicians from the eighteenth century was calomel in the form of blue pills.[86] Ipecac mixed with various wines and syrups became ipecacuanha wine and was a well-known emetic (inducing vomiting). Similarly, sweet spirits of nitre were a distillation of alcohol with nitric and sulphuric acids that worked as a diaphoretic (inducing perspiration), diuretic (inducing urination), and antispasmodic (used to treat gastrointestinal spasms, including diarrhoea, or bladder spasms). Castor oil and colocynth both worked as laxatives. Sedatives were also important, and for this MacKay had both paregoric elixir (liquid opium) and colchicum. Both could be used treat other symptoms: paregoric elixir also served to treat diarrhoea, and colchicum to

[83] Hardisty to The Governor etc., 2 Dec. 1867, fo. 2.

[84] Wm. C. King to William Hardisty, 4 Feb./1 Mar. 1867, B.200/b/36, fo. 80, HBCA. King told his life story to Mary Weekes in the 1930s, eventually published as *Trader King: The Thrilling Story of Forty Years' Service in the North-West Territories* (Calgary: Fifth House, 2007). See also 'I Became a Medicine Man', *The Beaver* (Dec. 1939): 24–6.

[85] E. E. Rich, 'The Fur Traders: Their Diet and Drugs', *The Beaver* (Summer 1976), 48.

[86] Roy Porter, *The Greatest Benefit to Mankind: A Medical History of Humanity* (New York: W.W. Norton, 1998), 269.

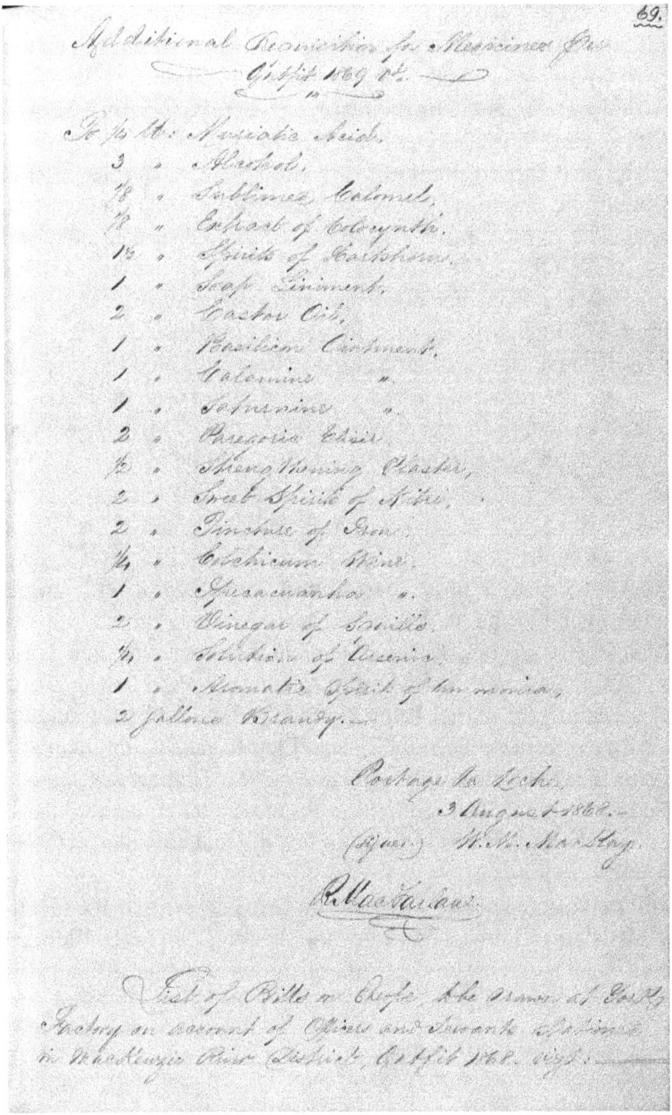

69.

Additional Requisition for Medicines for Outfit 1869 &c.

To ½ lb: Muriatic Acid.
3 " Alcohol.
⅛ " Sublimed Calomel.
⅛ " Extract of Colocynth.
1½ " Spirits of Hartshorn.
1 " Soap Liniment.
2 " Castor Oil.
1 " Basilicon Ointment.
1 " Calomine "
1 " [illegible] "
2 " Paregoric Elixir.
½ " Strengthening Plaster.
2 " Sweet Spirit of Nitre.
2 " Tincture of Iron.
¼ " Colchicum Wine.
1 " Ipecacuanha "
2 " Vinegar of Squills.
¼ " Solution of Arsenic.
1 " Aromatic Spirit of Ammonia.
2 gallons Brandy.—

Portage la Loche,
3 August 1868.—
(Signed) W. M. MacKay.

R. MacFarlane

List of Bills on Europe, the drawn at York Factory on account of Officers and Servants serving in MacKenzie River District, Outfit 1868. viz:—

Figure 3.1 William MacKay's medicines. B.200/b/37, fo. 69, Hudson's Bay Company Archives, Archives of Manitoba.

assist with problems with urination and to induce vomiting. Many of these medications had therapeutic properties, when used in moderation, but are otherwise more familiar as poisons. Calomel, for instance, was derived from mercury. MacKay's requisition included as well muriatic acid (another name for hydrochloric acid) and arsenic in solution. Both were used therapeutically to help with psoriasis and other skin irritations and with syphilis. Brandy, wine, and alcohol were essential medicines even when liquor was otherwise prohibited in shipments into the Mackenzie River District.[87]

MacKay also carried first-aid treatments for wounds (basilicon ointment), burns (saturnine ointment), or sprains and bruises (soap liniment). Injury and accidents were commonplace in the northern fur trade and could be so severe as to cause death. Of the 288 causes of death identified between 1862 and 1900, 8 per cent were from accidents including injuries from falls, burns, and drowning. McDonald recorded an accident in his diary on 6 September 1870. James McDougall, the clerk at Rampart House, was loading his gun when it 'went off accidentally and the charge lodged in the head of the boy in front of him. In half an hour the poor boy ceased to breathe.'[88] Mishaps with guns, if not fatal, led to awful wounds that required care. Adding in injuries from hunting, butchering animals, and travelling over the land, as Blondin observed, even if the Dene were healthy otherwise, 'people still hurt themselves in accidents'.[89] Notwithstanding his training under the distinguished surgeon Lister, 'surgery was not Dr. MacKay's forte', according to one biographer.[90] Instead, when confronted with closing an abdominal gash, MacKay turned to his wife, Jane Flett MacKay, to use her skills to complete the procedure. Jane was the same daughter of James Flett and Mary (a Gwich'in woman) who witnessed her mother's death from scarlet fever in 1865. She worked as a nurse and occasional surgeon in her own right.[91] Jane Flett MacKay complained about the paucity of imported medicines available at Fort Chipewyan when they were stationed at that post. She used Indigenous medicines and shared these with her husband as well. And it was Indigenous healing that prevailed in the north-west interior in this period.

Northern medicine power was much more expansive than the 'medicine' that in the Western idiom was used for healing. George Blondin offered a description of medicine power, while acknowledging the difficulty in defining the subject:

> The best I can do is say that medicine power is a spirit, with a mind of its own, and it attaches to us or, to see it another way, we borrow it. A person can't control this spirit. It

[87] Robert Hamilton to W. L. Hardisty, 12 Jun. 1871, B.200/b/38, fo. 118, HBCA.

[88] McDonald Diary, 6 Sept. 1870. [89] Blondin, *Yamoria*, 159.

[90] Robert Lampard, 'William Morrison MacKay', in *Alberta's Medical History: Young, Lusty, and Full of Life* (Red Deer: R. Lampard, 2008), 37.

[91] Lampard, 'William MacKay', 37; Jane Flett MacKay spoke with Heber Jamieson, recalling her own contributions to medical practice as well. See Heber C. Jamieson, 'The Pioneer Doctor of Alberta: William Morrison MacKay', *Canadian Medical Association Journal* (Oct. 1937): 388–93.

comes with its own rules or policy, so the owners have to follow these orders and live carefully by them, or they could be killed by their own medicine powers.[92]

Inuvialuk Elder Ishmael Alunik described the main purpose of an *angatkuq* (a medicine man or woman, or shaman) as seeking 'spiritual help in times of sickness or hunger'.[93] The role of medicine and medicine men and women in providing food and good hunts was part of good health in the late nineteenth century. Medicine power was essential to the interwoven spiritual and material worlds of humans and other-than-human animals that prevailed before the arrival of Europeans. Northern Indigenous conceptualizations of health enveloped right relationships with animals, spirits, and the land in ensuring well-being. Medicine power was used in times of war, for travelling, and to predict the arrival of visitors.[94]

The other great challenge to understanding medicine power was that one of the most common rules to accompany this power was, in Blondin's words, 'that the owner does not talk about his abilities'. As Blondin emphasized, 'that is why we know so little about medicine and, even today, I found it hard to talk to elders about the subject because they were instructed not to say anything about it'.[95] Such prohibitions kept medicine men and women in the nineteenth century and after from communicating about their medicine. Medicine power was firmly embedded in the spirit world. And these spiritual aspects of northern medicine power overlapped much more with the work of missionaries than with the work of someone like MacKay. For missionaries, their role was to minister to the body and soul. McDonald, Petitot, Séguin, and others visited with the sick, gave them medicines, and prayed with them. Thus the role of missionaries in healing was a greater challenge to Indigenous cultures than biomedicine, because wedding religious beliefs and spirituality with cures resonated much more with the medicine power found in nineteenth-century northern communities.[96]

Healing practices found among northern Indigenous peoples resemble folk medicine practised historically around the globe. Rooted in intimate knowledge of local plants and animals, empirical healing arose from generations of trial and error that involved as well rituals in preparation and administration that were essential to successful remedies. When collecting plants for medicine, Gwich'in and Dene women would leave a gift to acknowledge their gratitude. To omit this essential step 'might rob the plants of their special power'.[97] Using a plant for

[92] Blondin, *Yamoria*, 51–8; for discussion of Indigenous theories of disease, see Waldram, Herring, and Young, *Aboriginal Health*, chapter 5.

[93] Alunik, *Ishmael*, 5. [94] Heine et al., *Gwichya Gwich'in Googwandak*, 98–101.

[95] Blondin, *Yamoria*, 51; Heine et al., *Gwichya Gwich'in Googwandak*, 97.

[96] Blondin, *Yamoria*, 161–2.

[97] Heine et al., *Gwichya Gwich'in Googwandak*, 154; see also Marie Adele Rabesca, Diane Romie, Martha Johnson, and Joan Ryan, *Traditional Dene Medicine*, part 1 (Lac La Martre: Govt. of the NWT, 1994), 19.

medicine was part of the reciprocal relationships maintained with other-than-human nature and required respect and spiritual acknowledgement.[98] Women were primarily responsible for practical healing, although both men and women could have medicine power. Just as some people had stronger medicine power, there were more and less skilled healers, women and men with greater experience who had seen more and knew more ways to heal. Alunik was thankful that an old Gwich'in woman was present at his birth when he stopped breathing. 'She said some babies breathe again, and she used a small feather and started to put it in my nose. It didn't take long, my mother said, before I sneezed and started to breathe. The old lady saved my life.'[99] Care was also collective, in the ways that it connected Indigenous northerners not just to their lands, but also to each other. When people fell ill, they were cared for by others. When Pagot'ine received an awful head wound, Blondin tells how he was unconscious for two weeks 'and people had to stay with him all the time. They took turns.'[100] Healing was rooted in skill, knowledge, spirituality, culture, and community.

There are extensive bodies of work that have documented the breadth and depth of northern Indigenous ethnobotany.[101] *Gwichya Gwich'in Googwandak* identified a few of the most important plants Gwichya Gwich'in used for healing. Black spruce branches could be boiled to treat colds and bronchitis, while the inner layer of bark was used for cuts and wounds. Red willow was used for skin ailments including rashes and burns, green willow leaves worked for skin rashes and bee and wasp stings. Gastrointestinal ailments could be treated with white birch and juniper berries, while liquorice or bear root would cure diarrhoea. Right relationships with the land brought forth plants and animal products that provided first aid – treating wounds, sores, and broken bones – that worked to heal and treat chronic ailments, and even served to facilitate surgery.[102] Trees, plants, roots, and berries, and all parts of these might have different preparations (boiled, chewed into a paste, turned into a powder and applied directly) that worked for different purposes, including in the same way as the laxatives, sedatives, and purges employed by MacKay. Parts of otters, hares, beavers, dogs, bears, pike, trout, caribou, whitefish, loons, and ducks were all used. The practical, empirical aspect of Indigenous healing is also apparent in the value of rotten wood and soot or ashes from the

98 Rabesca et al., *Traditional Dene Medicine*, part 1, 18.

99 Alunik, *Ishmael*, 36.

100 Blondin, *When the World Was New*, 163.

101 Rabesca et al., *Traditional Dene Medicine* parts 1 and 2; Alestine Andre and Alan Fehr, *Gwich'in Ethnobotany: Plants Used by the Gwich'in for Food, Medicine, Shelter and Tools* (Tsiigehtchic: Gwich'in Social and Cultural Institute, 2001); Inuvialuit Elders with Robert W. Bandringa, *Inuvialuit Nautchiangit: Relationships between People and Plants* (Inuvik: Inuvialuit Cultural Resource Centre, 2010); Robin James Marles, *Aboriginal Plant Use in Canada's Northwest Boreal Forest* (Vancouver: UBC Press, 2009).

102 For surgery see Rabesca et al., *Traditional Dene Medicine*, part 2, 288–91; A. G. Morice, 'Déné Surgery', *Transactions of the Canadian Institute* 7 (1904), 15–28.

stovepipes. The former was used to treat rashes and to help the umbilical cord fall off after birth, and the latter was identified, along with rat root, as an effective treatment for pinworms.

Looking more closely at MacKay's medicine chest, we see that his elixirs and potions were at once remarkably close to, and yet still distant from, the northern Indigenous medicines he encountered through his wife Jane Flett MacKay. Many of William MacKay's medicines were also derived from plants and animals and similarly worked to treat a range of ailments. Of the twenty or so items requisitioned for MacKay in the 1869 outfit, half originated in plants and animals, whether it was the opium from poppies in paregoric elixir, or the herb colocynth, or the plant from which colchicum wine was derived, *Colchicum autumnale*, which resembles a crocus. Castor oil was a vegetable oil derived from pressed castor beans, the tincture of iron was derived from herbs with high iron content, and the camphor used in soap liniments was extracted from the wood of camphor trees. The spirits of hartshorn took their name from the seventeenth century when harts' horns (a hart is an English name for a male deer) were distilled into ammonium carbonate or smelling salts.

Some treatments, like the rotten wood or soot used by Dene, drew from inorganic materials, although proportionately more of MacKay's had inorganic origins. Calamine ointment took its properties from zinc compounds that Pliny the Elder and Dioscorides in ancient Rome had described being collected from the walls of copper furnaces and which were used to treat the eyes and skin.[103] Basilicon ointment used resin from pines with wax, oil, and pitch (from tar) to encourage the production of pus and the extraction of thorns and splinters. Some of MacKay's inorganic compounds were notably more toxic, including mercury, arsenic, or the lead that was combined with beeswax and oil to make saturnine ointment.

Even if his medicine relied on the properties of plants and animals, MacKay's pharmacy was globalized, in sharp contrast to the ways in which northern Indigenous medicine was profoundly and intimately local. Gwich'in or Tłı̨chǫ or Inuvialuit were surrounded by and spiritually embedded in rich storehouses of healing. William MacKay, except when he turned to his wife Jane Flett MacKay for assistance, relied on imperial trade networks and the HBC's transportation routes to deliver medications. These medicines originated in the English countryside or the wider British Isles, while others came from farther afield. Castor beans are native to the Mediterranean basin and East Africa. Other medicines relied on global markets and the Columbian exchange.

[103] Gianna Giachi, Pasquino Pallecchi, Antonella Pomualdi, et al., 'Ingredients of a 2,000-y-old Medicine Revealed by Chemical, Mineralogical, and Botanical Investigations', *PNAS* 110, no. 4 (2013): 1193–6, https://doi.org/10.1073/pnas.1216776110.

Opium and camphor were traded with China and Japan in the nineteenth century. Ipecacuanha wine, or ipecac, was made from the dried root of *Cephaelis ipecacuanha,* a plant indigenous to South America, which had been first brought to Europe from Brazil by a Dutch physician in 1649.

Colonial networks of knowledge and exchange conveyed MacKay and his medicines into the north-west interior in the late 1860s and in so doing contributed to the new colonial ecologies of this period that connected the Mackenzie and Yukon rivers and their tributaries to lands and living things far distant and began to construct new social, cultural, and economic relationships. But, with one notable exception, MacKay's medicines did not change the material ecologies of the region. That is to say, he relied on processed imported products rather than seeds to plant poppies or castor beans (which would never have even sprouted in the subarctic interior). In this fashion, Indigenous medicines rooted – literally – in the land prevailed and endure into the present, where MacKay's extracts of colocynth and sublimed calomel have faded into obscurity.[104] The one notable exception – the one way in which MacKay and biomedicine did alter the ecology of disease in the north-west interior after 1868 – was with a specialized tool that the HBC procured from the London Vaccine Institute: smallpox vaccination lymph and tips.[105]

Vaccination

Pathogens circulated in the Mackenzie district and Yukon from 1870 through the 1890s. People fell ill, and some died in these outbreaks, although none can be characterized as regional epidemics or of severity comparable to the scarlet fever or influenza epidemics in the late 1860s. Arguably, the most important disease episode in these years was an outbreak of smallpox that went nowhere.

At Rampart House in October 1870, Robert McDonald 'visited three sick persons; their disease resembles chicken-pox'.[106] In his diary McDonald noted that people fell ill on Blackstone River and at Fort McPherson, and there were reports from the LaPierre's House people that the sickness was among them. The outbreak did not appear that virulent; although many fell ill, several recovered (including at least one man, Bechan, whom McDonald nursed). Some of the fatalities were recorded with sadness, including one 'excellent young man, named Abraham'.[107] The disease was most certainly smallpox, not chicken pox, which even in severe cases is rarely lethal.[108] According to

[104] Rabesca et al., *Traditional Dene Medicine*, part 1, 22; See Joan Nazon in *Gwichya Gwich'in Googwandak*, 156–7.

[105] Rich, 'The Fur Traders', 52. [106] McDonald Diary, 24 Oct. 1870.

[107] McDonald Diary, 11 Dec. 1870.

[108] Romola Davenport, Leonard Schwarz, and Jeremy Boulton, 'The Decline of Adult Smallpox in Eighteenth-Century London', *Economic History Review* 64, no. 4 (2011): 1289–314 (p. 1294).

Andrew Flett, the clerk at Peel River (and no direct relation to Jane Flett MacKay), 'Shortly after our boats returned from Fort Simpson, the small pox or something similar broke out first among the Fort people which spread rapidly among the Indians (of the latter 5 died). Our hunter caught the infection & failed entirely in the fall fresh meat hunt.'[109] Given McDonald's description, it is likely that more than five people perished in this outbreak, although no more than ten or fifteen total, as Flett's was the only post report that mentioned the outbreak at all and McDonald described more people recovering from, than succumbing to, their illness.

Why is an outbreak in which a handful of people died at one or two posts an important historical episode? Those familiar with the disease history of the North American plains will recognize that this outbreak occurred in the midst of the last, most devastating smallpox epidemic of the nineteenth century, one which James Daschuk described as 'catastrophic to the Niitsitapi and other First Nations on the plains' and in which over 3,500 Indigenous people died.[110] Beyond the North American west, 1869 to 1874 saw a smallpox pandemic across Europe that killed an estimated 500,000 Europeans.[111] The disease appeared first in the autumn of 1869 amongst French soldiers fighting in the Franco-Prussian War. At the time, the French Army had low rates of vaccination in its ranks as compared to other European armies. Writing on the outbreak in 1933, J. D. Rolleston observed that the war combined with the unvaccinated soldiers meant that 'a vast amount of susceptible material was thus provided and resistance to infection was considerably lowered by the stress and privations of active service'.[112] Michael Bliss described how the pandemic crossed from Europe to North America, although in his attention to Canada's urban centres such as Montreal, Bliss did not connect that pandemic to smallpox on the plains.[113] Nevertheless, the larger history of the *Variola* (smallpox) virus and efforts at treating this highly disfiguring and destructive disease are essential to our story.

By the late nineteenth century, effective vaccination against *Variola* was widely available and used. As early as the 1820s, contrary to Jenner's original claims, it became clear that a single vaccination did not confer lifelong

[109] Andrew Flett to William Hardisty, 19 Jan. 1871, B.200/b/38, fo. 77, HBCA.

[110] Daschuk, *Clearing the Plains*, 81–2. [111] Bliss, *Plague*, 50.

[112] J. D. Rolleston, 'The Smallpox Pandemic of 1870–1874', *Proceedings of the Royal Society of Medicine* 27, no. 2 (1933): 177–92 (p. 179), https://doi.org/10.1177/003591573302700245; see also Matthew Smallman-Raynor and Andrew D. Cliff, 'The Geographical Transmission of Smallpox in the Franco-Prussian War: Prisoner of War Camps and Their Impact upon Epidemic Diffusion Processes in the Civil Settlement System of Prussia 1870–71', *Medical History* 46 (2002): 241–64.

[113] Ryan Eyford discusses smallpox in 1876 in the context of settler colonialism on the prairies, see 'Quarantined within a New Colonial Order: The 1876–1877 Lake Winnipeg Smallpox Epidemic', *Journal of the Canadian Historical Association* 17, no. 1 (2006): 66–71.

immunity and that re-vaccination was needed to ensure ongoing protection. Europe and the United States had early on introduced vaccination campaigns to protect their citizens against smallpox, and several European states even introduced compulsory vaccination, although without the necessary enforcement measures. The implementation of effective vaccination campaigns struggled in this period of nascent public health structures. It was not just the treatment of the disease that was evolving but also the pathogen itself. As historian Anne Hardy notes, 'it is often assumed that vaccination measures were the means by which the disease was brought under control', as when these measures were introduced in the early nineteenth century, this coincided with a period of decline for smallpox in Europe.[114] However, detailed studies of smallpox in England after the eighteenth century show that the range of factors at play included changing virulence (lethality), inoculation and vaccination rates, and urban–rural relations, including most significantly migration.[115] After the 1860s, the character of the disease shifted. Thereafter – in the UK at least – 'each successive smallpox epidemic in the nineteenth century [was] more severe'.[116] Certainly, one of the distinguishing features of the 1870–4 European pandemic was the intensity of the disease: the high levels of mortality and the appearance of the haemorrhagic form of smallpox in cities and European armies.[117] There were also references to 'black smallpox' (another term for haemorrhagic smallpox) on the western plains in the 1860s, although none, it seems, from 1869 to 1870.[118] The appearance of more virulent forms of *Variola major* (if not necessarily haemorrhagic smallpox) would help account for the high mortality rates among some of the plains Indigenous peoples, as does the prevalence of famine and malnutrition on the plains in the wake of the collapse of bison populations.

And what of the role of vaccination on the western plains and to the northwest? The HBC, after all, had introduced inoculation and later vaccines to the fur trade in the late eighteenth century with varying degrees of success.[119] Traders brought vaccines to Fort Simpson in 1838.[120] Vaccination was critical in helping to check the course of the 1869–70 epidemic in some parts of western Canada. Moreover, both McCarthy and Daschuk, where they describe the outbreak to the north, argue that it was vaccination by Oblate missionaries and the HBC that kept the virus in check. However, it is not quite so

114 Hardy, *Epidemic Streets*, 111.
115 Davenport, Schwartz, and Boulton, 'Decline', 1310.
116 Hardy, *Epidemic Streets*, 115.
117 Rolleston, 'Smallpox Pandemic', 180.
118 See Appendix IV, Blood Winter Count, in The R. N. Wilson Papers, ed. Philip H. Godsell, R. N. Wilson Fonds, GM.
119 Hackett, 'Averting Disaster', 575–609. for an important comparative perspective on smallpox inoculation in colonial Guatemala, see Martha Few, 'Medical Humanitarianism and Smallpox Inoculation in Eighteenth-Century Guatemala', *Historical Social Research* 37, no. 2 (2012): 303–17.
120 Yerbury, *Subarctic Indians*, 156.

straightforward as all that, and the fuller story illuminates weaknesses in medical responses in this period, as well as the importance of local conditions and the character of disease itself in abruptly truncating the outbreak.

Robert McDonald described the first cases in October of 1870, and Andrew Flett similarly noted the disease appeared 'after our boats returned from Fort Simpson'.[121] Unsurprisingly, *Variola* reached the Mackenzie district along the open water route that connected the district to global networks of trade and disease. However, unlike influenza or measles, smallpox does not spread as quickly as it is not contagious during the incubation period (seven to seventeen days after exposure), but only after a fever develops. Once someone fell ill, not only were they then contagious, but also at that point they were less likely to travel far, and thus the long-distance transmission of the disease was somewhat curtailed.[122] Although the virus can be airborne and spread by clothes and touch, it was transmitted mainly 'by droplet infection to very close contacts'.[123] Crowding, close quarters, and malnutrition (all of which were found in the Franco-Prussian armies and in late nineteenth-century urban centres) provided ideal conditions for smallpox to spread. But the winter of 1870–1 along the Peel River and Nagwichoonjik was not an especially difficult one. This was not a crowded place. There was little violence in the northlands at this time, in contrast to the south. Although Flett described the failure of the Peel River autumn meat hunt, this was because of the sickness of the fort hunter; elsewhere hunts were good and the summer and autumn fisheries had been a success.[124] Although people continued to travel and move about the land, no effort was made to erect a quarantine: Peel River people (Teetł'it Gwich'in) joined with those from Nagwichoonjik for a hunt, and Inuvialuit came and went in the autumn and winter months that year, according to Flett. There were, though, fewer contacts with places outside of the North where the virus was circulating. The disruption to the trade that year, arising from the continued unrest in Red River, briefly disconnected the Mackenzie district from the Western trade. Movement never stopped in winter, but it did slow, and a virus that appeared after the end of the open-water season had fewer opportunities for travel. When the virus appeared at Peel River and in the vicinity, it burned out quickly, and, after the river closed in November, it was less likely that it would be reintroduced from the south.

At this point, the role of vaccination became important. Although the disease first broke out on the plains in August of 1869, the conflict in Red River disrupted the shipment of fresh vaccine supplies throughout the

121 Flett to Hardisty, 19 Jan. 1871. 122 Fenn, *Pox Americana*, chapter 1.
123 Hardy, *Epidemic Streets*, 113; Fenn, *Pox Americana*, 15.
124 See for example the report from Fort Rae, W. C. King to William Hardisty, 30 Nov. 1870, B. 200/b/38, fo. 70; from Fort Nelson, William Brass to William Hardisty, 10 Feb. 1871; Flett to Hardisty, 19 Jan. 1871, all HBCA.

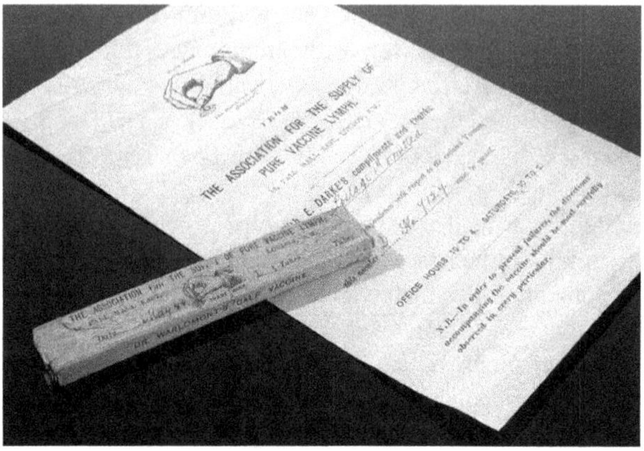

Figure 3.2 Wooden box containing tube of calf lymph, England, 1888. Science Museum, London. Attribution 4.0 International (CC BY 4.0).

country.[125] It was not until December of 1870 – after the disease had already appeared in the Mackenzie – that Donald Smith, as head of the Northern Department, wrote from Fort Garry to his brother-in-law, William Hardisty, describing the epidemic in the Saskatchewan District and expressed his 'hope that it is abating'. Nevertheless, Smith added, a package of 'Vaccine Lymph sent from England by the Governor & Committee' would be forwarded to the Mackenzie district 'with the view of having vaccination very generally introduced throughout the country'.[126] The lymph, 'said to be of the best quality & put up to keep', was sent with the regular packet that arrived three months later.[127] The precise form and origin of the vaccine lymph is not detailed in the HBC records. However, the production and global dissemination of smallpox vaccine was well established by 1869 (Figure 3.2). Vaccination material could be preserved by drying and then sent long distances.[128] Sometimes when the lymph arrived it was no longer infectious, hence the need for assurances of quality in the HBC correspondence. How much vaccination material was sent is unknown. John McIntyre and Stuart

125 Hackett, 'Averting Disaster', 609.

126 Donald A. Smith to William Hardisty, 15 Dec. 1870, B.200/b/38, fo. 69, HBCA.

127 J. H. Mactavish to William Hardisty, 15 Dec. 1870, B.200/b/38, fo. 95. The packet arrived at Fort Resolution in March, Thomas Swanston to William Hardisty, 26 Feb./2 Mar. 1871, B.200/b/38, fo. 89, HBCA.

128 Donald A. Henderson and Bernard Moss, 'Smallpox and Vaccinia', *Vaccines*, 3rd ed., ed. S. A. Plotkin and W. A. Orenstein (Philadelphia: Saunders, 1999), www.ncbi.nlm.nih.gov/books/NBK7294/; see also Lydia Murdoch, 'Carrying the Pox: The Use of Children and Ideals of Childhood in Early British and Imperial Campaigns Against Smallpox', *Journal of Social History* 48, no. 3 (2015): 511–35.

Houston indicate that arm-to-arm transfer was employed by the HBC on the plains in this epidemic as in previous ones.[129] In arm-to-arm transfer, new serum was harvested from people who had been vaccinated several days earlier. Given that other pathogens, including syphilis, could be transmitted using this approach and given that new vaccination material could be grown using calves, arm-to-arm transfer ceased to be practised in the late nineteenth century. By 1885, a vaccine manufacturing farm was operating in Ottawa.[130] Locally though, William MacKay used his children (the first was born in 1875) as passive vaccination instruments. He vaccinated them and then sent them to reserves to spread the attenuated smallpox virus.[131] These methods enabled a relatively small amount of vaccination material to be magnified in its dissemination.

Alison Bashford writes, 'As technology and as matter, vaccination was part of what connected Empire.'[132] Lymph came into the Mackenzie district along the fur-trade network, and its distribution was prompted by established HBC responses to smallpox outbreaks in combination with its reaction – including hiring William MacKay – to recent ill health in the region. Nevertheless, missionaries more than traders or MacKay were the ones who vaccinated people.[133] The interchangeability of colonizers in the role of 'public vaccinator' made vaccination a tool and symbol of colonization and control, as much as a medical technology requiring specific expertise or a measure exclusively adopted by the HBC. As the HBC's physician in the district in 1870, MacKay was based at Fort Simpson, and he travelled from there to other posts. Indeed, he annoyed Thomas Swanston at Fort Resolution by suggesting that he had the authority to use 'men & dogs' from Resolution, or any post for that matter, whenever necessary. Swanston grumbled about this to Hardisty in February 1871, and we also learn from this letter that MacKay did not vaccinate anyone in the Mackenzie before leaving the district that same month.[134] MacKay left to travel south to Peace River, where smallpox had broken out with greater severity and from there participated in the HBC's vaccination campaign.[135] Petitot described MacKay as having 'refused his duty', in a letter to Archbishop Taché, although Petitot did so primarily to bolster the significance of his own and Séguin's work as vaccinators. Petitot had procured lancets and lymph two years previously, and they used this (and possibly also the

[129] John W. R. McIntyre and C. Stuart Houston, 'Smallpox and Its Control in Canada', *Canadian Medical Association Journal* 161 (1999): 1543–7.

[130] William B. Spaulding, 'The Ontario Vaccine Farm, 1885–1916', *CBMH/BCHM* 6, no. 1 (1989): 45–56.

[131] Lampard, 'William Morrison MacKay', 36. [132] Bashford, *Imperial Hygiene*, 24.

[133] Cody, *Apostle of the North*, 388. [134] Swanston to Hardisty, 26 Feb./2 Mar. 1871, fo. 87.

[135] Daschuk, *Clearing the Plains*, 86, 90.

material from the HBC) to vaccinate 1,704 people between Portage La Loche and downstream of Fort Good Hope.[136]

In the spring of 1871, William Bompas, at the time a travelling preacher for the Church Missionary Society, vaccinated 'about 500' people at Fort Vermillion, Fort Chipewyan, and Fond du Lac. He offered some insight in the response of Indigenous northerners to the vaccination campaign: 'Knowing the danger of the smallpox to the Indians, it has been a pleasure to me to vaccinate them, though rather troublesome sometimes to persuade them to submit to the operation.'[137] Séguin described some ambiguity in the Dene response to the vaccination campaign. In writing about his efforts at Fort Good Hope, Séguin noted that the work was continuous because he basically had to catch people when they appeared from their lodges, a description that suggests that the practice was coercive.[138] Further on, though, Séguin noted that families who had not returned to the post for three or four years now travelled there because they had heard that the missionaries had medicine to prevent a dangerous disease.[139] We should not assume that Indigenous northerners had a single response to the vaccination campaign, particularly given that uneven attitudes to vaccination can be seen in many different contexts and endure into the present. Vaccinating approximately 2,200 people from Fort Chipewyan and points north would have represented perhaps a tenth of the population of the Mackenzie district and Yukon in this period. Moreover, vaccination followed *Variola* into the north-west. Nevertheless, it helped to ensure that a further outbreak of smallpox would not appear in the midst of a larger pandemic.

Vaccines are a technology – a form of artifice – that reproduces the biological consequences of a first, authentic historical encounter between an individual and a virus, or a community and a virus, by means of large-scale vaccination campaigns. The smallpox outbreak in 1870 went nowhere and caused only few deaths because of the circumstances in which it appeared combined with the character of the disease itself: the pathogen arrived after freeze-up, when movement had slowed and connections to the south had closed for the season. The subsequent vaccination campaign was a contributing, but not necessarily the determining, factor in the history of that outbreak, illustrating how colonial ecologies of infectious disease in the nineteenth-century north-west interior were closely tied to climate and ice. But the presence of the vaccine did alter the ecology of disease along the Mackenzie and Yukon rivers and their tributaries. In the wake of the vaccination campaign, smallpox antibodies had an established presence in the region – a presence which had no historical precedent

[136] Jean Séguin to sister, 1 Jun. 1871, 71.220 / 7344, OMI, PAA.

[137] Cody, *Apostle of the North*, 131–2.

[138] Séguin to sister, 1 Jun. 1871.

[139] Séguin to sister, 1 Jun. 1871.

given the absence of evidence for earlier smallpox epidemics. In this regard, the vaccination campaign contributed to the good health of the district in the late nineteenth century. However, the vaccination campaign was also the exception that proves the rule. For otherwise, colonial ecologies in the north-west interior created pockets of ill health: among the boat crews that carried trade goods across the land, in the newly opened residential schools, and with time at the missions and trade posts.

There is a genealogy connecting late twentieth-century 'virgin soil' models and their application to northern history with older colonial discourses of epidemics and their effects. These discourses exaggerated the scale of sickness and mortality, while displacing responsibility for epidemics onto indifferent pathogens, harsh environments, and the assumed weakness and vulnerability of Indigenous bodies. The fabulations examined here, Petitot's epidemics or Dall's extinctions, were important but exceptional instances within a larger body of evidence – of trader, explorer, and missionary accounts of disease – that must be read discursively *and* literally. For these are detailed accounts that have survived and can, in spite of their fictions, allow later readers to discern important moments in the history of northern epidemics. Oral histories endure that share an alternate version of the nineteenth century, one in which Indigenous health and strength prevailed. This perspective is critical to guiding interpretation of colonial sources, and the example of smallpox shows us why. Smallpox arrived eventually in the Yukon and Mackenzie district; when and under what circumstances meant that it played a very different role in the colonial project compared to its impacts in the Pacific Northwest or the Western Plains, not least because of the history of the virus itself and the availability of vaccines. By the late nineteenth century and into the twentieth century, not only was vaccination more effective in the North, but it was used against a less virulent pathogen. Smallpox would go on to have an important part to play in the rise of public health as a tool of colonial control, but that is the subject of a later chapter.

4 The Gold Rush and After

In early 1900, John Ttssietla prepared to travel south to the Stewart River to hunt and share the gospel. Robert McDonald outfitted Ttssietla and saw the reverend and others off to ascend the Peel River on 17 July. When they reached the Hart River, the group split up and went different ways. Bella Alexie's father Martin and her brother-in-law George Robert were in one camp along with Sam Smith and Andrew Deya. Bella herself stayed with Ttssietla, her uncle Amos Njootli, Simon Cho, Neesheh, Vittsee-Yune-Jik, and Tsit, a 'Slavey Indian'. Bella was to help care for her infant cousin Thomas, Amos's son. The families stayed in their camps through the late summer and autumn and had success hunting caribou and moose. Then, after the families in Bella's camp built moss houses and settled in for winter, 'a terrible thing happened. There was a bad sickness in our camp. The minister, John Chee Akla [Ttssietla], and his wife both died, also Simon Cho, Vittsee-Yune-Jik's wife, Mary, and this man called Tsit. These were the only ones I remember passing away but if there was more I don't remember.'[1] Johnny Kyikavichik (Kaye) was not there but was told the story of this epidemic. He shared that it was Martin and Andrew Deya who came to visit and found 'to their surprise, everyone in the camp was suffering terribly from a sickness unrecognizable. Many were already dead.'[2] The people all gathered together to help, 'the dead were buried and the sick looked after'.[3] Those who survived joined up again and continued to travel, while grieving for those who had died. As Bella Alexie remembered, 'Sometimes you'd think a kid was crying; it was one of the widows mourning for her deceased man. Those times were very sad.'[4]

1 Bella Alexie, 'Early 1900s as I Remember It', in 'Gwich'in COPE stories', 13.
2 Johnny Kaye [Kyikavichik], 'An Epidemic among Our People', in 'Gwich'in COPE Stories', 279.
3 Kaye [Kyikavichik], 'An Epidemic', 279; Black City was a major traditional settlement at the junction of the Blackstone River and the East Blackstone River used into the 1920s. See Sheila Greer, 'Place Names in Heritage Site Research, Dempster Highway Corridor, Yukon', *Canoma* 16, no. 2 (Dec. 1990), 3–4; See also Alfred Semple, interview, 19 Jul. 2000, GSCI, Gwich'in Elders' Biographies Research Project, tape 13.
4 Alexie, 'Early 1900s', 14.

Teetł'it Gwich'in hunters carried the news back to Fort McPherson by mid-June 1901, and the deaths were recorded in the parish register. In all, twenty-eight Gwich'in had died. In their seventies, John Ttssietla and Alice Bitsikotrig were among the oldest. Twelve children died, and the others were adults, men and women of different ages. McDonald noted in his diary that 'some died of measles, others of la grippe, and some it is said of smallpox'.[5]

The winter of 1899–1900 had been very hard for some families, including Ttssietla and Bitsikotrig living near Zheh Gwitsal. McDonald described 'cold . . . so intense that hunting of the reindeer was almost an impossibility'.[6] The deepest cold at Fort Good Hope came at the end of December and again a month later, when it was colder than it had been in a decade.[7] Dogs perished. Ttssietla and Bitsikotrig both suffered frostbite on their faces. Although they met with caribou later in January, the cold and hunger they experienced weakened Ttssietla's and Bitsikotrig's health in the summer to come when they and the other Gwich'in families travelled into a hornet's nest in 1900. In those days, according to Johnny Kyikavichik, 'the people never knew of Dawson yet', and they were not headed to that place but to the Stewart River.[8] The story that Annie Henry knew was that the Tukudh (Dagoo) and Blackstone people had heard of Dawson and were looking for it. When they found it, they also found sickness.[9]

Dawson and the gold rush created this epidemic. Whether they came from the east, the north, the west, or the south, 50,000 men and women converged on the creeks of the Klondike after 1896. Within two years, the population of Dawson peaked at 30,000 people.[10] With the gold rush, the numbers of people travelling across northern lands increased dramatically, including greater travel by Indigenous peoples looking for new trade opportunities. With this increased movement came a marked change in the intensity and frequency of epidemic disease, not only on the creeks of the Klondike, but also across the Mackenzie district, Yukon, and beyond. This change and its effects are the subject of this chapter. On 16 July, the day before Ttssietla and the others had set off in 1900, McDonald posted letters with miners passing through McPherson en route to Dawson City. Bella Alexie recalled that after the sickness had passed, she and the others moved on, 'I don't remember where to but do recall meeting up with strange men. They wore Stetson hats.'[11] These strangers were Na-cho Nyäk Dun wearing the quintessential cowboy

[5] McDonald Diary, 17 Jun. 1901; Sax and Linklater, *Gikhyi*, 59.
[6] McDonald Diary, 30 Jan. 1900.
[7] Canada, *Historical Climate Data*, daily data for Fort Good Hope 2, NWT, 1897–1966.
[8] Kaye [Kyikavichik], 'An Epidemic', 279.
[9] Joe and Annie Henry interview, translated by Percy Henry, Dawson City, YT, Jan. 1992, Tape/Transcript #92–03, Tr'ondëk Hwëch'in Heritage Department.
[10] Charlene Porsild, *Gamblers and Dreamers: Women, Men, and Community in the Klondike* (Vancouver: UBC Press, 1998), 8.
[11] Alexie, 'Early 1900s', 13.

hat of the western plains. The sickness in 1900 was tied in Gwich'in history both to the passing of Ttssietla, an important leader in a time of great turmoil, and to the profound changes that came to the people on the cusp of the twentieth century.

The Great Sickness

Bad sickness, sickness unrecognizable, 'Discovery Flu' – these were names given to this epidemic by the Gwich'in.[12] From the west and north came other names: the Big Death and the Great Sickness. This last was the English translation of *quserpak*, the Yup'ik name for the epidemic and the one by which it is best known.

In the spring, summer, and autumn of 1900, a vicious epidemic crossed from Siberia over to Alaska, appearing first near Nome and on St Lawrence Island before moving along the mainland coast and into the interior. Historians Robert Fortuine and Robert Wolfe described the path and intensity of the Great Sickness. Fortuine characterized it as influenza accompanied by measles, smallpox, 'and possibly other diseases'.[13] In places, entire communities fell ill with measles, and although people recovered from the first infection, they then perished from subsequent infection with influenza or other complications including pneumonia and bronchitis. Where the epidemic hit suddenly, 'with lightning force', some communities were left unable to get food, to nurse the sick, or to bury the dead. Elsewhere, the epidemic came in waves that caused extended suffering over the spring and summer months of 1900. Conservative estimates are that 2,000 people lost their lives in Alaska, between 25 and 50 per cent of the total population. Fortuine described the Great Sickness as 'probably the most calamitous event in the history of the Alaska Native people since the smallpox epidemic of 1835–40'. The epidemic reshaped historical memory for some Alaskan communities who, for years to come, reckoned events from that date.[14]

Wolfe characterized the Great Sickness as a 'virgin soil epidemic'.[15] Fortuine eschewed this language and placed greater interpretive weight on the chaos of multiple infections at the individual and community level. The impact of measles in particular was significant. There were communities, including on St Lawrence Island, where 'the attack rate was nearly one hundred percent'.[16] Measles is not only highly infectious and potentially

[12] Semple interview, Gwich'in Elders' Biographies. [13] Fortuine, *Chills and Fever*, 215.
[14] Fortuine, *Chills and Fever*, 226.
[15] Robert J. Wolfe, 'Alaska's Great Sickness, 1900: An Epidemic of Measles and Influenza in a Virgin Soil Population', *Proceedings of the American Philosophical Society* 126, no. 2 (1982): 91–121.
[16] Fortuine, *Chills and Fever*, 217.

fatal, but it also has dramatic effects on the body's immune system. The virus lives in the nose and mouth of an infectious person and can persist in the air for two hours. An infectious person might sneeze and then leave a room. Should a susceptible person then enter, they can inhale the virus and fall sick. Once infected, the incubation period is ten to twelve days until the first symptom appears, typically a fever. The distinctive measles rash arises around two weeks after exposure and lasts for five or six days. Infection with measles confers immunity against the disease in future. Complications from measles are most common in children under five and adults over twenty. Diarrhoea and middle-ear infections commonly follow measles, but the most significant complications include rapid swelling of the brain (acute encephalitis), which can lead to death or permanent neurological damage; infection with viral or bacterial pneumonia, which can cause death particularly in very young children; and for pregnant women a greater chance of premature labour and miscarriage. On St Lawrence Island in 1900, about half of those infected experienced respiratory complications and others had encephalitis, although only two babies died of measles.[17]

Measles infection can create vulnerability to other diseases by erasing the immune system's 'memory' of previous illness, destroying as much as 73 per cent of a child's protective antibodies in one study.[18] This provides a mechanism by which to understand the observed vulnerability of communities in the wake of measles infections; even if measles did not kill people, it left them highly vulnerable to subsequent infection. Epidemiological reports have demonstrated that infection with measles can activate a latent tuberculosis infection (convert the underlying infection to an active disease) or aggravate an active tuberculosis infection.[19] On St Lawrence Island in 1900, after the measles passed, influenza arrived, and 'within a short time virtually every individual was [again] sick'.[20] Forty-four people died in this one community alone from pneumonia and influenza in the wake of measles, and then, in the year to come, another twenty perished from tuberculosis.

Wolfe and Fortuine outlined the path of the epidemic in Alaska, delimiting its northernmost reach as Point Hope on the north-west tip of the Alaska coast, 1,175 km west from Herschel Island by water. Inland, along the Yukon River, the epidemic went as far as Big Bend, a village about 840 km downstream from Dawson. Fortuine and Wolfe assumed that the Great Sickness stopped well

[17] Fortuine, *Chills and Fever*, 217.

[18] Michael J. Mina, T. Kula, Y. Leng, et al., 'Measles Virus Infection Diminishes Preexisting Antibodies That Offer Protection from Other Pathogens', *Science* 366, no. 6465 (1 Nov. 2019): 599–606, http://doi.org/10.1126/science.aay6485.

[19] Chang-Hoon Lee, E. G. Lee, J. Y. Lee, et al., 'The Incidence of Tuberculosis after a Measles Outbreak', *Clinical Infectious Diseases* 46, no. 6 (15 March 2008): 902–4, http://doi.org/10.1086/528856.

[20] Fortuine, *Chills and Fever*, 217.

before reaching the Yukon or Mackenzie. As Fortuine noted, 'further upriver' from Big Bend, by about 275 km, 'there were scattered cases of both influenza and measles but not in epidemic proportions except perhaps around Dall River (near present-day Stevens Village)', where the US Revenue department steamship *Nunivak* tied up for the winter.[21]

Beyond Big Bend, across the Canada–United States border, what happened to the epidemic? There is no existing scholarship on the Great Sickness per se in the Yukon and Mackenzie, but the history of pandemics is a history of border-crossing pathogens, and, as we have already seen with the Gwich'in who fell sick and died in the central Yukon, those pathogens that circulated in 1900 were no different.

In September 1900, North West Mounted Police (NWMP) Constable Herman Fisher was diagnosed with measles.[22] At twenty-four years old, Fisher was fortunate to avoid serious complications and, after a month in hospital, he fully recovered. The availability of hospital treatment helped ensure Fisher's recovery. Dawson at the time had two general hospitals, St Mary's and the Good Samaritan Hospital – Roman Catholic and Protestant institutions respectively – in addition to several private hospitals. Many nurses and doctors lived in town. Outside of the Klondike, however, such a concentration of institutional medical care was rare. There were other hospitals in Alaska at this time, but few of those who fell ill with measles in 1900 received institutional medical treatment.

More unusual was that Fisher fell ill with measles in the first place. Originally from Ontario, Fisher signed up to serve with the NWMP in London six months earlier.[23] By 1900, measles was a common childhood disease in Canada. It spread rapidly through communities and, as Mona Gleason has noted, was the target of hygienic education measures directed at children across the country. Even in a smaller city like Kingston, measles made up a significant number of hospital admissions for children under fourteen years of age.[24] That Fisher made it to adulthood without previous exposure was uncommon. According to his thin NWMP personnel file (which mostly includes charges against him for insolence and sleeping on the job), Fisher

21 Fortuine, *Chills and Fever*, 224.

22 Canada, Parliament, *Sessional Papers*, 'Report of the North-West Mounted Police, Part III, 1900' (Ottawa: S. E. Dawson, 1901), 67.

23 LAC, *North West Mounted Police (NWMP) – Personnel Records, 1873–1904*, www.bac-lac.gc.ca/eng/discover/nwmp-personnel-records/Pages/north-west-mounted-police.aspx.

24 See Mona Gleason, *Small Matters: Canadian Children in Sickness and Health, 1900–1940* (Montréal: McGill-Queen's University Press, 2013), 88, 105. In the United States, by 1917 measles 'developed in 2–3 year cycles in large cities and irregularly in rural areas'. See David M. Morens and Jeffery K. Taubenberger, 'A Forgotten Epidemic That Changed Medicine: Measles in the US Army, 1917–18', *Lancet Infect Diseases* 15, no. 7 (July 2015): 852–61, http://doi.org/10.1016/S1473-3099(15)00109-7.

had been previously employed on a farm near Stratford. A rural upbringing may have shielded Fisher from measles until he reached his twenties and found himself stationed as a police officer in the instant, cosmopolitan city of Dawson.[25]

McDonald attributed the Gwich'in deaths not only to measles, but also to influenza and smallpox. Smallpox arrived in the gold fields in June 1900 and spread up the creeks and as far away as Whitehorse.[26] No deaths, aside from those in Ttssietla's camp, were attributed to smallpox in 1900. Given the size of the population at Dawson, that neither measles nor smallpox produced major outbreaks or significant mortality in that community in 1900 and in the context of the Great Sickness tells us something important about the geographies of immunity and disease as part of the transformative effects of the gold rush. Scholarship on the history of HIV has demonstrated the role of urban centres in central Africa, in colonial context, as sites that amplified infection.[27] The opposite happened in Dawson in late 1900. Even as the draw of gold brought new people and new pathogens through the Mackenzie district and into the Yukon, in Dawson itself, the character of the population acted to hinder measles and smallpox viruses, serving to slow and stall the spread of disease, rather than encourage its spread.

Viruses are in constant search of susceptible hosts to survive. As John McNeill aptly put it, 'they cannot reproduce on their own, but must seize control of cells in other creatures and convert them into copying machines'.[28] Once infected with a virus, there are two outcomes for a person: either their body's immune system will successfully fight off the virus, in the process producing immunity that will then offer varying degrees of defence against future reinfection, or they will die. Either way, for the virus to persist it needs to find a new host and quickly. At the level of a community or population, if in its search the virus encounters mostly immune bodies, then it will die out. This is the logic behind 'herd immunity' as well as present-day vaccination programmes, which aim to vaccinate enough people (between as much as 80 or 95 per cent, depending on the contagiousness of a virus) so that even if some cannot be vaccinated, and therefore remain susceptible, they are protected by the fact that they are surrounded by other (mostly) immune bodies.

In Dawson, contact tracing led authorities to believe that Constable Fisher was infected by a man also in contact with Tr'ondëk Hwëch'in in Moosehide, where there was an outbreak of measles.[29] Given the infectiousness of measles, that Fisher was the only reported case in Dawson that year – particularly where he apparently got the disease via at least one other person, and given the

[25] Porsild, *Gamblers and Dreamers*, 191, for Dawson as an 'instant' city.
[26] 'Report of the NWMP 1900', 73.
[27] Jacques Pepin, *The Origins of AIDS* (Cambridge: University of Cambridge Press, 2011).
[28] McNeill, Mosquito Empires, 32. [29] 'Report of the NWMP, 1900', 4, 67.

number of cases reported elsewhere – suggests that there were a high number of immune people in Dawson – enough, that is, to check the pathogen's spread. Looking at the remarkable demography of Dawson in 1900 shows how this may have worked.

In March 1900, twelve-year-old Annie O'Brien won a dancing prize at the Orpheum Theatre in Dawson, where she performed in an act with her parents.[30] Some children accompanied their parents to Dawson, others joined after a period of time (most often the wife and children joined their husband). And, from the outset, men and women established families together, or at least reproduced, bringing new children into the community.[31] Nevertheless, Dawson City – like any mining boom town – had a very skewed population distribution, with adult men between the ages of fifteen and sixty-four making up a vast majority of residents. Historical census data from 1901 for the Yukon as a whole shows boys made up less than 4 per cent of males; 96 per cent of males were over the age of fifteen. For Canada in this year, these same proportions were 34 per cent boys and 66 per cent adult men. The proportion of girls to women in the Yukon was not quite so extreme (17 per cent girls to 83 per cent adult women), but females made up only 15 per cent of the total population.[32] In Dawson, an 1898 census taken by the NWMP counted 400 children from a total population of 15,000 people.[33] In 1900, there was a small pool of children susceptible to measles surrounded by thousands of adults, many of whom were immune. The measles virus found it difficult to reach susceptible hosts in Dawson in the summer and fall of 1900, disrupting rather than amplifying the Great Sickness in the Yukon.

We know more about smallpox immunity in Dawson at the turn of the century by virtue of the medical examinations required of new NWMP recruits. When young men signed up with the NWMP, they were required to pass a medical examination that documented general health (including an assessment of temperament: 'bilious', 'sanguine', or 'cool') and recorded whether the new recruit had vaccine marks.[34] From a sample of twenty personnel files among NWMP officers stationed in Dawson in 1900–2, all but one – Herman Fisher again – had been vaccinated, some more than once (their forms noting as many as three vaccine marks, or giving the general

[30] Michael Gates, 'History Hunter – Children in Klondike Theatre', *Yukon News*, 28 Mar. 2019, www.yukon-news.com/opinion/history-hunter-children-in-klondike-theatre/.

[31] Porsild, *Gamblers and Dreamers*, 20–3.

[32] Statistics Canada, Historical Age Pyramids, 'Yukon', www12.statcan.gc.ca/census-recensement/2016/dp-pd/pyramid/pyramid.cfm?geo1=60&type=1.

[33] Charlene Porsild, 'Klondike Family Life', *BC Studies* 123 (Autumn 1999): 59–68 (p. 66); Porsild, *Gamblers and Dreamers*, 201.

[34] As of 1900, although vaccines existed for rabies, typhoid, cholera, and plague, none were in widespread use, only smallpox vaccines. John Duffy, *The Sanitarians: A History of American Public Health* (Urbana: University of Illinois Press, 1990), 195.

assessment, 'well-vaccinated').[35] Assistant Surgeon L. A. (Louis Alphonse) Paré confirmed the generally high level of vaccination among NWMP officers. Among the 'new men' he observed at the post, most had previously received a vaccine. Fisher appears to have been particularly immunologically naïve – a sheltered young man, that is, when it came to infectious pathogens.

Medical reports are not available for the vast majority of the Dawson population; however, we know that many came from or passed through urban centres where, in Paré's words, 'there is always a case or two' of smallpox.[36] San Francisco had a major smallpox epidemic in the 1870s, as did Montreal in 1885, both significant points of origin for men and women who found their way to the Klondike. Calixte-Aimé Dugas and Osias Dugas (no relation) represented two ends of the class spectrum within the French-Canadian community that flourished in Dawson. Calixte-Aimé Dugas was formerly a Montreal police magistrate and was appointed to one of two positions on the new Yukon Territorial Court in 1898. Osias Dugas was a miner, born in Montreal in 1860. Magistrate Dugas appears fleetingly in the pages of Michael Bliss's account of Montreal's 1885 epidemic.[37] Few details of Osias Dugas's life appear in the archival record, but he may well have lived through the smallpox epidemic in Montreal too. Both or either may have survived smallpox in that previous encounter or were vaccinated as part of epidemic control measures. Previous vaccination offered some protection against infection. In his first semi-annual report, the Medical Health Officer for the Yukon John Hardie MacArthur observed that there was 'nothing extraordinary' among the smallpox cases in 1900: '27 or 64% were vaccinated; 13 or 31% were vaccinated in childhood ... no case had been previously re-vaccinated'.[38] Vaccination against smallpox was not a single event that conferred immunity – it offered some protection but required revaccination. This prompted a wider policy of vaccination in the months and years to come, which is discussed in Chapter 6.

The Great Sickness in Alaska included influenza. In the Yukon, there were reports of influenza among the Gwich'in in Ttssietla's camp, as well as deaths from 'chest complaints' and pneumonia at Moosehide and elsewhere. It is striking, though, that in the excess mortality from Dawson in 1900, the primary cause (where attributed) was not measles but pneumonia. Pneumonia was a relatively common cause of death throughout this period. In the burial records

[35] LAC, *NWMP Personnel Records*. Sample used registration numbers of NWMP personnel identified in the annual reports for 1900, 1901, and 1902. See also Rod Macleod, *The NWMP and Law Enforcement 1873–1905* (Toronto: University of Toronto Press, 1976), 84, 95–6.

[36] Extract forwarded by P. C. H. Primrose [Aug. 1900], GOV 1677, file 7, YRG 1, Series 1, Central Registry Files, YA.

[37] Bliss, *Plague*, 162, 181.

[38] John Hardie MacArthur, 'The Semi-Annual Report on the Sanitary Condition of the Dawson Health District', for the half year ending December 31, 1900, p. 9, in RG 29 vol. 2, file 937013, part 1, LAC.

from Dawson, there was a marked increase in the number of deaths from pneumonia in December 1900, through January and February and lingering as late as April (see also Figure 8.2). Meghan Highet noted that in 1900 and 1901, people in Dawson were significantly more likely to have died or sought medical care in hospital from pneumonia than from any other single cause.[39] NWMP Assistant Surgeon W. E. Thompson reported a 'sharp epidemic of pneumonia', including cases in the NWMP barracks and deaths reported in the hospitals.[40] The majority of deaths in Dawson were among adult men (unsurprising given the town's demography and a common pattern in pneumonia mortality). They included Osias Dugas, who died in January 1901 at the age of forty-one. The NWMP reported on the death of a child from pneumonia in February 1901. The body was taken to Tagish for burial.[41]

Thompson attributed the pneumonia outbreak to environmental causes. He observed that 'during the months of December, 1900, and January and February, 1901, the weather was very trying; a dense fog hanging around town'.[42] Inspector Cortlandt Starnes, in his assessment, similarly ascribed the epidemic to 'the extreme cold weather we experienced last winter'.[43] Even though they were new to the region, Thompson and Starnes were right to consider the weather that winter as unusually cold. Colder-than-average temperatures were recorded in Dawson, Fort Good Hope, and on Herschel Island, with marked cold spells from late November to early December, mid to late January 1901, and in the first half of February.[44] Thompson and Starnes's emphasis on environment and miasma (the 'dense fog') reflected contemporary medicine which, as late as 1928, connected epidemic pneumonia to climate and environment.[45] Highet agreed with the assessment of the role of extreme cold, alongside working conditions in smoky and damp mines, aggravated by the recent introduction of steam engines underground.[46] She suggested further that poor nutrition among townspeople would have been a contributing factor in the outbreak. These interpretations do not wholly satisfy, however, for while environmental conditions can aggravate chest infections and contribute to fatalities, they do not cause pneumonia, which is an infectious disease.

[39] Megan J. Highet, 'Gold Fever: Death and Disease during the Klondike Gold Rush, 1898–1904'(MA thesis, University of Manitoba, 2008), 91–4.

[40] Canada, Parliament, *Sessional Papers*, 'Report of the North-West Mounted Police, 1901, Part III Yukon Territory' (Ottawa: S. E. Dawson, 1902), 78.

[41] 'Report of the NWMP 1901', 16. [42] 'Report of the NWMP 1901', 16.

[43] 'Report of the NWMP 1901', 64.

[44] Canada, *Historical Climate Data*, monthly data for Dawson, Hay River, Herschel Island, Fort Chipewyan, Fort Good Hope 2, Fort McPherson, Fort Simpson, 1893–1921.

[45] See Hilda M. Woods, 'On the Statistical Epidemiology of Respiratory Diseases', *The Lancet* (17 March 1928): 539–43.

[46] Highet, 'Gold Fever', 95–8.

Physicians attending those who died Dawson in the winter of 1900–1 were sufficiently skilled to diagnose influenza and measles – both of which can lead to a secondary fatal infection with pneumonia – and yet they did not. In other words, Dawsonites were not getting measles or influenza and then dying of pneumonia. But epidemic pneumonia in that year cannot be solely ascribed to environmental conditions, notwithstanding the severe cold that descended on the townsite or the conditions underground. Was it simply a coincidence that Yup'ik, Inupiat, and Gwich'in perished from measles and influenza in the Great Sickness, while Dawsonites hailing from the United States, Europe, Canada, and elsewhere died from pneumonia? Or were these epidemics connected?

A 1917–18 a measles outbreak in US army camps offers insight into the ways different pathogens, including those that cause measles and pneumonia, interact to cause heightened mortality.[47] The 1917–18 outbreak saw widespread infection with measles, with the rates highest in the camps that recruited predominantly from rural and remote areas – recruits like Herman Fisher. As adults, many of these cases were severe or fatal. As many as 50 per cent of the soldiers who contracted measles developed subsequent bacterial complications including pneumonias and died at rates much higher than were normally seen in measles outbreaks. In addition to high rates of 'post-measles pneumonias', there was also a parallel epidemic of 'severe and fatal primary pneumonia'.[48] In other words, alongside those who contracted measles, there were some who contracted measles and then developed pneumonia, and still more who developed severe and fatal pneumonia independent of any other disease. There were high levels of fatalities across the board. This pattern resonates with what we see during the Great Sickness in 1900, where there were those who perished from measles, those who died from measles and a subsequent infection, and then the epidemic of fatal pneumonias in Dawson.

In the 1917–18 army outbreak, the predominant cause of post-measles pneumonia and of primary pneumonia was bacteria, specifically *Streptococcus pyogenes* (at the time known as *Streptococcus haemolyticus*) – the same bacteria we encountered in Chapter 2, responsible for scarlet fever, erysipelas, acute tonsillitis, and other sickness. Medical researchers at the time determined that the epidemics of severe measles and of primary pneumonia 'coincided temporally with so-called carriage epidemics of asymptomatic *S. haemolyticus* colonisation'. When new army recruits arrived in barracks, they were soon infected or colonized by *Streptococcus* bacteria (and could remain colonized for months). These infections only rarely produced sickness (there were cases of scarlet fever and erysipelas in the camps) but were mostly asymptomatic and thus invisible in the absence of fluid samples and

[47] Morens and Taubenberger, 'A Forgotten Epidemic'.
[48] Morens and Taubenberger, 'A Forgotten Epidemic'.

microscopes. Nevertheless, the *Streptococcus* bacteria were the main cause underlying the deadly pneumonias and the severe cases and fatal complications from measles. Researchers at the time and since have described the 'viral-bacterial co-pathogenesis' or the way that the effects of the measles virus interacted with the effects of the *Streptococcus* bacteria on susceptible bodies to produce fatal synergies.[49]

The similarities between these two epidemics are striking. In both 1900 and in 1917–18, we see epidemic measles alongside epidemic pneumonia, each causing high mortality. Influenza was also reported in 1900 and would have been an additional contributing factor, although it is also clear that many reports of respiratory illness and death from lower respiratory infections (e.g. pneumonia and bronchitis) were generally classed as 'influenza', even though there may have been a different contributing cause.[50] Among the Yup'ik, Fortuine noted that 'pneumonia was the immediate cause of death in many cases'.[51] Pneumonia is grouped by Wolfe into the 'secondary infections precipitated or exacerbated by the measles and influenza' along with gastrointestinal disorders and tuberculosis.[52] Contemporary observers like D. H. Jarvis, who travelled that year along the Seward Peninsula and Yukon delta, estimated that 25 per cent of the regional population had died of 'measles, influenza, pneumonia, and starvation'.[53] If we start paying attention to pneumonia, we see that it was very much a defining feature of the Great Sickness in Alaska as well. *Streptococcus pyogenes* was also present in the Yukon and Alaska in 1900. MacArthur reported four cases of scarlet fever in Dawson between July and December 1900.[54] The mechanism of an underlying bacterial infection facilitating infection with measles and pneumonias allows us to understand what was going on better than any other hypothesis, including the model of 'virgin soil epidemics' used to describe the Great Sickness by Wolfe.[55]

Thus the Great Sickness may have also involved widespread infection with a colonizing *Streptococcus* bacteria. These bacteria are easily transmitted in close quarters like mines or through small, close-knit communities. This bacterial infection would have facilitated subsequent infection with measles among those who had not previously had the disease (including Herman Fisher as well Yup'ik, Inupiat, Tr'ondëk Hwëch'in, Gwich'in, and others) and possibly also infection with influenza (Map 4.1). The severe outcomes from

[49] Morens and Taubenberger, 'A Forgotten Epidemic', 853, 857.

[50] Fortuine, *Chills and Fever*, 220, 224; John F. Brundage and G. Dennis Shanks, 'Deaths from Bacterial Pneumonia during 1918–19 Influenza Pandemic', *Emerging Infectious Diseases* 14, no. 8 (Aug. 2008): 1193–9, http://doi.org/10.3201/eid1408.071313.

[51] Fortuine, *Chills and Fever*, 225. [52] Wolfe, 'Great Sickness', 94.

[53] D. H. Jarvis, Letter to the Secretary of the Treasury, 14 Feb. 1901, Senate Document No. 178, 56th Congress, 2nd Session, as cited in Wolfe, 'Great Sickness', 98–9.

[54] MacArthur, 'Sanitary Report', p. 10.

[55] Morens and Taubenberger, 'A Forgotten Epidemic', 858.

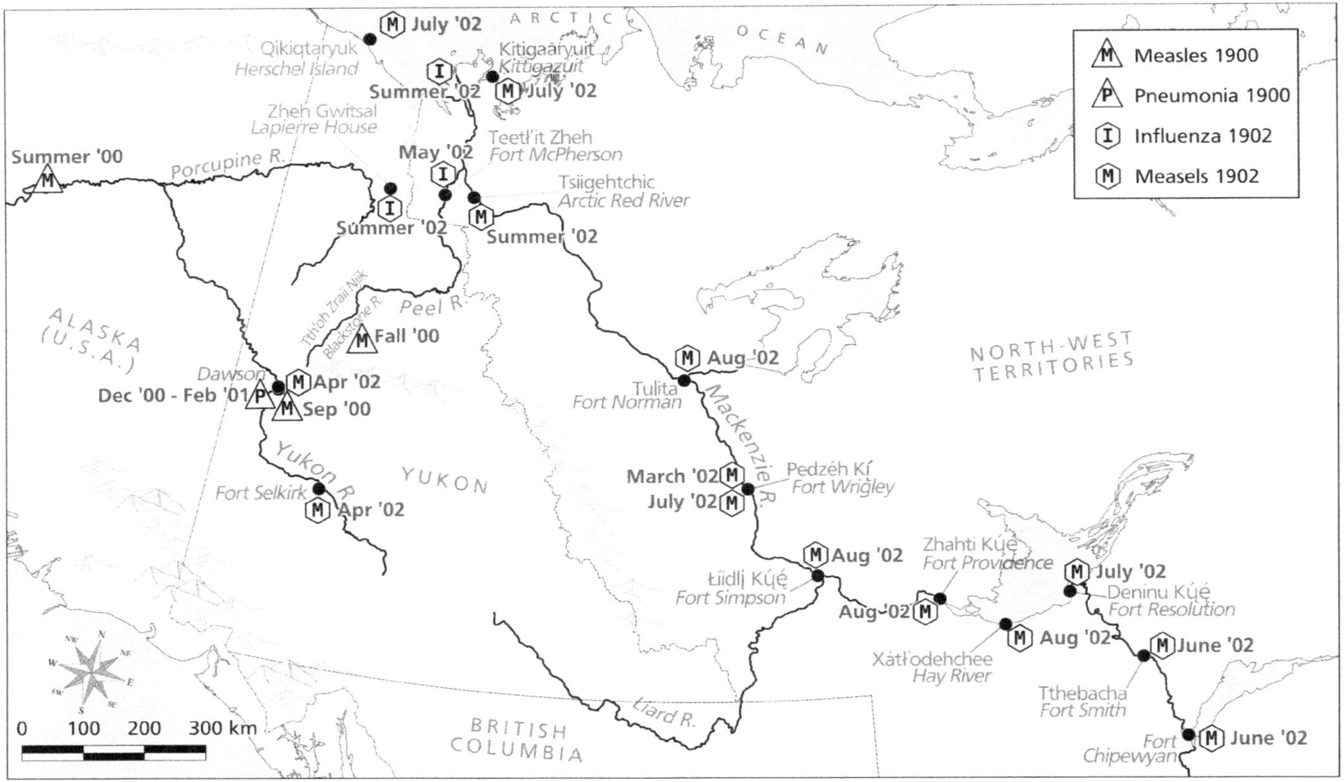

Map 4.1 Map of measles and influenza, 1900–2.

complications of measles, including pneumonia, as well as separate primary pneumonias that caused disproportionate high fatalities across Alaska, into the Yukon as far as the Stewart River, where Ttssietla and others camped, were a product of the co-pathogenesis of viruses and bacteria in human bodies with a range of immunities to infection. Dawsonites were not spared by the Great Sickness. Even if the town site acted as a sink for measles, it offered no protection against either initial streptococcal infection or subsequent pneumonia.

Cosmopolitan Pathogens

The Great Sickness did not reach communities to the east of the Mackenzie Mountains, along Dehcho, in the delta, and along the coast in 1900–1. Influenza did spread that year, with reports of *la grippe* in Fort Chipewyan, Fort Resolution, and Tulita, but measles did not. Stripped of its companion pathogen, influenza alone was less lethal, highlighting the significance of syndemics to the concussive impact of the Great Sickness.[56] But families along Dehcho were not safe from the effects of cosmopolitan pathogens arriving with sojourners and settlers (Figure 4.1, Table 4.1). As the Oblate missionary at

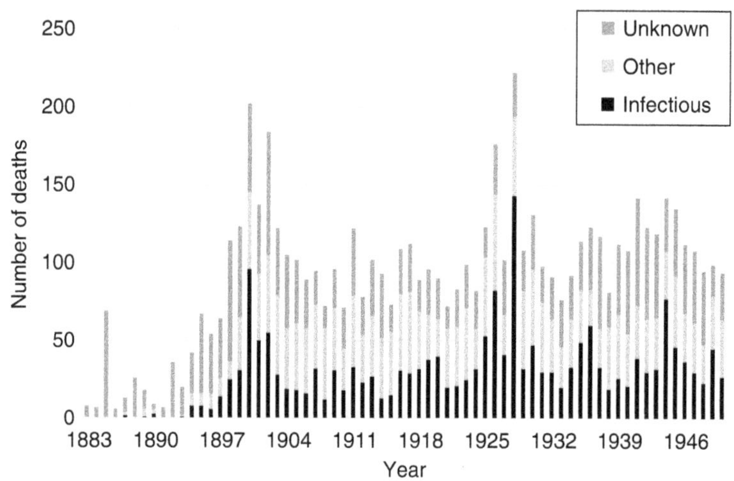

Figure 4.1 Deaths from infectious disease, other causes, or unknown cause 1883–1950. Source: COD Database.

[56] Newfield, 'Syndemics'.

Table 4.1 *Infectious disease as cause of death, ranked*

Year	Most frequent cause of death	No. of deaths	Second most frequent cause	No. of deaths	Third most frequent case	No. of deaths	Fourth most frequent cause	No. of deat
1898	Typhoid	9	Pneumonia	6	Influenza	4	Tuberculosis	4
1900	Dysentery	51	Measles	29	Pneumonia	22	Tuberculosis	14
1901	Pneumonia	30	Tuberculosis	8	Typhoid	6	Meningitis	3
1919	Whooping cough	13	Pneumonia	12	Influenza	11	Tuberculosis	9
1920	Pneumonia	18	Tuberculosis	17	Influenza	9	Typhoid	2
1924	Tuberculosis	25	Pneumonia	5	–	–	–	–
1926	Influenza	60	Tuberculosis	12	Whooping cough	5	Pneumonia	3
1927	Tuberculosis	22	Influenza	11	Pneumonia	6		
1928	Influenza	105	Tuberculosis	32	Pneumonia	3		
1935	Tuberculosis	38	Pneumonia	5	Diphtheria	3	Meningitis	2
1936	Tuberculosis	37	Pneumonia	11	Influenza	8	Syphilis	6
1937	Tuberculosis	25	Pneumonia	4	Influenza	3		
1941	Tuberculosis	18	Influenza	17	Meningitis	3	Dysentery	3
1944	Tuberculosis	31	Influenza	25	Pneumonia	11	Meningitis	8
1946	Tuberculosis	19	Influenza	10	Pneumonia	3	Diphtheria	2
1949	Influenza	24	Tuberculosis	18	Cold	2		

Source: COD Database.

Fort Chipewyan observed in 1900, 'This year, there was great mortality across the north west.'[57] To what exactly he was referring is unclear: he likely heard reports from places hit by the Great Sickness but added to these was a different pathogen, the principal cause of mortality along Dehcho and its tributaries in 1900 – *Shigella dysenteriae*, the bacteria that causes dysentery.

Shigella bacteria are ancient human pathogens. Human-adapted clones of the better-known *Eschateria coli* (*E. coli*), the *Shigella* strains that have caused great human suffering and death are thought to have affected human populations earlier than the bacteria and parasites responsible for tuberculosis, bubonic plague, and malaria.[58] Dysentery is among the diarrhoeal diseases that have persisted into the twenty-first century as major global causes of mortality. *Shigella* bacteria are a virulent enteric pathogen that cause endemic or epidemic dysentery – a disease characterized by bloody diarrhoea with high

[57] Codex Historicus, Fort Chipewyan, 1900, vol. 1, p. 66, PR2001.1181/1, OMI, PAA.

[58] Gulietta M. Pupo, Ruiting Lan, and Peter R. Reeves, 'Multiple Independent Origins of Shigella Clones of *Escherichia coli* and Convergent Evolution of Many of Their Characteristics', *PNAS* 97, no. 19 (September 12, 2000): 10567–72, http://doi.org/10.1073/pnas.180094797.

death rates (in contrast to cholera, a disease characterized by watery diarrhoea). Helene Castenbrandt, who has examined epidemic dysentery in Sweden between 1750 and 1900, notes that while it cannot have been easy for the general public, priests, and doctors to distinguish dysentery from other diarrhoeal diseases in the eighteenth and nineteenth centuries, 'dysentery was considered a recognizable disease, and there appears to have been consensus as to its nature'.[59] This recognition of dysentery as its own disease is apparent in missionary writings (Catholic and Anglican) from the Mackenzie in the late nineteenth century. Beyond the unmistakable bloody diarrhoea, those infected with dysentery also suffered fever, abdominal cramps, and rectal pain.

Where laboratory facilities existed, dysentery could be identified with greater certainty after Japanese bacteriologist Shiga Kiyoshi isolated the *Shigella* bacterium during a severe outbreak in Japan in 1897 that saw 90,000 cases and 20,000 deaths.[60] Historical samples, including a collection gathered from Allied forces fighting at Gallipoli in the First World War, have shown that the *Shigella* type (Sd1) isolated by Shiga in 1900 existed since at least the eighteenth century and 'swept the globe at the end of the nineteenth century'.[61] Sd1 spread globally in the years before the First World War.[62] Northern North America was tied into global movements of people at this moment – particularly those drawn to the region heading to the goldfields of the Klondike. Given the transcontinental circulation of an especially virulent *Shigella* type, the outbreaks in the Mackenzie district were part of a global experience with dysentery in the decades immediately preceding the First World War.

There were occasional reports of 'dysentery' dating back to the 1820s in the Mackenzie district. More detailed reports came from Jean Séguin at Fort Good Hope of outbreaks in 1867, 1876, and 1891.[63] In each instance children perished from the disease, and in 1876 – the most severe outbreak – all of the Dene, including adults (but none of the whites or Métis), fell ill.[64] The pattern of mortality reported by Séguin at Good Hope is consistent with the disproportionate impacts of dysentery and other diarrhoeal diseases on the very young. Each time the disease broke out, it was in late July or August, and Séguin attributed the outbreaks to heatwaves.[65] The seasonal recurrence of the disease

[59] Helene Castenbrandt, 'A Forgotten Plague: Dysentery in Sweden, 1750–1900', *Scandinavian Journal of History* 39, no. 5 (2014), 612–39 (p. 616); http://doi.org/10.1080/03468755.2014.953199.

[60] E. Njamkepo, N. Fawal, A. Tran-Dien, et al., 'Global Phylogeography and Evolutionary History of *Shigella dysenteriae* Type 1', *Nature Microbiology* 1 (April 2016), http://doi.org/10.1038/nmicrobiol.2016.27.

[61] Njamkepo, Fawal, Tran-Dien, et al., 'Global Phylogeography'.

[62] Njamkepo, Fawal, Tran-Dien, et al., 'Global Phylogeography'; see also Hackett, *Remarkable Sickness*, 211.

[63] Krech, 'Influence of Disease', 127, 129.

[64] McDonald reported dysentery on 18 Jul. 1877 and 6 Jul. 1892.

[65] Jean Séguin to his sister, 2 Jul. 1879, 71.220 / 7345, OMI, PAA.

was apparent in Sweden as well. There, in 1857, an epidemic of dysentery was worst in districts where the summer had been very warm and dry, leading to water shortages. Castenbrandt describes how 'trusted sources of drinking water ran dry, forcing people to drink unsafe water and travel long distances when their wells dried up'.[66] Drinking water at Tulita would have been taken from creeks and streams flowing into Dehcho. When dysentery appeared in 1891, the mercury did not reach into the thirties (Celsius), but it was hotter than normal for the late nineteenth century, with daily temperatures in the twenties for most of the month.[67] Summer heat could have dried up safer water sources or otherwise altered local drainage in such a way that drinking water became contaminated.

The nineteenth-century outbreaks at Fort Good Hope were minor compared to those which hit Fort Simpson and Fort Wrigley in 1900. In notes attached to the St David's mission register at Fort Simpson, Emily Reeve, wife of Anglican bishop William Day Reeve, described the dysentery outbreak that year as 'the most fatal sickness which has visited the place since 1865'.[68] Surviving burial registers record fifty-two deaths from dysentery in those two communities in this epidemic: thirty-seven in Wrigley and fifteen in Simpson. The experience of the community at Wrigley is particularly striking, given that it was one of the smallest posts in the Mackenzie district; in 1911, its total population according to the federal census was only seventy-nine people. To suffer more than thirty deaths from dysentery in 1900 would have been devastating and had enduring consequences. Fort Simpson was a mid-sized post, with a total population tallied at 375 in 1911. Dysentery also broke out that year in Fort Providence and Tulita, with twenty-four deaths in the latter community attributed to various causes including dysentery and influenza.[69]

On June 5, 1900, there was only a small attendance at prayers at St David's, the Anglican church at Fort Simpson. William Day Reeve recorded 'several people sick with "sore bellies"' that kept them away. From there the outbreak intensified. William departed for Peel River on 14 June, and his wife, Emily, kept the mission diary in his absence. More than that, through much of June Emily Reeve cared for the children who fell ill and suffered enormously. Dysentery is an awful disease. One child was described as having 'incessant diarrhea for fifteen hours', another suffered diarrhoea for three days, with her 'her bowel protruding after every stool'. One adult who fell ill was 'passing pure blood'. Along with these most severe and dramatic experiences of

66 Castenbrandt, 'Forgotten Plague', 624.

67 Canada, *Historical Climate Data*, daily data for Fort Good Hope 2, NWT, 1897–1966.

68 St David's Mission, Fort Simpson, Burial Register – Notes, Diocese of the Arctic, MF 84–1, GSA.

69 Most of the deaths in Providence and Tulita in 1900 do not have an identified cause of death. The Tulita records include only the year of death, not the month. See also Abel, *Drum Songs*, 173.

suffering, many had fevers, stomach cramps, and no appetite. Some died, others were sick, most for several days, one or two for weeks, but then recovered. The girl who had suffered for three days turned a corner on 23 June and was 'beginning to talk as usual for which God be thanked', wrote Emily.

Twenty-three years earlier, Robert McDonald was travelling with Julia and others in July. They had just passed the mouth of the Blackstone River when dysentery broke out in their camp. McDonald lamented that 'nearly all the medicines I had for the trip are spent – so that we can not do much to remove the cause of the disease. All took a dose of rhubarb'.[70] Rhubarb (*Rheum rhabarbarum*) was native to southern Siberia and northern and central China, where it was used from the third millennium BCE for its medicinal properties as a purgative (or laxative) and a bactericidal agent for dysentery.[71] Europeans imported rhubarb seeds, and the plant thrived in gardens and became a popular food in the nineteenth century. Back in Fort Simpson, in mid-July 1900, while the outbreak still raged, Emily Reeve gathered rhubarb to make jam and perhaps take advantage of its medicinal properties as well. This was imported rhubarb, planted along with other seeds in the gardens maintained by missionaries and traders.[72] There were a range of plant medicines used by Gwich'in, Dene, and Inuvialuit that helped with gastrointestinal problems, including the stomach cramps, loss of appetite, and diarrhoea that came with dysentery.[73] To treat stomach problems, including pain and diarrhoea, Dene Elders emphasized the value of gooseberries, tamarack, and – when herbal medicines did not work – grouse intestines.[74] These medicines would have been used by families to help those who fell ill in 1900 along the southern reaches of Dehcho.

Rhubarb jam aside, Emily Reeve made no mention of any medicine – herbal or otherwise – during the epidemic. She closely attended those who were ill, staying up with them during the night. Managing constant diarrhoea in children in the absence of indoor plumbing would have been very challenging. She kept them comfortable with hot water bottles, while other women in the community brought fresh milk and eggs. The epidemic lasted for weeks and notwithstanding

[70] McDonald Diary, 18 Jul. 1877.

[71] Donald G. Barceloux, 'Rhubarb and Oxalosis (*Rheum* Species)', in *Medical Toxicology of Natural Substances* (Hoboken: John Wiley and Sons, 2008), 84.

[72] Wild rhubarb (*Koenigia*) grows on steep riverbanks north on the Mackenzie River. An important foodstuff for the Gwich'in, wild rhubarb is a different species from the imported variety and did not have medicinal uses. Gwich'in Social and Cultural Institute, *Nan Srìdatr 'igwijìinlik Gwà 'àn Nin Duulee Nìinjìi / Species at Risk in the Gwich'in Settlement Area*, pamphlet.

[73] See descriptions of Arctic willow leaves (to treat upset stomach), berries (to combat diarrhoea and as a strong laxative), and spruce sap (to give appetite) in Inuvialuit Elders with Bandringa, *Inuvialuit Nautchiangit*, 138–9; liquorice root was used by Gwichya Gwich'in for diarrhoea: see Heine et al., *Gwichya Gwich'in Googwandak*, 156.

[74] See section on 'Stomach Problems', in Rabesca et al., *Traditional Dene Medicine*, part 2 (Database).

the injustices and inequities wrought by colonial relations in Fort Simpson, as elsewhere in the Mackenzie district and Yukon in this period, Emily Reeve did her utmost to care for the children and others who fell ill during this time. When the epidemic first hit, she got so little sleep that she confided in the mission register, 'I am afraid I shall break down if the children are not better soon'.[75] As the epidemic wore on, towards the end of June and early July, she was able to get some rest as others (mostly from the main Métis and white families in Simpson) stayed with the sick through the night. She was very attentive to those who were sick, writing in one entry, 'A quieter night with Eliza, for which I am very thankful. A change is coming over the poor child. Time will show whether it is for better or worse.'[76] In this instance, it was for the better, and Eliza recovered.

The outbreak in Fort Simpson was intense and persisted through June and July, drawing to a close in early August. The last death from dysentery was recorded on August 1 in Fort Simpson's register. Throughout this time, outsiders arrived in the community and people embarked on the boats – the HBC's steamer *Wrigley*, the Oblate Mission schooner the *St Alphonse*, and a small steam-powered boat operated by the Anglican mission out of Hay River, the *Ella Ya*, initially purchased from miners and used to ferry children to the school – headed up and down the Mackenzie River. No quarantine was established. The *Wrigley* had started off for Fort Good Hope two days after the sickness appeared at Simpson and passed through the community four times, in each instance stopping over for a couple of days, while the epidemic raged. Although there was no formal quarantine, Emily Reeve chose not to send the children from Fort Simpson to the Anglican residential school in Hay River is mid-June. In justifying her decision, she wrote, 'the *Wrigley* is crowded with miners and others and the children are too unwell'.[77] Hay River recorded no deaths from dysentery that year thanks to Emily Reeve's precaution. Unaware of the dire situation in Fort Simpson, her husband failed to exercise the same good judgement. On his return to Fort Simpson on 21 July, William Day Reeve brought 'half a dozen more children for the Hay River school, one of whom is sick'.[78] The sick child, Annie, had tapeworms. She soon contracted dysentery, against which she would have had few defences, and died a week later. It was not just little Annie. The arrival of children en route to residential school provided a new cohort of susceptibles for the epidemic to persist. As Emily Reeve put it several times during the course of the epidemic, 'more fresh cases'.

The coming and going of the *Wrigley* and other boats also brought news that the outbreak had spread. The first deaths from Fort Wrigley were reported in mid-July, and the epidemic peaked there in August. As late as November there

[75] St David's Mission Journal, 20 Jun. 1900, Fort Simpson, Diocese of Mackenzie River, II 5 a vol. 2, GSA.

[76] St David's Mission Journal, 17 Jul. 1900.

[77] St David's Mission Journal, 20 Jun. 1900.

[78] St David's Mission Journal, 21 Jul. 1900

were still deaths attributed to dysentery. By August, travellers on the *Wrigley* brought word of 'five deaths in two days at Providence'.[79] The burial record at Providence shows eight deaths clustered in a three-week period between 22 July and 11 August, most likely deaths from dysentery when the epidemic reached that place.[80]

When *Shigella* bacteria infect the body they damage the colonic epithelium (the tissues lining the colon), leading to the characteristic bloody diarrhoea. This can produce a range of complications that arise from the damage to the gastrointestinal system, from the Shiga toxins and from dehydration, which is the most direct cause of death. Given their susceptibility to dehydration, dysentery is most dangerous to the very young.[81] This was apparent in the mortality associated with dysentery between 1860 and 1940 and in the 1900 epidemic. For all the dysentery cases where an age was known, 74 per cent were infants (up to two years old) or children (three to fifteen years old). In Fort Wrigley and Fort Simpson in 1900, the percentage of children who died rose to 81 per cent. In 1900, seven adults died and no elders, although in the larger period (from 1860 to 1940) there were deaths in each age group.[82] As Castenbrandt found, deaths appear to have been evenly distributed between the genders, although in 1900 more women and girls died (57 per cent of the total deaths where gender was known).[83] More illuminating as to the character and effect of this epidemic were the two groups that were most significantly affected. First, the children in Fort Simpson, those being sent to the residential school at Hay River, and those at the residential school in Fort Providence made up a significant number of deaths in this outbreak. Second, in Fort Wrigley especially, many members from the same family died. In the burial registers, immediate family relationships were often described with a person identified as the father, son, wife, daughter, child, or sibling of the deceased. Of the thirty-seven deaths in Fort Wrigley, all but six involved families where more than one person perished. For three families, both parents and one or more children died in this outbreak. In other families, one parent and one or more children passed away.

Exposure to *Shigella* bacteria can produce immunity against reinfection. Notwithstanding its potential to spread through poor sanitation, dysentery was not a major source of either endemic or epidemic disease in nineteenth-century

[79] St David's Mission Journal, 10 Aug. 1900.

[80] These deaths are not counted as 'dysentery' though in the quantitative analysis below, as is the consistent methodology for this work. Of the eight deaths listed, five were in children under the age of fifteen. The other three had no age or identifying information.

[81] Beatrix S. Traa, Christa L. Fischer Walker, Melinda Munos, and Robert E. Black, 'Antibiotics for the Treatment of Dysentery in Children', *International Journal of Epidemiology* 39, suppl. 1 (Apr. 2010): i70–i74, http://doi.org/10.1093/ije/dyq024.

[82] Where 'elders' is used without capitalization in this book, it refers to an age category.

[83] Castenbrandt, 'Forgotten Plague', 618. All statistics from COD Database.

urban centres. Castenbrandt's work showed that dysentery primarily affected rural areas, appearing as an outbreak then disappearing, where cholera mostly affected towns.[84] Settlers born in Europe or southern Canada were therefore rarely protected from the disease through acquired immunity, and they too fell ill. Emily Reeve herself fell ill on 30 June, and was 'hors de combat' for several days suffering diarrhoea, pain, fever, and a bad cough. She recovered, but then Stanley Soanes – the schoolteacher who had given her some respite – also fell ill. In late July, Bishop William Reeve ended up in bed 'with the prevailing sickness'.[85] It was not only settler adults who survived; the mission register commented on Dene adults doing 'very poorly', but who later recovered. This included the poor soul who had passed nothing but blood for days. Healthy adults had greater resources to survive and recover from the ravages of this disease, although some suffered future health effects. A week after Bishop Reeve fell ill, he complained that he was 'scarcely able to move on account of rheumatism'. Serious arthritis has been found as a side effect in a minority of those infected with *Shigella*.[86] We only know of the ongoing effects of the disease in Reeve's body because he was keeping the mission register at that time. As with other epidemics, the unchecked course of pathogens in the Mackenzie and Yukon would have had much wider health repercussions than those that can be closely documented.

The infection of caregivers reflects the ease with which the bacteria could spread directly from those who were sick to the healthy and through contaminated food and water. It helps to account for the patterns of family mortality apparent in Fort Wrigley. Parents caring for their children may have caught the disease thus, and some died as a result. Yet Fort Wrigley stands out for the severity with which dysentery affected that community as compared to Fort Simpson, Fort Providence, or Tulita, the villages that recorded deaths from this disease in 1900.

Charles Camsell and George Blondin offer two perspectives on the sickness at Fort Wrigley. Although his name is now most closely associated with the Indian Hospital in Edmonton, Alberta, Charles Camsell was born in Fort Liard in 1876. He was one of eleven children of Julian Stewart Camsell and Sarah Foulds, who was the daughter of a Red River Métis family.[87] Charles travelled to Winnipeg for school in 1884, at the height of Métis resistance, and stayed for

[84] Castenbrandt, 'Forgotten Plague', 634. [85] St David's Mission Journal, 28 Jul. 1900.

[86] St David's Mission Journal, 2 Aug. 1900; Aldo A. M. Lima, Cirle A. Warren, and Richard L. Guerrant, 'Acute Dysentery Syndromes (Diarrhea with Fever)', in *Mandell, Douglas, and Bennett's Principles and Practice of Infectious Diseases*, ed. John E. Bennett, Raphael Dolin, and Martin J. Blaser, 9th ed. (Philadelphia: Elsevier, 2020), 1358.

[87] Charles Camsell, *Son of the North* (Toronto: The Ryerson Press, 1954); Margaret Mason Shaw, 'Charles Camsell (1876–1958)', *Arctic* 37, no. 1 (1984): 76–7; 'Camsell, Julian Stewart [born Onion]', Biographical Sheet, HBCA; 'Foulds, Sarah', M-7144–496,000, Charles Denney fonds and Métis genealogy files, Series 1, GA; 'Camsell, Charles [application for scrip]' file no. 950834, RG 15-D-II-8-c, vol. 1339, container: C-14955, LAC.

ten years to complete his education, returning to Fort Simpson in 1894. Charles never worked for the Hudson's Bay Company, taking instead odd jobs, fishing and trapping, and teaching at Tulita until the gold rush when he turned to prospecting and geological exploration. Charles's familiarity with northern life and languages made him indispensable to James Mackintosh Bell of the Geological Survey of Canada during a survey in 1900. This role as a 'son of the North' – an insider with expert northern knowledge and roots – would go on to shape his professional and political successes in the years to come.

In 1900, Charles was twenty-four years old. His older brother, Fred, was the HBC post manager at Fort Simpson and with his wife, Margaret Sibbeston, helped out Emily Reeve during the dysentery epidemic.[88] Charles passed the winter of 1899–1900 in Fort Wrigley, although he was off surveying with Bell in the summer of 1900 when the epidemic hit. Charles never mentioned the epidemic in his memoirs, but he described Fort Wrigley thus:

> Old Fort Wrigley was the meanest and most undesirable trading Post in the whole Mackenzie River district. It was perched on a sloping swampy bank, and was hidden behind an island on the east shore of the river with a small rapid in the channel alongside. There was nothing to commend the place, either as a strategic location for the fur trade or as a place to live. There was neither good hunting nor good fishing anywhere near.[89]

The poverty of local resources had led to starvation at that post in the 1880s. George Blondin also observed that along that stretch of Dehcho, the river was not good for fish and the people of Fort Wrigley 'travelled inland to hunt moose, woodland caribou, and snare rabbits. There was a smaller river not too far away that the people liked for fishing. There, the women gathered brush for the tepees and wood for the fires'.[90] Dene had camped on the island in the river, not on the shore. The HBC chose the land on the shore for their post, which proved so ill suited with its 'sloping swampy bank' which encouraged the dissemination of *Shigella* and other bacteria.

Blondin wrote about sickness in Fort Wrigley around 1900, in 'The Story of Bahwar and Yendee'. This is not a recounting of the epidemic, but rather a story in which Blondin tells about the changes underway in Dene life in this period. His story centres on two Fort Wrigley medicine men and brothers, Bahwar and Yendee. Bahwar led a group of men across the mountains to the Yukon to buy rifles, a much-prized commodity at that time, made readily available as a result of the gold rush. This journey led to a medicine war and from that, sickness among the people at Fort Wrigley. The main themes are most meaningful in the context of Dene laws and understanding medicine power – the central subject of Blondin's *Trail of the Spirit*, the book in which the story appears. Among these themes are Bahwar's dishonesty and arrogance, which ran contrary to

[88] St David's Mission Journal, 5 Jul. 1900. [89] Camsell, *Son of the North*, 107.
[90] Blondin, *Trail of the Spirit*, 74.

Dene values, and which lead to a crisis among his people. In this way, Blondin is writing to share Dene laws and to point to the historical changes that remade Dene lives and culture with the gold rush.[91] Yet there are also elements of the story that speak more closely to the experience of sickness in Fort Wrigley. In Blondin's telling, the sickness arises from Bahwar and the others visiting and trading with Dene and whites in the Yukon. An Elder who wonders if there is a medicine war that has 'to do with Bahwar's trip to the Yukon Territory. If it is, we have not seen the end of our troubles yet.' Blondin continues his story, 'Soon afterward, the wise Elder's words came true. A sickness spread throughout the community. Many people fell ill and soon died. Even the medicine people were dying.'[92] Only a few survived the sickness, and Yendee also sent the sickness back as well to the people in the Yukon, so that 'they will know what it is to lose so many relatives in a medicine war'. Blondin closes the story by emphasizing that 'of the many stories about medicine power, this is the cruelest story told about the work of medicine power'.[93] Rather than emphasize the swampy ground or poor conditions at Fort Wrigley, Blondin points to other key themes in this experience: the cruelty of the disease, the many who died at Fort Wrigley, and the connections between that place and the arrival of 'a mass of prospectors, Indian trappers and hunters', as part of the gold rush and the changes it brought to Dene life.[94]

The gold rush created new ties between distant places and peoples: thousands arrived in the Mackenzie district and Yukon heading to the gold fields near the confluence of the Yukon and Klondike rivers, while others already long familiar with these lands like the Gwich'in among whom Bella Alexie travelled, the Na-cho Nyäk Dun they met with, or the Dene from Fort Wrigley also sought opportunities with new people. The moral communities defined in these years were, as in the 1860s, never simply delineated along colonial lines. Even amid the cruelty of sickness apparent in Blondin's story, Emily Reeve's account, or the webs of relations illuminated in the burial registers from Fort Wrigley, there was empathy and care as people contended with the arrival of cosmopolitan pathogens.

Coda 1902

Fort Selkirk, the site of a fur-trade post, had been one of the most important settlements in the Yukon territory until it was dwarfed by Dawson with the gold rush. Construction on a winter trail from Whitehorse to Dawson began in the summer of 1902. This trail would remove Fort Selkirk from the main flow of people travelling around the territory. When it comes to infectious disease,

[91] Blondin, *Trail of the Spirit*, 67.
[92] Blondin, *Trail of the Spirit*, 76
[93] Blondin, *Trail of the Spirit*, 77.
[94] Blondin, *Trail of the Spirit*, 67.

timing can be everything. In the spring of 1902, three men made their way to Dawson from the south. Had the trail been completed a year earlier, they might have taken the winter route instead and bypassed the community. As it was, they arrived in Fort Selkirk, one after the other, each sick with measles.[95] With no hospital in town, the hotel proprietor nursed the men through their sickness. According to the NWMP Assistant Surgeon G. Madore, measles spread to the Northern Tutchone people while they were in Selkirk. The main king (chinook) salmon fishing camp of the Selkirk people was located about two kilometres below the community at Thi Ts'ach'än (Victoria Rock). The trade post was situated in the larger traditional territories where they travelled to hunt, fish, gather berries, trade, and meet with kin and friends.[96] Twenty-eight of the Selkirk people fell sick with measles. They were given nursing care, but many developed serious complications including bronchitis, pneumonia, and conjunctivitis. Three adults and at least four infants died.[97]

On the western tip of Lake Athabasca in the expansive Peace-Athabasca delta, lies Alberta's oldest settlement, Fort Chipewyan. In many ways a maritime community in the northern reaches of a landlocked province, Fort Chipewyan had important boat-building and fishing industries, as well as serving as an essential node in the geography of the fur trade. In her rich examination of the history of the community, Patricia McCormack showed Fort Chipewyan as a dynamic plural society situated at a crossroads: a meeting place for Indigenous and international cultures and economies.[98] The community, as the entry point for goods and people en route to the Mackenzie River District further north, was also a gateway for infectious disease as we saw with the flu in 1867. Major twentieth-century epidemics, including measles in 1902 and influenza in 1928, first appeared in Fort Chipewyan before moving down the Slave River and Dehcho. Fort Chipewyan was also an important Catholic centre in the North. Émile Grouard, after 1891 the Bishop of Athabasca-Mackenzie, was based at the Mission de la Nativité. In 1909, Grouard would direct the construction of a church in Fort Chipewyan, helping Sister Default, a Grey Nun, to decorate the murals inside using a paint made from fish oil and berries.

In June 1902, the Oblate missionary responsible for the Codex Historicus (possibly Grouard or another person at the mission) recorded the appearance of measles. 'All of a sudden' it appeared in epidemic form, and within weeks all in the community were sick including forty-four children at the 'orphelinat'

[95] Canada, Parliament, *Sessional Papers*, 'Report of the North-West Mounted Police, 1902, Part III Yukon Territory' (Ottawa: S. E. Dawson, 1903), 118. For a minor outbreak of measles in 1901 at Whitehorse, see 'Report of the NWMP 1901', 28.

[96] Hare and Gotthardt, *A Look Back in Time*, 12; *Fort Selkirk Elders Oral History Project* (1987).

[97] 'Report of the NWMP 1902', 118; COD Database; Highet, 'Gold Fever', 89.

[98] McCormack, *Fort Chipewyan*.

(residential school). The intensity of the epidemic owed to the fact that what started as measles was soon complicated with scarlet fever and severe diarrhoea, while many cases developed into bronchitis and tuberculosis.[99] Fifty people died at Fort Chipewyan, although the author of the Codex entries felt certain that without the ministrations of the Grey Nuns, who nursed everyone – Protestant and Catholic – that death toll would most certainly have doubled.

Fort Smith also saw cases in June and six deaths in one week. By July, measles appeared in Fort Wrigley and Fort Resolution, where it hit the Métis community especially hard and killed sixty people, 'chosen especially from among the children' as was recorded by the Oblate missionary at that place.[100] The pathogen continued downriver with the open-navigation season and the coming and going of the HBC and mission steamships, the *Wrigley* and the *St Alphonse*, among others. Tulita, Fort Simpson, and Hay River each saw deaths from measles in August. Fort Providence recorded seven deaths within a two-week period (five in five days after 20 August). The epidemic reverberated into autumn.

Even as measles travelled downriver from Fort Chipewyan after June, the virus had also reached Fort McPherson from the west – most likely from the earlier outbreak in Fort Selkirk and Dawson. Robert McDonald reported fevers and sickness in late May, before confirming 'nearly all around suffering from measles', on the 22nd of the month. Measles arrived in Fort McPherson along with the uptick in movement and travel that attended springtime, when the snow came off the land and frozen rivers broke up.[101] The outbreak peaked from late May through early July, and in these weeks, Inuvialuit travelled to Fort McPherson from the coast. This was not their first visit that spring. Two Inuvialuit had come from the 'East Coast' on 4 May. However, between April and early June, reports from Herschel Island and the coast made no mention of sickness. After 17 June was another matter. The Inuvialuit arrived in Fort McPherson a second time at the height of the measles outbreak. Within a few weeks, some fell sick with the disease, McDonald noting that on 8 July one Inuvialuk man and his son were 'well of measles', meaning they had fallen ill but thankfully recovered.[102] Kax'alik, the most important chief or *umialik* at Kitigaaryuit, arrived with a group of Inuvialuit on 9 July while the disease continued to circulate.[103] Whether from this later group or the earlier one,

[99] Codex Historicus, Fort Chipewyan, 1902, vol. 1, pp. 75–9. Dysentery here probably referred to severe diarrhoea.

[100] Codex Historicus, Fort Resolution, Aug. 1902, vol. 1, p. 32, PR1997.0109/2048, OMI PAA.

[101] McDonald Diary, 22 May 1902. [102] McDonald Diary, 8 Jul. 1902.

[103] Alunik, Kolausok, and Morrison, *Across Time and Tundra*, 86; Kax'alik was variously spelled, also Kakhilik, Kokhlik, etc. McDonald called him 'Kuglik Esqx chief', Diary, 9 Jun. 1902; he appears as Kokhlik in Frank A. Peake, *The Bishop Who Ate His Boots: A Biography of Isaac O. Stringer* (Toronto: Anglican Church of Canada, 1966), 27. The spelling here is taken from Alunik et al. Note 'Kitigaaryuit' not Kittigazuit is used throughout this book, as is consistent with Alunik and other recent publications on Inuvialuit history.

McDonald records Inuvialuit dying beginning in July 1902. On 18 July, he read a burial service at an Inuvialuit grave, and, two days later, a child of Kax'alik died.

For the Inuvialuit, this was the beginning of what would be among the most significant epidemics in the past 200 years. Some died in Fort McPherson, others returned to Herschel Island, Kitigaaryuit, and other whaling camps on the coast and perished there. Well-known Inuvialuk storyteller Felix Nuyaviak had many stories about epidemics.[104] He was ten years old in 1902 and recalled the epidemic as an old man in the 1970s:

> I remember in 1902 when this tribe of Eskimos was staying at Kittigaryuit and this big flu came on. . . . It hadn't been long after the flu arrived that the people began to die off. People died in their tents. People died while they were working on the whales. This was a dreadful sight. I remember though I was very small.
>
> All along the beach at Kittigaryuit and the tents up on the hill, people dying everywhere. Everywhere you looked people died . . . Most of the older people died off and the middle-aged. We also heard that in other whaling camps people were dying off too. . . .
>
> There was silence all over. This is something people will not forget for a long time.[105]

Charles Whittaker, an Anglican missionary stationed at Herschel Island that year, similarly observed that in the epidemic, 'older people took the disease more severely ... [it] carried away many of the middle-aged and elderly [Inuit]'.[106]

The 1902 measles epidemic was not the same epidemic as the Great Sickness in 1900, but there is some evidence to suggest that its severity among the Inuvialuit along the coast and in communities along the Mackenzie could have involved co-pathogenic infection, or a syndemic (Map 4.1). There were Elders, like Felix Nuyaviak, who referred to the epidemic as the flu, although they used that word in a general sense. Given the impact of subsequent influenza epidemics, 'flu' became synonymous with 'epidemic' in northern communities in the twentieth century.[107] Hope (Ayagutauraq) Shingnatuq Gordon, born in 1912, heard of the epidemic from her father Erwin Shingnatuq from Port Hope. She clarified how, 'Everyone was red. There was lots sick with flu. It was measles, you know. It was that, everyone got it'.[108] However, there were other reports of influenza that year too. At Tsiigehtchic, the Oblate missionary described the Gwich'in as having carried 'la Grippe' back from Herschel Island, from whence it spread among everyone in the community. Paul Vaudrack, from Fort Good

[104] Gruben interview, *Kitigaaryuit Oral Traditions Project 1996*, 244.

[105] Felix Nuyaviak in Murielle Ida Nagy, *Yukon North Slope Inuvialuit Oral History*, Occasional Papers in Yukon History No. 1 (Yukon Heritage Branch, 1994), 55–6.

[106] C. E. Whittaker, *Arctic Eskimo: A Record of Fifty Years' Experience & Observation Among the Eskimo* (London: Seeley, Service & Co., 1937), 109 and 225–6.

[107] See also Frank Cockney, interview with Florence Nasogaluak and Cathy Cockney, 13 Jul. 1996, Kitigaaryuit, tape 12A, transcript, in *Kitigaaryuit Oral Traditions Project 1996*, 172.

[108] Hope Gordon in *Yukon North Slope*, 56.

Hope, recalled losing his mother to influenza (brought back from Herschel Island) in 1901, and 'again in 1902 another flew run among the people, and my eldest sister died'.[109] As we will see in Chapter 8, influenzas circulated frequently in these years. After spreading independently between 1900 and 1902, influenza may have joined again with measles in the Mackenzie delta and along the Arctic Coast.

In 1902, pneumonia and other complications again followed on measles, particularly among older people, and led to greater mortality.[110] McDonald described diarrhoea and three miscarriages 'of women ill of measles', both of which are common complications. This report was made mid-summer to McDonald from Gwich'in travelling from LaPierre's House, who described as well the death of an adult man and woman and seven children.[111] In Fort McPherson itself, McDonald first recorded the appearance of the epidemic in late May: 'It seems to resemble measles, some are very suffering.'[112] Two days later, everyone in the mission house except McDonald was 'prostrated with measles'. Soon thereafter he developed a bad headache and by the following Monday had developed a severe case of erysipelas. McDonald stopped visiting, to prevent the spread of disease, until the rash was no longer visible and he felt better.[113] McDonald's erysipelas shows that *Streptococcus pyogenes* was in the community at the same time as measles and may have acted – as in 1900 in Alaska and the central Yukon, and as in 1917–18 in the US army camps – to cause greater mortality.[114]

The severity of the 1902 epidemic was apparent in the numbers who died and in the swiftness with which many of them were overcome by the disease. Felix Nuyaviak was not the only one to describe people who 'died while they were working on whales'. Frank Cockney also shared stories he had learned from the epidemic: 'Many of them working. When they're tired, go home maybe to their little shelter or something; never wake up, never get up and die there, nothing.'[115] There were stories about how some of those who survived were overwhelmed with the work of burying the dead. Cathy Cockney's grandfather, Bob Cockney or Nuligak, who was at Kitigaaryuit that summer, recounted that 'corpses were set on the ground uncoffined, just as they were'.[116] Nuligak did

[109] Paul Vaudrack [Voudrach] Manuscript, René Fumoleau Fonds, N-2004–031, NWTA.

[110] Whittaker, *Arctic Eskimo*, 226.

[111] McDonald Diary, 13 Jul. 1902; other reports from Hay River, Wrigley, Norman, and Dawson in this outbreak include deaths from pneumonia, bronchitis, premature birth/stillbirth, and middle-ear infection.

[112] McDonald Diary, 21 May 1902. [113] McDonald Diary, 7 Jun. 1902.

[114] In addition to Fort McPherson, there were also reports of scarlet fever or erysipelas from Dawson and Fort Chipewyan.

[115] Cockney interview, *Kitigaaryuit Oral Traditions Project* 1996, 172.

[116] Nuligak [Cockney, Bob], *I, Nuligak*, trans. M. Metayer (Toronto: P. Martin Associates, 1966), 27.

not have a number of how many died, 'but I know that when the people left for Kiklavak (Richardson's Island) they were but a handful compared to the number they had been'. In early December, news reached Fort McPherson from the coast that seventy-two Inuvialuit ('Eastern Esquimaux') had died in the epidemic 'among others Kuglik [Kax'alik] the chief and all his children'.[117]

Similar to the scarlet fever epidemic of the 1860s, stories of depopulation and inevitable decline swirled in the aftermath of 1902, complicating our understanding of the effects of this epidemic. Police reports of the number of people living at Kitigaaryuit suggested dramatic depopulation. NWMP Superintendent Charles Constantine prefaced his 1903 report of the measles epidemic with the comment 'The numbers are decreasing very fast', before attributing the high mortality among Gwich'in and Inuvialuit to their responses to the disease, a motif we have heard before.[118] In 1910, Inspector Jennings narrated a similar trajectory, reporting only fifty Inuvialuit living at Kitigaaryuit that summer: 'less than 20 years ago there were some 400 here, but native customs killed off some and many died of disease'.[119] These numbers are frequently lined up against population counts offered by John Franklin in 1825 and extrapolated to a larger population in the thousands in the nineteenth century, from which there were only a few hundred survivors in the early twentieth century.[120] Constantine or Jennings felt themselves superior to Inuvialuit and other northern Indigenous people, an attitude rooted in the racist ideas they shared with other colonizers about the inevitable and appropriate success of 'civilization' and the concurrent disappearance of 'savagery' as more people of Euro-Canadian ancestry moved north. These ideas shaped how they interpreted disease and its effects. Police, like many missionaries as well, *anticipated* the absence and decline of Indigenous northerners as a consequence of disease. Unfortunately, therefore, their reports and writings cannot be interpreted as unbiased empirical evidence of population decline or even population size. As Cathy Cockney expressed to archaeologist Natasha Lyons in the 1990s, there is good reason to doubt the estimates of major population decline as a direct consequence of the 1902 epidemic. 'Her sense', wrote Lyons of Cockney 'is that, at the time, a lot of people were out on the land, and not in the centres where the censes were taken, at places such as

117 McDonald Diary, 7 Dec. 1902.

118 Canada, Parliament, *Sessional Papers*, 'Report of the North-West Mounted Police, 1903, Part I North-West Territories' (Ottawa: S. E. Dawson, 1904), 49–50; Whittaker offered similar commentary, *Arctic Eskimo*, 226.

119 Canada, Parliament, *Sessional Papers*, 'Report of the Royal Northwest Mounted Police, 1910' (Ottawa: C. H. Parmelee, 1910), 151.

120 See Peter Usher, 'The Canadian Western Arctic: A Century of Change', *Anthropologica*, new series, 13, no. 1/2, 'Pilot, Not Commander: Essays in Memory of Diamond Jenness' (1971): 169–83 (p. 175).

Kittigaryuit and Herschel Island, which were hit especially hard.'[121] The nineteenth-century HBC censuses were flawed, incomplete records. But the two from 1858 and 1871 spanned a major epidemic and offered a reasonably consistent methodology. No equivalent census records exist for the turn of the twentieth century, and understanding the demographic impact of the epidemics between 1900 and 1902 must rely on estimating the number who died.

Conclusions

Many more died in this epidemic than were recorded as 'measles' deaths in the burial registers. Across the Mackenzie district and Yukon, using available source materials (mission journals, NWMP reports, diaries, and correspondence), between 222 and 267 people had their deaths recorded in 1902 from measles 'and its complications', including the seventy-two Inuvialuit.[122] For the twenty-one cases where the cause of death was listed as measles and an age was recorded, nine were adults (most in their twenties), eight were infants, and four were children. The significant number of children who died is consistent with anecdotal evidence from Fort Selkirk, Fort Resolution, and Tulita that reported greater mortality among infants and children. Of the adults who died, most deaths were attributed to measles and tuberculosis.

The severity of these epidemics was more than simply a product of measles infection in previously immunologically naïve populations. The disproportionate mortality among children and infants is consistent with measles mortality in an immunologically mature population. Prior to the development of an effective vaccine in the 1960s, measles was a deadly disease of childhood. In the 1910s, the first decade in which measles deaths were recorded in the United States, an average of 6,000 measles-related deaths were reported each year.[123] The Oblate missionary at Fort Chipewyan said that measles was endemic in that community but that the experience of 1902 was far worse than in recent memory. Children and babies were vulnerable to infection, injury, and malnutrition well before the arrival of Europeans. This should not obscure how high levels of infant and childhood mortality were a direct consequence of

[121] Natasha Lyons, 'Quliaq tohongniaq tuunga (Making Histories): Towards a Critical Inuvialuit Archaeology in the Canadian Western Arctic' (PhD diss., University of Calgary, 2007), 225.

[122] Notation used by J. R. Lucas at Hay River and Wrigley. The range from 222 to 267 includes 45 deaths in the cause of death database that overlap in time with the outbreak in each community and for which either no cause of death was listed, or the cause (tuberculosis, stillbirth, premature childbirth) is a known complication of measles infection. There is an outlier of 100 deaths at Rae reported in a secondary source, but it cannot be confirmed. RT and Associates, 'Fort Rae and Area 1789–1972', p. 15, HBCA.

[123] Centers for Disease Control and Prevention, 'Measles History', www.cdc.gov/measles/about/history.html.

colonialism with the arrival of infectious diseases such as scarlet fever, dysentery, and measles that caused disproportionate mortality in the very young.

The rush of people into and around the Yukon and Mackenzie district between 1896 and 1903 produced severe epidemics. People came from around the globe on whaling crews, in search of gold, as independent traders taking advantage of the end of the HBC's monopoly, as missionaries to proselytize and to staff schools and hospitals, and as police to secure the interests of the colonial state. They brought with them an array of pathogens, some of which moved with vicious intensity, others of which became established in communities and environments across the region, causing pain and ill health for years to come. In communities where there had been no measles reported for thirty-five, or as long as fifty years, between 1900 and 1902, there were two major epidemics originating from multiple outside sources.[124] The wide geographic reach of measles between 1900 and 1902, and of other cosmopolitan pathogens, was a consequence of the new patterns of mobility produced by the Klondike gold rush that brought more people in, via more different paths, than ever before. Severe epidemics and syndemics were a direct consequence of the twentieth-century face of resource and settler colonialism in the North.

[124] McCarthy, *Great River*, appendix B; COD Database first measles is in 1900. For measles in Saskatchewan and Alberta, see Canada, Parliament, *Sessional Papers*, 'Report of the North-West Mounted Police, 1902, Part I North-West Territories' (Ottawa: S. E. Dawson, 1903), 24, 68, 84. For outbreaks in Boer War concentration camps (1900–2), see G. Dennis Shanks, Zheng Hu, Michael Waller, et al., 'Measles Epidemics of Variable Lethality in the Early 20th Century', *American Journal of Epidemiology*, 179, no. 4 (February 2014): 413–22.

5 Infrastructures of Extraction, Sanitation, and Care

In the wake of epidemics, people moved away. Frank Cockney shared stories he had heard from Felix Nuyaviak about Inuvialuit families in the delta who had chased the sickness out by singing. Cockney recounted how, 'None of them families, the one they surround them, never get sick. Never die. . . . Like missed out whole thing [the epidemic], eh? Atukyuk, she sing a spirit song and chase out the sickness. Made sure it could not reach them.'[1] Those who survived left Kitigaaryuit and moved on. Nuyaviak emphasized this, that even those younger people who continued whaling 'did not remain at Kittigaryuit. They moved to the other camp.'[2] Inuvialuit understood that with so many deaths at that place, Kitigaaryuit was now haunted.[3] Nuligak described seeing a huge pack of wolves after he and his family left Kitigaaryuit: 'There were so many of them that the last ones were still in front of us when the leaders had disappeared on the eastern horizon.' Caribou no longer came to that place.[4] Later in the 1940s, when Anthony Apakark Thrasher camped at Kitigaaryuit as a child, he knew it as a haunted place.[5] The loss of so many at Kitigaaryuit, their bodies buried nearby, made it impossible to remain at that site.

Kitigaaryuit ceased to be the centre of Inuvialuit whaling, although it endured as an HBC trade post, opened in 1912 as an outpost to Aklavik. Willie Gruben, born at Kitigaaryuit in 1917, recalled how in his childhood people spent the summers there and continued to come through winter to get goods at the store.[6] Laura Raymond remembered families who lived at the site up to 1934, when the HBC moved their trading operations to Tuktoyaktuk.

[1] Cockney interview, *Kitigaaryuit Oral Traditions Project 1996*, 173.

[2] Felix Nuyaviak in *Yukon North Slope*, 56. Stefansson observed this as well. See *The Stefansson–Anderson Arctic Expedition*, 24.

[3] It was Dene custom, similarly, to move away from the places where people died. Blondin, *When the World Was New*, 193.

[4] Nuligak, *I, Nuligak*, 27.

[5] Anthony Apakark Thrasher, *Thrasher . . . Skid Row Eskimo*, ed. Gerald Deagle and Alan Mettrick (Toronto: Griffin, 1976), 19–20; see also Keavy Martin and Sam McKegney, 'Inuvialuit Critical Autobiography and the Carceral Writing of Anthony Apakark Thrasher', *Canadian Literature* 208 (Spring 2011): 65–83.

[6] Gruben interview, *Kitigaaryuit Oral Traditions Project 1996*, 217.

Raymond recalled the warehouse and store being taken down. She watched a whole house moved by barge.[7] Inuvialuit leadership had long since moved to Tuktoyaktuk. With Kax'alik's death from measles, Ovayuak 'was the boss after him' in Nuyaviak's words.[8] Ovayuak, pictured dancing in the foreground of Figure 5.3, was Nuligak's uncle, and while he was the most important man at Kitigaaryuit after Kax'alik's death, he also stayed in Tuktoyaktuk with its excellent harbour for fishing.[9] Leadership passed from Ovayuak to William Mangilaluk who, in 1905, 'tired of drifting here and there', decided to settle down in Tuktoyaktuk, building the first log house at that place.[10] In this way, the survivors from 1902 and others moved to Tuktoyaktuk, which grew thereafter in importance.[11]

Many people came east from Alaska in this period, before and after the 1902 epidemic. Abraham Okpik's family came because of the Great Sickness in 1900, which they called 'the Big Death'.[12] In his memoir, Okpik described camps at Utqiarvik (Barrow) and Nuwuk (Point Barrow) where 120 people died from measles. For Okpik's great-grandfather, 'we couldn't live in this cursed land'. And so they went east. Okpik's parents were both born around the time their families moved, on the way to Herschel Island.[13] Others came east pursuing opportunities created by whaling and access to diverse resources. Martha Harry said that her parents came before the whalers did, 'they all come from there 'cause there is no muskrats, no rabbits that's why they come this way'.[14] Caribou 'disappeared' from their normal routes in northern Alaska, prompting famine and migration.[15] Many who came did not stay at Herschel

7 Laura Raymond, interview with Florence Nasogaluak, Elisa Hart, and Cathy Cockney, 10 Aug. 1997, Kitigaaryuit, tape 11b, in Cathy Cockney, *Kitigaaryuit Oral Traditions Research Project 1997* (Inuvik: Inuvialuit Social Development Program, 1998), 354–6; See also Peter J. Usher, *Fur Trade Posts of the Northwest Territories 1870–1970* (Ottawa: Northern Science Research Group, Dept. of Indian Affairs and Northern Development, 1971), 106.

8 Sometimes also spelled Ovayoak. 'Boss' here refers to *umialik* or 'leader in the old tradition', see Alunik, Kolausok, and Morrison, *Across Time and Tundra*, 120; *MVPI Tuktoyaktuk, NWT* (8 and 9 March 1976), vol. 44 (testimony of Felix Nuyaviak), 4170–1; see also Vilhjalmur Stefansson, *Hunters of the Great North* (New York: AMS Press, 1922), 142–4.

9 Nuligak, *I, Nuligak*, 84; Alunik, Kolausok, and Morrison, *Across Time and Tundra*, 69, 119.

10 'Felix Nuyaviak: Mangilaluk Adrift on the Ice', in Penny Petrone, ed., *Northern Voices: Inuit Writing in English* (Toronto: University of Toronto Press, 1988): 183–9 (p. 183).

11 Cockney interview, *Kitigaaryuit Oral Traditions Project 1996*, 174; Arnold et al., eds., *Taimani*, 81.

12 Abraham Okpik, *We Call It Survival: The Life Story of Abraham Okpik*, ed. Louis McComber (Iqaluit: Nunavut Arctic College, 2005), 71.

13 Okpik, *Survival*, 71–2.

14 Martha Harry, interview with Renie Arey and Murielle Nagy, 5 Jul. 1991, Inuvik, tape 16B, transcript, in Murielle Nagy, ed., *Yukon North Slope Cultural Resources Survey*, book 1, 4; Bessie Wolki, interview with Agnes Gruben White and Murielle Nagy, 23 Jun. 1991, Tuktoyaktuk, tape 4A, transcript, in *Yukon North Slope Cultural Resources Survey*, book 1, 9.

15 Ernest S. Burch, Igor Krupnik, and J. Dau, *Caribou Herds of Northwest Alaska, 1850–2000* (Fairbanks: University of Alaska Press, 2012), 108.

Island, central to whaling activity and with plentiful driftwood. They moved elsewhere along the coast, for example to Tikiraq, where there were 'a lot of seals, different types of seals, and there's also caribou hunting'.[16] Albert Oliver's parents came as hunters for whalers but stayed after the whalers left because the land 'had lots of animals. ... There is muskrat, rabbits, ptarmigan, all kinds of animals to hunt that is why they stayed and claimed the land when they finished with the ships and when they didn't hunt for them anymore.'[17]

Turn-of-the-century epidemics prompted the HBC to move two trade posts in the Mackenzie district. Around 1902, Fort Wrigley was relocated forty-eight kilometres downstream to a site near Wrigley Rock. Severe hunger in the 1880s and the devastating dysentery epidemic in 1900 had laid bare the unsuitability of old Fort Wrigley. Around the same time, between 1905 and 1909, the HBC also moved their post from Nishì (Old Fort Rae) to Behchokǫ̀. Like Fort Wrigley, there were multiple problems at the Old Fort Rae site. In 1894, post manager Joseph Hodgson complained about the poverty of fuel in the vicinity of the post.[18] The end of the HBC monopoly led to Hislop and Nagle establishing a trading post nearby at Willow River in 1895.[19] More independent traders and the arrival of more white and other non-Indigenous trappers in the North altered long-standing trading practices and relations with the ever-dominant HBC. In the case of Old Fort Rae, competition from Hislop and Nagle forced up the prices the HBC had to pay for furs and meant less trade. This decline deepened with deaths from measles among families who traded at the post, so the HBC sought out a better location.

Trade posts moved for environmental reasons, at the request of Indigenous trade partners, to secure fish and game, or in response to the ravages of epidemic disease.[20] There were also satellite posts – these were very small and rarely lasted more than a year – that contributed to the changing geographies of the nineteenth-century fur trade. Moving Old Fort Rae and Fort Wrigley was part of this long-standing process. Spatial fluidity persisted in the twentieth century. Chapter 9 describes villages and trade posts that flourished in the 1920s

[16] Lily Lipscombe, interview with Renie Arey and Murielle Nagy, 7 Jul. 1991, NiVi-6 at Arvaqvik, tape 24A, transcript, in *Yukon North Slope Cultural Resources Survey*, book 2, 12.

[17] Albert Oliver, interview with Renie Arey, Murielle Nagy, and Bill Schneider, 11 Jul. 1990, Aklavik, tape 11B, transcript, in Murielle Nagy, ed., *Qikiqtaqruk (Herschel Island) Cultural Study* (Inuvik: Inuvialuit Social Development Program, 1994), 6.

[18] As cited in Shannon Hayden, 'One Land, Many People: Archaeology, Agency, and Landscape at Old Fort Rae, Northwest Territories' (MA thesis, University of Leicester, 2010), 38.

[19] Hislop and Nagle were active in the Mackenzie Valley as early as 1882 and were bought out by the Northern Trading Company in 1913. See Arthur J. Ray, *The Canadian Fur Trade in the Industrial Age* (Toronto:University of Toronto Press, 1990), 104.

[20] See, for examples, Mélanie Fafard and Ingrid Kritsch, *Yeenoo Daì' Gwatsat Teetł'it Zheh Googwandak: The History and Archaeology of Fort McPherson* (Tsiigehtchic: Gwich'in Social and Cultural Institute, 2005), 12; Yerbury, *Subarctic Indians*, 99; Robert McGhee, *Beluga Hunters: An Archaeological Reconstruction of the History and Culture of the Mackenzie Delta Kittegaryumiut* (St John's: Institute of Social and Economic Research, 1974), 91; Alunik, Kolausok, and Morrison, *Across Time and Tundra*, 15–17.

and 1930s, although many later declined. New extractive operations came and went. Such fluidity was possible with very small villages and hamlets, and new transportation technologies – namely bush planes – fit easily into this dynamic environment. Most important, though, were the ways in which people continued to live out on the land and did not stay in place. This chapter turns on the tensions that arose between *settler* colonialism and the persistently unsettled geographies of the Mackenzie and Yukon. Although many of those who came north from the turn-of-the-century onwards did not stay and 'settle', colonialism exerted new gravitational forces on families and ways of life. Treaties sought to organize relations with Indigenous peoples and facilitate access to resources, and they were integral to new infrastructures of extraction that appeared from 1900 on. This chapter examines the treaty agreements to consider their relationship to land and health, from both Dominion and Indigenous perspectives. With large numbers of new arrivals and the waste they created, exemplified in the instant city of Dawson, sanitary infrastructures – physical and bureaucratic – became critical for health. Lastly, this chapter considers the infrastructures of care erected in the early decades of the twentieth century. These infrastructures – of extraction, sanitation, and care – were in response to and would go on to create more fixed geographies, integral to the processes of northern colonialism. But this chapter opens by following people out on the land, to see how mobility and travel defined northern ways of life in the early twentieth century.

Busy Trails

Gwich'in, Inuvialuit, Dene, and other northern people lived their lives on the land. This was expressed in countless different ways by Elders born after 1885, who were children and young adults in the first two decades of the twentieth century.[21] 'People never stayed in one place, they travelled all the time to find meat', Albert Fabien, born in Fort Resolution in 1916, recalled in the 1980s.[22] Philip Simba (Chųą), in his July 1976 testimony to the Berger Inquiry at Kakisa Lake, described it thus: 'There was a set place I guess for the trading post. Everybody wandered around after the game. Whenever somebody shot a moose or anything, they all would go over there and live there.'[23] Persis Gruben, born on the Peel River in 1918 and who later moved to Tuktoyaktuk, spoke about how 'Inuit, Inuvialuit, and Nunataarmiut they never stayed in one place. Always moving every year looking for a good place or spot where there's

[21] See Julienne Andre and Eliza Andre, chapters 19 and 20 in *Gwichya Gwich'in Googwandak*; and 'Life Lived from the Land', in part 2: 'The First Generation', Vuntut Gwitchin First Nation and Smith, *People of the Lakes*, 64–118.

[22] Albert Fabien in *That's the Way We Lived*, 10.

[23] *MVPI Kakisa Lake, NWT* (17 July 1976), vol. 69 (testimony of Philip Simba), 7932.

a good fishing and meat hunting right there.'[24] Pierre Wedzin of Behchokǫ̀ recalled relations between the land, people, and villages:

At the start of 1900 there were people scattered everywhere in the bush. Behcho Ko was our home community but hardly anyone ever stayed there. . . . The fur trader and first missionaries each had a family staying with them to provide them with wild meat and fish, but everyone else was in the bush.[25]

As a Gwich'in minister, Amos Njootli held services out on the land, in bush camps, and in the community (Figure 5.1). Helen Rabesca told how women 'would often stay home on the treeline while our husbands and older sons made the one hundred-mile trip to Behcho Ko in the fall. It would take them a month or so to get there and back.'[26]

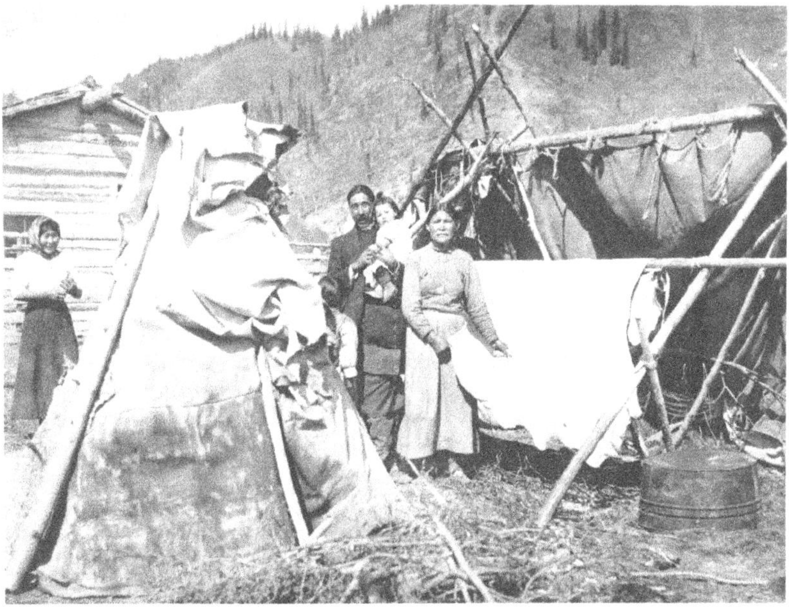

Figure 5.1 Amos Njootli, Eunice Njootli, and family at Rampart House. Dan Cadzow Papers, UAF-1965–31–54, Alaska and Polar Regions Collections and Archives, University of Alaska Fairbanks.

[24] Persis Gruben and Charlie Gruben, interview with Agnes Gruben White and Murielle Nagy, 22 Jun. 1991, Tuktoyaktuk, tape 2A, transcript, in *Yukon North Slope Cultural Resources Survey*, book 1, 3.

[25] Pierre Wedzin, 'Working to Live', in Blondin, *Yamoria*, 201–2.

[26] Helen Rabesca, 'One Hundred Years in Denendeh', in Blondin, *Yamoria*, 207.

Lives lived out on the land found expression in the ways that people described themselves and their relations with others. Simba spoke of how 'he lived among a lot of people and he travelled with all of them'.[27] Pascal Baptiste, born in 1898, testified before the Berger Inquiry at Tsiigehtchic. Using an interpreter, Baptiste's testimony opened with the statement, 'He's travelled quite a bit.' Baptiste went on to say how when he was with his parents, all they did was travel around: 'we never stayed one place. We were forever travelling.'[28] This travelling was over long distances. Baptiste described going 135 kilometres up the Arctic Red River and staying all winter, travelling in the mountains. Madelaine Simba (Philip's wife), born in 1897, 'used to love to travel all the way to Trout Lake' 200 kilometres distant from Fort Providence. 'Can you imagine anyone walking that far nowadays?', she added.[29]

People walked, paddled, and used sleds. Charlie Thomas, born at Rampart House in 1916, recalled 'there were no such things as rubbers or hard-soled shoes so everyone wore skin moccasins. They travelled long distances and those moccasins didn't last very long.'[30] In long-ago days, in the words of Neil McDonald (son of Robert and Julia), 'long before the white man came, the way I hear it, they had no dogs. They had no toboggans, but they used sleighs. They had to pack their stuff and pull their sleighs.'[31] By 1900, dogs were commonplace (Figure 5.2).

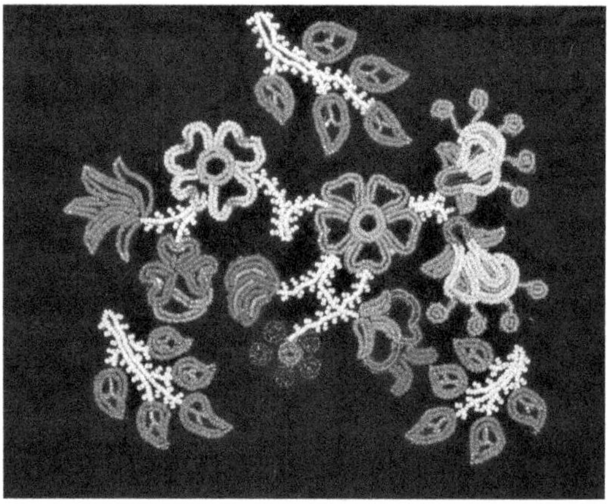

Figure 5.2 Dog blanket beaded by Julia (Kutug) McDonald, used for decoration. Artefact 1984.154, Old Log Church Museum.

[27] Simba in *MVPI Kakisa Lake*, 7932.
[28] *MVPI Arctic Red River, NWT* (13 March 1976), vol. 47 (testimony of Pascal Baptiste), 4643–4.
[29] Madelaine Simba in M. M. Thom and E. Blondin-Townsend, eds., with Tessa Macintosh Wah-See (photography), *Nahecho keh/Our Elders* (Fort Providence: Slavey Research Project, 1987), 39.
[30] Charlie Thomas interviewed by Louise Profeit-Leblanc, in *Rampart House*, 27.
[31] Neil McDonald in *People of the Lakes*, 67.

They were good draught animals but required a lot of fish and care to keep up their strength. People paddled. Tłįchǫ Elders described how they and their ancestors travelled long distances by birchbark canoe. Joan Nazon (Gwichya Gwich'in born in 1913) put it thus: 'people never stayed quiet, they paddled all the time'.[32]

Some of the travelling around was on major routes and timed to key events in the annual calendar. Charlie Thomas spoke about how they spent time in summer and winter in Crow Flats, but 'when the caribou came we spent a lot of time in the mountains'.[33] People would come to trade posts (town) to pick up gear or to trade their furs. They came as well for big gatherings and celebrations at Christmas and New Year's, at Easter, and in summer timed around treaty gatherings, or the 15 August feast of the Immaculate Conception (in the Catholic calendar), depending on the community.[34] These gatherings lasted for days and often included big tea dances that continued through the night, as well as handgames and competitions (Figure 5.3). Rivers and trails served as

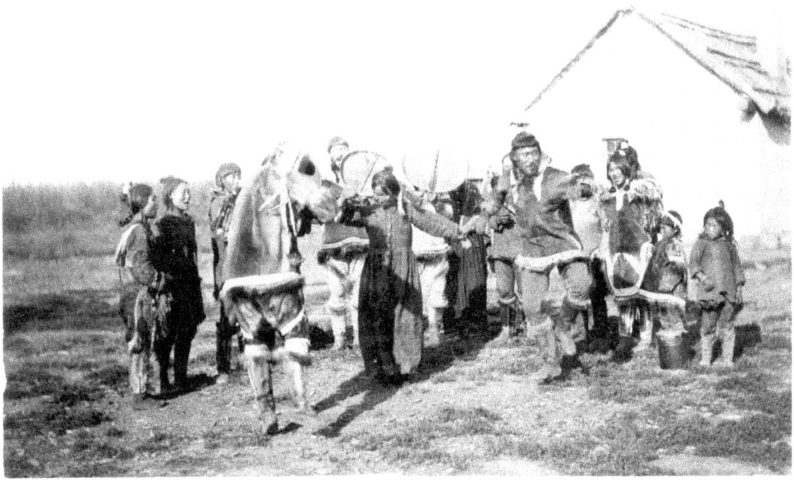

Figure 5.3 Inuit dancing at Fort McPherson, 1893–4. Photograph by James McDougall. HBCA 1987/13/210, Hudson's Bay Company Archives, Archives of Manitoba.

[32] Joan Nazon in *Gwichya Gwich'in Googwandak*, 54. [33] Thomas in *Rampart House*, 27.

[34] See chapter 16 in Heine et al., *Gwichya Gwich'in Googwandak*; 'Chiefs and Treaty Days', in *That's the Way We Lived*; Suzie Bruno, 'Living the Dene Laws', in Blondin, *Yamoria*, 215.

major thoroughfares that brought people together and connected distant places across the land. Moses Tizya, born in 1900, spoke about his father's time when 'they made four roads to move one camp to the other'.[35] Tłı̨chǫ Elders interviewed in the 1990s emphasized the importance of Biati and Ek'ati as 'places where the several major trails come together'.[36] Gwich'in Elder Sarah Abel spoke of how, as a child, 'In those days, they moved in the early morning while it was still dark. Then they set the camp before it got dark in the evening.'[37] With all of that movement, trails could get busy. Julienne Andre recalled her travels: 'From long ago, there was a road from there made by Slavey Indians. There was a good trail.' She spoke of meeting people on the trail. They stopped near Fort Good Hope, then 'we left and followed someone's trail. We met lots of people . . . When we got back, our people came back from the mountains.'[38] George Blondin similarly described the trails between Whitehorse and Fort Good Hope: 'it was a very long journey to get home, with many opportunities to meet people along the way'. He went on to tell of a time when a group of Dene from Fort Good Hope met with Yukon Dene and they played handgames together.[39] Fort Selkirk people hosted Dene from Dehcho in the early decades of the twentieth century and would hold stick-gambling competitions that could last many days.[40]

This movement shaped the immeasurable knowledge and expertise that Indigenous peoples had about the land – never just in one place, but at great distances as well. As Tłı̨chǫ Elders said in the 1990s, 'it is impossible to talk about one place, such as Ek'ati without discussing the total Dogrib territory. Knowledge of where the ancestors travelled provides a blueprint on how places are connected.'[41] As Charlie Peter Charlie, born in Crow Flats, said, this was 'their country, so since they were small they travel with their parents. Nobody really (got lost).'[42] Tony Andre, born in the Yukon at Nihtavan Diniinlee in 1924, remembered learning about important trails and places from his parents, who would test his knowledge. This education meant that 'Even if I were half blind, I'd still remember, because my dad taught me all of these trails and lakes'.[43] Edward Ruben (Angusinauq), born in 1917 at Nuvuraq, spoke about how he formed geographical knowledge: 'When you travel through an area then maybe in one year you pass

[35] Moses Tizya in *People of the Lakes*, 70.
[36] Arrowmaker et al., *We Know and Love Tłı̨chǫ̀ Ndè*, 13–14.
[37] Sarah Abel in *People of the Lakes*, 66–7.
[38] Julienne Andre in *Gwichya Gwich'in Googwandak*, 268.
[39] Blondin, *Trail of the Spirit*, 129–30. [40] Hare and Gotthardt, *A Look Back in Time*, 27.
[41] Arrowmaker et al., *We Know and Love Tłı̨chǫ̀ Ndè*, 13.
[42] Charlie Peter Charlie, interviewed by Veronica Germaine and Georgina Griffith in *Rampart House*, 47.
[43] Tony Andre in *Gwichya Gwich'in Googwandak*, 56, 250–1.

through it again, you use your mind, your memory.' He emphasized how he learned from others:

> you hear what people see, the first time you travel maybe you don't remember it except what you recognize . . . By hearing what the people tell you about what the country looks like . . . When you get there you look for what people tell you about the area, the lakes, streams, rivers and you can recognize the land.[44]

Travelling shaped knowledge, practice, and material life. Many Elders spoke of how life was hard work at this time, but no one complained.[45] Travelling was hard work; so too was setting up and moving camp. Mary Evik Ruben, born across from Tuktoyaktuk in 1925, recalled her mother, when they would camp: 'we put up tent, she start doing all the laundry, you know like bedding and everything. She leave it outside, you know clean rocks, ah? Really so nice. We live long ago clean ah?'[46] Moving camp and travelling solved problems of sanitation that would otherwise arise in longer settled places. Myra Moses, born in 1884, remembered her childhood when there were no towels and she washed herself using rabbit feet.[47] Travelling meant that the moccasins Charlie Thomas described wore through quickly, 'but there was a good supply of skins so they had a lot of moccasins'.[48] Martha Tizya, a Dagoo Gwich'in woman born in 1898, described how long ago they sewed ten caribou skins together to make a tent, 'just like a house, they made it really big'. And then when it was time to move camp, they used caribou skins for toboggans, shaping the skins while they were wet.[49] The need for lightweight, readily available materials influenced how people used what they harvested from animals and what they traded for. Skin tents were light and, with a fire inside, they kept people warm. Heavier canvas tents and woodstoves, introduced by traders, trapped less smoke inside, making them warmer and more comfortable than skin tents even though they created a greater burden when travelling (Figure 5.4). This was a trade-off that many found worthwhile.[50]

Canvas tents were an architecture that helped to constitute an infrastructure. As an introduced trade good, canvas tents were fairly neutral compared to, for instance, new foodstuffs or guns that effected more dramatic change over short and long terms. Much like twine, adopted for its durability as fish netting,

[44] Edward Ruben Angusinauq, interview with Lena Ruben and Catherine Cockney, 26 Jan. 2000, in Parks Canada, *Paulatuuq Oral History Project: Inavialuit Elders Share Their Stories* (Inuvik: Parks Canada Western Arctic Field Unit, 2004), 175.

[45] 'At that time he said nobody was worried about a house. Nobody complained about the cold.' Simba in *MVPI Kakisa Lake*, 7932.

[46] Ruben interview in *Paulatuuq Oral History Project*, 244.

[47] Myra Moses in *People of the Lakes*, 66. [48] Thomas in *Rampart House*, 27.

[49] Martha Tizya interpreted by Alice Frost in *People of the Lakes*, 82.

[50] Alfred Charlie and Sarah Abel in *People of the Lakes*, 127–9.

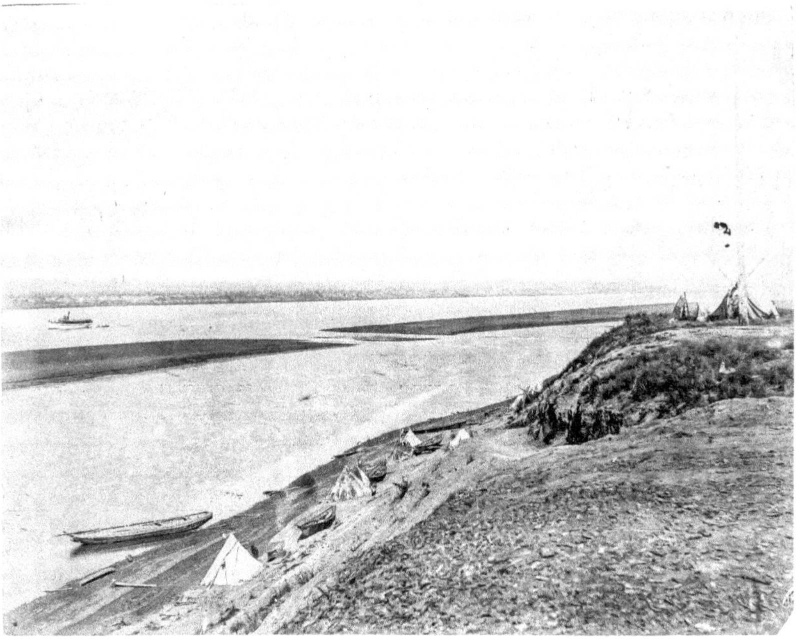

Figure 5.4 Canvas and skin tents at Fort McPherson, July 1892. Photograph by James McDougall. 1987/13/212, Hudson's Bay Company Archives, Archives of Manitoba.

canvas tents were widely taken up because the basic functionality of the object persisted – its Indigeneity endured – but a new material with new advantages was adapted to an Indigenous form. Tents were tents. They could be put up, taken down, and carried along; tents let in light, trapped warmth, and kept out weather. As a technology, canvas tents exemplify the persistence and adaptation of northern Indigenous cultures in the face of colonial pressure and trade opportunities in the nineteenth and early twentieth centuries. But that heaviness – that added weight of canvas and the woodstoves used to keep them warm – draws our attention to the gravitational forces that colonialism exerted in the Mackenzie district and Yukon territory. Colonial power aimed to delineate boundaries, channel movement, and get people to stay in place. The persistence of people travelling all over, being on the move all the time, came only in the face of an assertive, southern-based colonial state that, in the words of Tłįchǫ Elder Margaret Lafferty, 'made us sit still'.[51]

[51] Margaret Lafferty in *We Know and Love Tłįchǫ̀ Ndè*, 8.

Census Records

From the late nineteenth century on, the evolving colonial bureaucracy attempted to tie people who lived on the land down to specific trade posts in a settled, capitalist geography and used census making to these ends.[52] The oldest HBC censuses tallied adult male hunters or counted families that traded at their posts, rather than recording individuals organized into households in the manner of federal census records. On lands both governed by and outside of treaties, the DIA relied on missionaries, traders, and Indian Agents to estimate the number of 'Indians', a category defined using the restrictive criteria set out in the Indian Act.[53]

The first federal census of Canada's northern territories was taken in 1881. Julian Camsell, HBC district chief, gathered information from the posts along the river in June and July 1882. While he provided detailed tallies of post residents, with each family member and individual identified, for the Indigenous population Camsell filled in a form headed 'Indians (Not being in Treaty Lands)' with the total numbers that traded at each post. These numbers implied precision: from the 141 'Tukudh or Mountain Indians' who frequented Rampart House to the 616 'Dog Rib Indians' at Fort Rae. An even 350 'Esquimaux' recorded at Peel River is suggestive of the ways that census records persistently approximated Inuit populations, apparent also in later years when total Inuit population counts would be divided exactly in half between men and women.[54] The next census, in 1891, was the first that attempted to count individual Indigenous people and group them into families along the Mackenzie River. That year, traders at each post served as enumerators and in the spring and summer of 1892 counted HBC employees, religious personnel, domestic servants, and Indigenous families with varying degrees of precision. Fred Camsell, son of Julian and older brother of Charles, conducted the census at Fort Rae. He dutifully recorded names, ages, family relationships, and religion. Birthplaces were recorded simply as 'McK River', and Camsell organized people into nuclear family groups (W[ife], S[on], D[aughter]). Sam Scott, a forty-six-year-old Presbyterian fur trader originally from Quebec, served as enumerator at Fort Providence and was less attentive. He listed the names of adults, whether they were married, and their religion. But then everyone was simply 'Ind[ian] Hunter' and children were left unnamed,

52 Bruce Curtis, *The Politics of Population: State Formation, Statistics, and the Census of Canada, 1840–1875* (Toronto: University of Toronto Press, 2002), 33.

53 Michelle A. Hamilton, '"Anyone Not on the List Might as well Be Dead": Aboriginal Peoples and the Censuses of Canada, 1851–1916', *Journal of the Canadian Historical Association* 18, no. 1 (2007): 57–79 (pp. 62, 79); See also Maggie Walter and Chris Andersen, *Indigenous Statistics: A Quantitative Research Methodology* (Walnut Creek, CA: Left Coast Press, 2013), 28–33.

54 Canada, *Sixth Census of Canada, 1921*, vol. 1 (Ottawa: F.A. Acland, 1924), 380–1.

grouped under their parents: '2 boys', '3 girls'. William Irvine, the forty-seven-year-old clerk at Tulita, explicitly acknowledged on the forms he completed the distance between the logic of the census and the reality of Indigenous life along Dehcho. Irvine filled one page with the information on Tulita residents (trade-post employees, including labourers and fishermen, and missionaries). Over the next thirteen pages, filled with the names of Indigenous people in the area, Irvine noted in the margins of each page, 'All these live in Moveable Wigwams. Ages only Conjecture.'[55]

Federal census makers appeared to forget these earlier enumerations, claiming in 1901 that this was the 'first time' the northern territories were counted.[56] That year, the Dominion designed special schedules for use in the Unorganized Territories, one for the Yukon (with ninety-seven census divisions) and another for the Mackenzie, Athabaska, Ungava, Franklin, and Keewatin districts (with no more than eight divisions apiece). The economic conceptualization of value to the settler state inherent in the census were exemplified in these schedules, which used different categories to record occupation, profession, labour, and earnings compared to the south. These categories were eliminated altogether on the Mackenzie schedules and reconstituted for the Yukon to include real estate, claims, personal property, horses, cows, and dogs. The Yukon schedules also asked for new information about naturalization in Canada, highlighting the cosmopolitan character of the gold rush. The North was implicitly claimed for English Canada with these census forms: they were exclusively in English, while southern forms were bilingual. And this notwithstanding that the pages returned from Fort Providence were completed in French and, as noted by enumerators, the vast majority of people living in the Northwest Territories spoke Indigenous languages.[57]

Racial constructions shifted between different census years. In 1881, Julian Camsell had distinguished between missionary Robert McDonald as 'Scotch', his twenty-one-year-old wife Julia McDonald as 'Indian', and their two children aged three and one also as 'Scotch'. François Boucher, who had been troublesome to James McDougall at Fort Yukon fifteen years earlier, was described as French Canadian, with his wife Eliza Boucher as 'Indian'. Their six children, ages three to twelve, were described as 'Mixed'. Julian Camsell's wife was 'English', as were their seven children. In 1901, enumerators were instructed to strictly designate 'the races of men' with a w (white), r (red), b (black), and y (yellow).[58] White supremacist ideologies that ranked races

[55] See pages 2–14 of 'McKenzie River N.W.T.', *Census of Canada 1891*, LAC.

[56] Canada, *Fourth Census of Canada 1901*, vol. 1 'Population' (Ottawa: S. E. Dawson, 1902), xiii.

[57] Many people were multilingual, Heine et al., *Gwichya Gwich'in Googwandak*, 247, 216; interviews with Albert Lafferty, Beatrice Daniels, and Dora Tourangeau in Metis Heritage Association Fonds, N-1997–012, NWTA; Abel, *Drum Songs*, 182.

[58] Archibald Blue, *Fourth Census of Canada 1901: Instructions to Chief Officers, Commissioners, and Enumerators* (Ottawa: Government Printing Bureau, 1901), 13.

hierarchically and saw miscegenation as a threat informed Canadian politics and the census at that time.[59] Instructions emphasized that 'only pure whites will be classed as whites'. Children born to racially mixed parents 'will be classed as red, black or yellow, as the case may be, irrespective of the degree of colour'.[60] Fred Camsell, who served again as a census enumerator, tripped over this new 1901 classification system. When he entered his own information, Camsell originally described himself as W(hite). He then went back and corrected that to R(ed), a correction he made as well for a handful of others in the community. His own 'Racial or Tribal Origin' he kept as Eng(lish), even though the instructions for enumerators made provision for the description of different 'breeds' ('Persons of mixed white and red blood').[61]

That census records were rife with inaccuracies, inconsistencies, and omissions when it came to the Yukon and Mackenzie district at the turn of the twentieth century is characteristic of the colonial archive when it comes to northern Canada. By the next census, in 1911, the special schedules were abandoned, and the same forms used in the North as elsewhere. By 1921, the state struggled to count people who continued to be highly mobile and to assign them to particular locations. In the persistent use of the census as a tool for racial designation, whites and Indigenous people were enumerated separately and assigned to different subdistricts, albeit using the same schedules. H. A. Conroy enumerated the 'Slavey' and 'Hare Indians' at the trade post, Fort Norman (Tulita), while D. L. McKeand enumerated the whites at the post and at Norman Wells – the emerging industrial site – and on the HBC's *Mackenzie River* steamer. There is instructive irony that 'whites' could be counted on board a floating sternwheeler, while enumerators continued to try and tie Indigenous peoples to trade posts and not the land.

Infrastructure of Extraction

The possibilities for northern treaties had been discussed by those in government, by Indigenous leaders, missionaries, and fur traders in the years prior to 1898. But the most important trigger for Treaty 8 was the Klondike gold rush and for Treaty 11 the Norman Wells oil strike. Neither of these were single or solitary reasons for the government to seek to extinguish Indigenous title to northern lands. In the 1890s, there were the prospects for petroleum and bitumen in northern Alberta and down the Mackenzie, as well as promising mineral showings on the shores of Great Slave Lake. The oil strike at Norman Wells inaugurated a system of public ownership of petroleum in Canada and

[59] See Timothy J. Stanley, *Confronting White Supremacy: School Segregation, Antiracism and the Making of Chinese Canadians* (Vancouver: UBC Press, 2011).

[60] Blue, *Instructions*, 13–14. [61] Blue, *Instructions*, 14.

was part of broader geological explorations that led to major gold and uranium extractive operations.[62] From the government's perspective, even though Treaties 8 and 11 were part of the numbered treaty process, shaped on the moving edge of the agricultural settlement frontier in the west, these northern treaties were not made out of a concern for the welfare of northern Indigenous peoples, nor did they arise from settlement objectives or pressures.[63] The opportunities for non-renewable resource development that lay at the heart of the northern treaties (and this includes not just Treaty 8 and 11, but also 9, 10, and a major adhesion to Treaty 5) created circumstances that produced substantially different agreements from those made in the southern prairies.[64]

The political economy of resource development produced a rushed process. This put treaty commissioner H. A. (Henry Arthur) Conroy in a situation where, to get Treaty 11 signed, 'he purported the treaty to be one thing to the Dene and another to the government', according to Michael Asch.[65] The government of Canada wished to minimize its responsibilities to Indigenous peoples. While northern lands held resource potential, always exaggerated by boosters, potential alone did not suffice to overcome the hesitation in taking on new treaty responsibilities.[66] The gold find on Bonanza Creek in August of 1896 and the moment when Imperial Oil's crews struck oil at Norman Wells in August of 1920 set in motion the processes that culminated in Treaty 8 and Treaty 11. However, this sequence also meant the treaty processes happened alongside, if not actually trailing after, the circumstances that had created their need. As surveyor F. H. Kitto reported, 'the recent discoveries of oil at Norman have been made on lands virtually belonging to those tribes'.[67] But it is a limited vision if we believe that what the government wanted from the treaty process was control over lands which held minerals, oil, or gas. After all, the Klondike creeks where

[62] Philip A. Wight, 'The Militarized "Hydrocarbon Frontier": Petroleum Development and the State in Arctic North America, 1919–1977', in *Cambridge History of the Polar Regions*, ed. P. Roberts and A. Howkins (Cambridge: Cambridge University Press, 2023), 593–620.

[63] Dennis F. K. Madill, 'Treaty Research Report Treaty Eight (1899)', for Treaties and Historical Research Centre Indian and Northern Affairs Canada, 1986, www.rcaanc-cirnac.gc.ca/eng/1100100028809/1564415096517.

[64] Kenneth S. Coates and William R. Morrison, 'Treaty Research Report Treaty No. 11 (1921)', for Treaties and Historical Research Centre, Indian and Northern Affairs Canada, 1986, www.rcaanc-cirnac.gc.ca/eng/1100100028912/1564415459067.

[65] Michael Asch, 'On the Land Cession Provisions in Treaty 11', *Ethnohistory* 60, no. 3 (2013): 451–67 (p. 464).

[66] Charles Mair, *Through the Mackenzie Basin: A Narrative of the Athabasca and Peace River Treaty Expedition of 1899* (Toronto: William Briggs, 1908); *Report of the Select Committee of the Senate Appointed to Enquire into the Resources of the Great Mackenzie Basin* (Ottawa: Brown Chamberlin, 1888); Kenneth Coates, *Canada's Colonies: A History of the Yukon and Northwest Territories* (Toronto: Lorimer, 1985), 127; Coates, *Best Left as Indians*.

[67] As cited in René Fumoleau, *As Long as This Land Shall Last: A History of Treaty 8 and Treaty 11, 1870–1939* (Calgary: University of Calgary Press, 2004), 202.

gold was found, on the traditional territories of the Tr'ondëk Hwëch'in and Nacho Nyäk Dun, were not subject to treaty negotiations at this time.[68]

When the government of Canada sought the mineral wealth of the North, they were not so concerned to secure title to the deposits but rather, in the words of Patrick Wolfe, '*access* to territory'.[69] Non-renewable resources are of limited value in that they eventually run out. Once the oil well has run dry or the gold has been mined, that is it. There is no more. And, by and large, the land that remains is much the worse for wear: contaminated by toxic substances used or exposed in the processes of extraction, shorn of vegetation, and with fish and animal populations taxed if not extirpated by intensive hunting and fishing pressure from transient working populations.[70] The treaty process served not to secure specific deposits but to create an infrastructure of extraction: in the first instance, a safe (peaceful) pathway for people to travel as they sought out resources, and thereafter a transportation and commercial infrastructure to supply extractive operations and carry resources to outside markets. Where the state had already asserted control, as in the Klondike on the heels of tens of thousands of prospectors, there was no apparent need for a treaty. Infrastructural logic is readily apparent in the map of Treaty 8 signed in 1898–1900 with peoples in northern Alberta, British Columbia, Saskatchewan, and the southern Northwest Territories (see Map 5.1). As Dennis Madill noted, the factors that shaped the boundaries of Treaty 8 were 'the areas likely to be traversed by miners or settlers; the areas which could be reached in one summer; the reduction of expenses; and obligations of government'.[71] The boundaries extended to the southern shore of Great Slave Lake because of the interest in that locale from prospectors, headed overland to the Klondike. Treaty 11 covered the balance of the Mackenzie district, including the river and west to the Yukon border, Great Slave and Great Bear lakes and east to include most of the Mackenzie watershed. The Arctic Coast was also included within Treaty 11 territory, although the Inuit who lived there never signed a treaty.

The perspective of the government of Canada on treaty negotiations was transactional: treaties promised Indigenous signatories certain continued rights to the land alongside annuities, promises of relief, and material goods in

[68] Fumoleau, *As Long as This Land Shall Last*, 40–1; Paul Nadasdy, *Hunters and Bureaucrats: Power, Knowledge, and Aboriginal-State Relations in the Southwest Yukon* (Vancouver: UBC Press, 2003), 53; Ken Coates, 'Asking for All Sorts of Favours: The Anglican Church, the Federal Government, and the Natives of the Yukon Territory, 1891–1909', in *The Anglican Church and the World of Western Canada, 1820–1970*, ed. Barry Ferguson (Regina: Canadian Plains Research Centre, 1987), 126–42 (p. 130).

[69] Patrick Wolfe, 'Settler Colonialism and the Elimination of the Native', *Journal of Genocide Research* 8, no. 4 (2006): 387–409 (p. 388). Emphasis added.

[70] For an example from northern Alberta, see Hereward Longley, 'Bitumen Extraction, Indigenous Land Conflicts, and Environmental Change in the Athabasca Oil Sands Region, 1963–1993' (PhD diss., University of Alberta, 2021).

[71] Madill, 'Treaty Research Report Treaty Eight (1899)'.

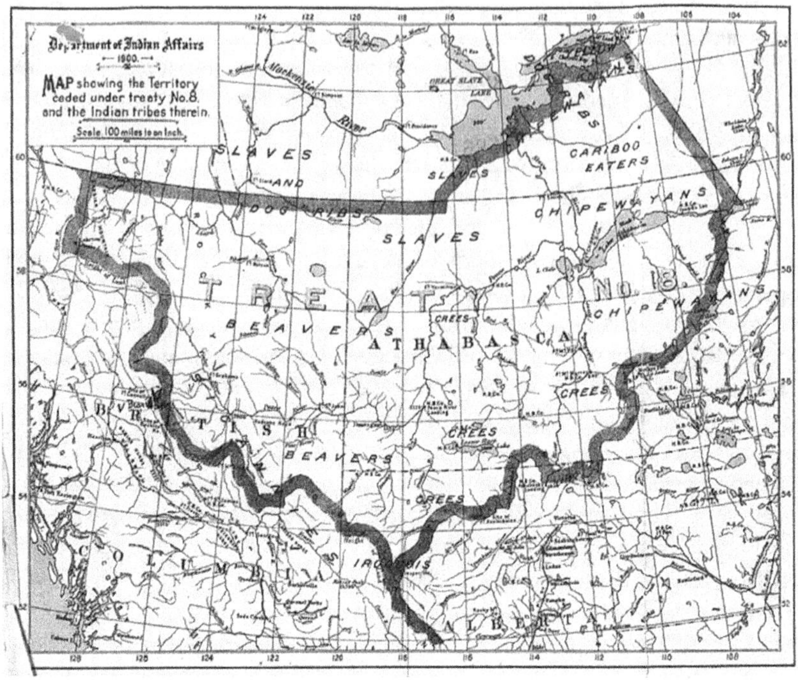

Map 5.1 Treaty 8 lands, 1900. Department of Indian Affairs, Library and Archives Canada.

exchange for title. Indigenous perspectives at the time and since emphasized that the treaties involved agreeing to a relationship in peace and friendship between the original inhabitants of the land and those who wished to join them. As Glen Coulthard has shown for the Dene and as Elaine Alexie has shown for the Gwich'in, this relationship was inseparable from the land.[72] Coulthard writes about Indigenous struggles as 'deeply *informed* by what the land as a mode of reciprocal *relationship* (which is itself informed by place-based practices and associated forms of knowledge) ought to teach us about living our lives in relation to one another and our surroundings in a respectful, nondominating and nonexploitative way'.[73] Coulthard refers to this ethical framework as

[72] Elaine Alexie, '"Nakhwanh Gwich'in Khehłok Iidilii – We Are Our Own People": Teetł'it Gwich'in Practices of Indigeneity: Connection to Land, Traditional Self-Governance, and Elements of Self Determination' (MA thesis, University of Victoria, 2011). See also Shelagh Marie Beairsto, 'Dinjii Kat Chih Ahaa: Gwich'in Notions of Leadership' (MEd thesis, University of Manitoba, 1999).

[73] Glen Sean Coulthard, *Red Skin White Masks: Rejecting the Colonial Politics of Recognition* (Minneapolis: University of Minnesota Press, 2014), 60. Emphasis in original.

'grounded normativity'. Using this framework, we can better understand how Dene signatories to Treaty 11 were articulating connections to the land in all aspects of the treaty relationship, not just those specific elements about hunting, trapping, and fishing. Moreover, this connection to the land was not a reaction to settler colonialism's singular, defining obsession with the same. Rather, the connections were rooted in Dene ethics, communicated in oral histories recorded with Elders where they articulate moral foundations that emphasize care for others in times of need and sharing what one had.

These values appeared in the discussions when treaties were signed and in the Indigenous histories of what was promised. Signatories to Treaty 8 asked for help in times of need and care for those who were too old to hunt and trap; they also expected to receive medicines and access to doctors. Treaty 8, unlike Treaty 6 with its medicine-chest clause, made no specific provisions regarding health and medical care. Nevertheless, the 1899 report of the Treaty 8 commissioners described promises made that medicines 'would be put in the charge of persons selected by the Government at different points, and would be distributed free to those of the Indians who might require them'. The commissioners 'explained that it would be practically impossible for the Government to arrange for regular medical attendance upon Indians so widely scattered over such an extensive territory. We assured them, however, that the Government would always be ready to avail itself of any opportunity of affording medical service.'[74] Medical doctors who travelled with the treaty party reinforced these promises. In 1900, Dr O. C. Edwards dispensed medicines and vaccinated people while travelling with the Indian Commissioner J. A. Macrae as he sought signatures to Treaty 8 south of Great Slave Lake.[75] In effect, the government understood it had promised that *when feasible* they would make medical care available – and that medical care would be free. According to Richard Daniel, 'the Indian people apparently understood this as a general commitment to provide health care. Today the Elders say that Indians should have doctors, medicine, hospital care, and medical aid free of charge as a treaty right.'[76]

Health and medicine figured similarly in the discussions and expectations around Treaty 11. Pascal Baptiste was present in Tsiigehtchic when H. A. Conroy came to arrange the signing of Treaty 11. 'I was among these people listening to what was said in this meeting', said Baptiste. He remembered Conroy saying, 'In a few years, there will be a hospital for you. If you get

[74] Report of Commissioners for Treaty No. 8, Sept. 22, 1899, available online 'Treaty Texts: Treaty No. 8', www.rcaanc-cirnac.gc.ca/eng/1100100028813/1581293624572.

[75] Fumoleau, *As Long as This Land Shall Last,* 138.

[76] Richard Daniel, 'The Spirit and Terms of Treaty Eight', in *The Spirit of the Alberta Indian Treaties*, ed. Richard Price, 3rd ed. (Edmonton: University of Alberta Press, 1999): 47–100 (p. 98).

into an accident or get sick in any way, you will be treated with care and if you stay in hospital you will not have to pay for all this.'[77] Baptiste shared this at the Berger Inquiry, emphasizing in his testimony that at that time (the 1970s) they had to pay for medicines and hospital bills when they sought treatment in Inuvik.[78] Peter Thompson, born in 1893, testified before the Berger Inquiry that 'Mr. Conroy told him straight from now on you people will be well looked after. You will get free hospital and he said that the Government will look after you good.'[79] Similarly at Behchokǫ̀, Tłı̨chǫ Elders had recorded their memories of the treaty discussions including the promise of free medicines and that 'the sick . . . will also be cared for'.[80]

Tłı̨chǫ, Dene, and Gwich'in treaty signatories placed great weight on promises of reciprocity and care. In his book *Trail of the Spirit*, Blondin imparted the laws that Yamoria brought to the Dene. The first was 'Share with your people. … Help the poor; help the Elders that are too old to work.' The second was 'Help each other as much as possible. Help the sick people who are in need.'[81] Elaine Alexie described how respect and sharing were 'key principles of Gwich'in leadership and self-government'.[82] Among Dënesųłıné Elders in Fort Resolution interviewed in the 1980s, Albert Fabien described how people cared for their parents into their old age when it was no longer easy to travel with them in the bush.[83] An ethic of care and sharing extended across lines of kin, culture, and language. Elders used stories to emphasize why it is so important to 'be kind to everybody and you can always get help' in the words of Pascal Baptiste.[84] In the 1990s, Tłı̨chǫ Elders 'emphasized that creating peaceful relationships brings co-operation', using the example of peaceful relations between Tłı̨chǫ and Inuit to illustrate the historical importance of good relations.[85] In testimony to the Berger Inquiry in the 1970s, witnesses emphasized that the moral community created in the wake of treaty promises extended to southern settlers and sojourners, creating new bonds of reciprocal obligation. In Aklavik, Archie (Headpoint) Erigaktuk, born near Carter River, Alaska, spoke of his sick wife. 'Today I am still praying that my wife will get better', Erigaktuk said, 'because when we were young we helped everyone that needed help, although we didn't have very much in those days. We always had a cup of

[77] Pascal Baptiste in *Gwichya Gwich'in Googwandak*, 376–7.
[78] Baptiste in *MVPI Arctic Red River*, 4644–5.
[79] *MVPI Fort McPherson, NWT* (10 July 1975), vol. 13 (testimony of Peter Thompson), 1168.
[80] *MVPI Rae/Edzo, NWT* (11 August 1976), vol. 72 (testimony of Jim Erasmus), 8120 and (testimony of Alphonse Eronchi), quotation page 8126. Eronchi presented a written brief to the Inquiry that drew on the recorded memories of Chief Jimmy Bruneau, Henri Lafferty, and Ned Heron.
[81] Blondin, *Trail of the Spirit*, 26. [82] Alexie, 'Nakhwanh Gwich'in Khehłok Iidilii', 100.
[83] Isidore Edjericon, Albert Fabien, and Pierre Hilaire in *That's the Way We Lived*, 14.
[84] Pascal Baptiste in *Gwichya Gwich'in Googwandak*, 376.
[85] Arrowmaker et al., *We Know and Love Tłı̨chǫ̀ Ndè*, 4–13 for treaty meanings.

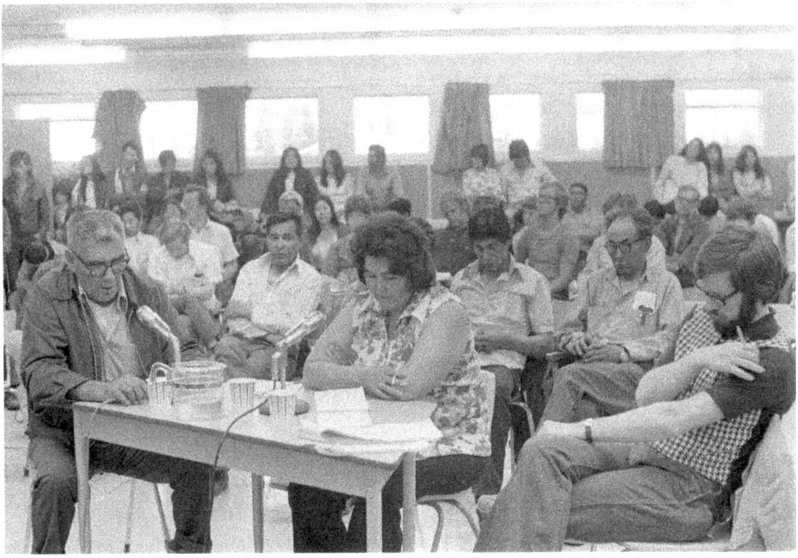

Figure 5.5 Bertha Allen (centre) at Mackenzie Valley Pipeline Inquiry community hearing at Old Crow, July 1975. © NWT Archives/NCS – Native Press photo/N-2018–010–02893.

tea for the white people when they came through our camp, and my wife was always ready to help anyone that came through our camp.' They gave food and drink freely 'because of our custom'.[86] Bertha Allen called Berger's attention to her grandfather and long-time chief of Old Crow, Peter Moses, who on two occasions collected money to send overseas, including to children left orphaned and homeless in England after the Blitz (Figure 5.5).[87] Allen showed the Inquiry how her people practised generosity and care as part of their treaty relationship.

The relationship as expressed here by the signatories to Treaties 8 and 11 and their descendants was one that extended a reciprocal responsibility of care, learned from relations with the land and animals, to the settlers and sojourners who now wished to cross and access their lands. But for the government it was *feasibility* (cost, resources, available personnel) that governed what aspects of healthcare would be made available in the territories. Feasibility is an elusive

[86] *MVPI Aklavik, NWT* (2 April 1975), vol. 1 (testimony of Archie Headpoint), 9. Abraham Okpik translated for Archie Headpoint at the inquiry.

[87] *MVPI, Old Crow, YT* (12 July 1975), vol. 15 (testimony of Bertha Allen), 1436; See also Minister of Mines and Resources to Chief Peter Moses, 1 Nov. 1941, *The Canadian Letters and Images Project*, www.canadianletters.ca/content/document-5453.

criterion. What is feasible is what is possible within the constraints that invariably limit the scope of action. There were constraints created by climate and distance from centres of biomedicine. There are also the very real limitations in treating sickness, 'the elusiveness of medical efficacy', in the words of David S. Jones. Even with a doctor's care, people still die. But, as Jones also emphasizes, when evaluating decisions made by bureaucrats or physicians with regards to Indigenous healthcare, the failure to provide care is measured by when 'they failed to provide the same care they would have sought for themselves'.[88] That is a yardstick to assess the infrastructure of care created in the wake of Canada's assertion of control over northern lands. Before turning to examine that infrastructure of care, we go first to the Klondike, where the surge of new arrivals made for filthy conditions on the ground, creating demand for hospitals, doctors, and nurses and prompting the creation of a sanitary infrastructure.

Sanitary Infrastructure

Among the pathogens carried into the Klondike was *Salmonella typhi* (*S. typhi*), the bacteria responsible for typhoid. In the dense settlements of the gold fields, the bacteria found ideal conditions. Medical Health Officer (MHO) John Hardie MacArthur observed that 'the only portions [of the Yukon territory] that could be called urban are White Horse, Dawson and Grand Forks, Bonanza'.[89] Grand Forks, formally known as Bonanza, was at the heart of the gold rush on the creeks outside Dawson but was abandoned in the early twentieth century. Sanitary issues could arise in smaller communities, but the only 'city' in the Mackenzie and Yukon at this time was Dawson. And it was there that typhoid – the classic filth disease of Victorian cities – took hold. Between 1896 and 1904, there were over 100 deaths from typhoid in Dawson, accounting for over 13 per cent of all mortality in the Yukon – second only to accidents (mine accidents, drowning, violence) as a cause of death in that period.[90]

The summers of 1897 and 1898 saw the worst typhoid epidemics in Dawson, described by W. E. Thompson (the first City Officer of Health) as 'one of the dirtiest places on Earth'.[91] An order of Grey Nuns, the Sisters of Ste Anne, arrived in the middle of the summer in 1898. Trained but not certified as nurses, these women staffed St Mary's Hospital, a Catholic institution opened the previous year by an American Jesuit priest, William Judge. St Mary's was

[88] Jones, *Rationalizing Epidemics*, 9–10. [89] MacArthur, 'Sanitary Report', 2.

[90] Highet, 'Gold Fever', 124; Megan J. Highet, 'Catching Gold Fever: A Social History of Typhoid Fever among the Klondike Gold Rushers, 1896–1904', *Alaska Journal of Anthropology* 15, nos. 1 & 2 (2017): 141–57 (p. 144). Maureen Lux, 'Disease and the Growth of Dawson City: The Seamy Underside of a Legend', *Northern Review* 3/4 (1989): 96–117.

[91] W. E. Thompson to Commissioner, 24 Jun. 1902, Gov 1624, Series 1, vol. 14, file, 2921, YA.

overwhelmed by the typhoid epidemic and employed just about anyone claiming medical training.[92] In 1898, Presbyterians rallied to raise funds to construct a second hospital for the community – what came to be the Good Samaritan Hospital, staffed by the Victorian Order of Nurses – where typhoid patients also received treatment and care, and which was also overwhelmed during the epidemics.[93] These were the two most significant institutions, although there were also a number of private hospitals including one at Grand Forks. St Mary's and the Good Samaritan Hospital both treated anyone regardless of religion or ability to pay. The institutions were funded by fees, donations, and modest support from the territorial council.

Dawson City was built on a swampy river flat.[94] In his inaugural sanitary report, MHO MacArthur noted that pollution in the Yukon River, 'need hardly be considered until we reach Indian (28 miles) and Klondyke (just) rivers above Dawson. These two tributaries drain the whole of the thickly populated Klondyke District and make these waters unsafe for domestic purposes.' And that was before the waters even reached the townsite.[95] Initially, human waste was dumped directly into the Yukon River to be washed downstream. The river was also the community's main water supply. In winter, when the river froze, the waste was dumped on the surface of the ice, which formed an imperfect barrier. The greatest risk from typhoid came in spring, when the thaw rotted the ice in the Yukon River, produced swampy conditions on land, and contaminated most local freshwater sources with human waste. Megan Highet looked at the role of saloons in the spread of typhoid, where 'what amounted to whisky-flavoured water', drawn from the Yukon River, was served to the clientele.[96] Men who passed their evenings drinking in Dawson's saloons were repeatedly exposed to *S. typhi*, and the more they consumed, the more severe their infection.[97]

Rasmus and Karl Karlson, brothers from Norway in their twenties, tragically exemplified this risk. After striking it rich on Bonanza Creek in 1896, they celebrated in Dawson, contracted typhoid fever, and died one within ten days of the other in July 1897.[98] They were buried in the city's first public cemetery, known variously as the Third Avenue Cemetery, Prospect Hill, and – after the epidemics of 1897 and 1898 – the typhoid cemetery (Figure 5.6). Given the significant mortality in this period, combined with the rapid growth of the city

[92] Porsild, *Gamblers and Dreamers*, 146, 151.

[93] Highet, 'Gold Fever', 126; Porsild, *Gamblers and Dreamers*, 150.

[94] Porsild, *Gamblers and Dreamers*, 146; Zaslow, *Opening*, 125; for similar problems at Nome, Alaska, see Kathryn Taylor Morse, *The Nature of Gold: An Environmental History of the Klondike Gold Rush* (Seattle: University of Washington Press, 2003), 164.

[95] MacArthur, 'Sanitary Report', 2. [96] As cited in Highet, 'Catching Gold Fever', 153.

[97] Highet, 'Catching Gold Fever', 154. [98] Porsild, *Gamblers and Dreamers*, 77.

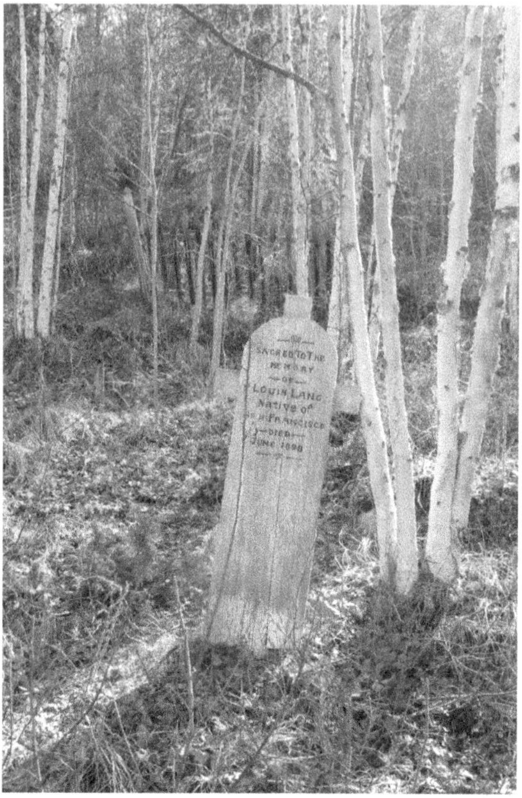

Figure 5.6 Grave marker in Dawson's typhoid cemetery. Photograph by L. Piper, 2013.

itself, the available ground at the cemetery soon filled up, with the last burial at that site in October 1898.[99]

The sanitary infrastructure that followed typhoid to Dawson was physical and bureaucratic. By 1900, the surface waters that had accumulated at the townsite were dispersed through open drains that emptied into the Yukon River. In short order, the townsite was rendered 'comparatively dry to what it was in 1898'.[100] A local drinking-water market emerged, with peddlers offering 'water, rendered pure and germless' for sale.[101] By 1900, the Dawson Water and Power Company had laid a network of pipes, drawing water 'of excellent quality for domestic purposes' from a well at the south end of town, which

[99] Ed and Star Jones, 'Third Avenue Cemetery (May 16, 1897–October 25, 1898)', research report, 2002–5.

[100] MacArthur, 'Sanitary Report', 11. [101] As cited in Highet, 'Catching Gold Fever', 146.

operated even at a temperature of -55 degrees Celsius, according to MacArthur.[102] (This was exceptionally cold even by Dawson standards.) Dawson Water and Power expanded their system, providing service to hillside settlements and, upon application, to home- and business-owners.[103] The provision of a clean water supply after 1900 unequivocally improved the typhoid situation, and the demands on the sanitary system also eased as the rush ebbed.

The other essential part of this work was administration and enforcement: the creation of a sanitary bureaucracy. In his first sanitary report, MacArthur compared the mortality data from London, England to the Yukon Territory, noting that the Yukon fared more poorly for respiratory diseases, accidents, and violent deaths, but better in all other categories, even 'zymotic diseases' or contagious diseases including typhoid and smallpox. Urbanized Western Europe informed the interpretation of healthy and unhealthy places – the creation of public health expertise – in the Yukon Territory at the turn of the century.

The Yukon's first public health ordinance was assented to in March 1899. It created the Dawson Health District, the position of Medical Health Officer, and the Board of Health. This Board could make regulations 'as may to them seem necessary to preserve the public health and comfort of the people of the Dawson Health District'.[104] The 1899 ordinance was substantially revised in 1902. The later Yukon Health Ordinance applied to the entire territory, included provisions for vaccination and quarantine and the inspection and regulation of steamships.[105] The MHO secured significant power under the 1899 ordinance that went unchanged in the 1902 revision. The ordinance required specified infectious diseases to be reported. The MHO inspected food and slaughter-houses, could enter and examine 'any premises' during the day, and could require the removal to hospital or isolation of people suspected to have an infectious disease, as well as the destruction of property. Expenses were borne by those who were sick. The MHO could appoint others as sanitary inspectors, and the police were at his command, when needed. The public health ordinance of 1899 was not unusual in the scope of powers given to the MHO, the use of police to ensure their enforcement, nor in the intrusions permitted to private property and private life.[106] This was perhaps especially so in the Yukon, where

[102] MacArthur, 'Sanitary Report', 11.

[103] Highet, 'Gold Fever', 149–52; the hydrant system installed in 1906 finally provided effective protection against fire in winter, Zaslow, *Opening,* 126.

[104] Yukon Local Ordinance No. 5 of 1899, Respecting the Public Health, Assented to March 3rd, 1899 [hereafter Public Health Ordinance 1899].

[105] Yukon Health Ordinance No. 20 of 1902, s. 1. There was a separate vaccination ordinance before 1902.

[106] J. N. Hays, *The Burdens of Disease: Epidemics and Human Response in Western History*, rev. ed. (New Brunswick, NJ: Rutgers University Press, 2009), 249–53.

the North West Mounted Police played a disproportionate role in erecting settler society.[107]

The swiftness of urbanization in Dawson City saw an unimaginably abrupt transformation in the lives of the Tr'ondëk Hwëch'in. Settlement displaced their ancient fish camp at Tr'ochëk, a gathering place at the confluence of the Klondike and Yukon rivers that had served as a base for hunting moose and processing hides. Tr'ochëk became the site of Lousetown (formally named Klondike City), an industrial area with a brewery, train yards, and a sawmill, as well as a thriving red-light district.[108] As the Tr'ondëk Hwëch'in emphasize, under the leadership of Chief Isaac they soon chose to leave Dawson altogether – aiming to keep a distance from the emergent settler society – and secured reserve lands three kilometres downstream at Moosehide, a traditional gathering place a little less than halfway to Fort Reliance. Tr'ondëk Hwëch'in, Teetł'it Gwich'in from Fort McPherson, Tutchone from Selkirk, Tlingit, and other Indigenous peoples continued to visit and travel through Dawson. Some lived in town and would have had to contend with the typhoid epidemics alongside the rest of the community.[109] Moosehide became the centre for community life with cabins, a school, and a church, while Tr'ondëk Hwëch'in continued to live on and harvest the lands across their traditional territories.[110]

Outsiders assumed that the sanitation in Moosehide was poor. These assumptions were rooted in the sanitary hazards created by downstream proximity to Dawson and in the racism baked into sanitary discourse.[111] Waste dumped into the Yukon River travelled past Moosehide, exposing the Tr'ondëk Hwëch'in to typhoid and other infectious pathogens. As Heather Green described, Bishop Stringer visited Moosehide in 1913 to lecture on sanitation and tuberculosis prevention, only to find Moosehide cleaner than Dawson.[112] His surprise was deemed worthy of reporting in the *Dawson Daily News*, speaking to assumptions made by the settler society about the cleanliness of Indigenous communities. The Tr'ondëk Hwëch'in had a clean source of water at Moosehide. Gerald Isaac, grandson of Chief Isaac, remembered packing water for drinking in pails, buckets, and five-pound lard cans from Moosehide

[107] Ken S. Coates and William R. Morrison, *Land of the Midnight Sun: A History of the Yukon*, 2nd ed. (Montreal: McGill-Queen's University Press, 2005), 99.

[108] Helene Dobrowolsky and T. J. Hammer, *Tr'ochëk: The Archaeology and History of a Han Fish Camp* ([Dawson City, Yukon]: Tr'ondëk Hwëch'in, 2001).

[109] Porsild, *Gamblers and Dreamers*, 54 notes that in the 1901 census only two Métis families lived in Lousetown.

[110] See Heather Green, 'The Tr'ondëk Hwëch'in and the Great Upheaval: Mining, Colonialism, and Environmental Change in the Klondike, 1890–1940' (PhD diss., University of Alberta, 2018).

[111] Kelm, *Colonizing Bodies*, 49; Anderson, *Colonial Pathologies*, ch. 4.

[112] Green, 'Mining, Colonialism', 160–1.

Creek. The creek flowed into the Yukon River, at no risk from the city's waste and far from the goldfields.[113] In winter, people in Moosehide melted snow and took water from the Yukon River through holes cut in the ice.[114] No deaths from typhoid or 'enteric fever' were reported from Moosehide between 1917 and 1958. Proximity to the boomtown brought health hazards – including measles, pneumonia, tuberculosis, and other pathogens. But when it came to cleanliness and sanitation, Moosehide was far better off than Dawson.

Infrastructure of Care

Constructing sanitary infrastructures could not wait, particularly at the site of the instant city of Dawson with its thousands of bodies that needed clean water and produced waste. Other health infrastructures, however, were slower to be built and more piecemeal in their distribution. In the first three decades of the twentieth century, the government, Christian missions, and private companies offered some institutionalized biomedicine – doctors, hospitals, and treatments rooted in the Western therapeutic tradition – as healthcare in the North. The limits of this care are readily apparent. There were those among the doctors, nurses, and missionaries who provided medical treatments but who failed to uphold an ethic of care. Others, who came with good intentions and delivered care to northerners in their times of need, were undermined by the inadequacies of the larger infrastructure essential to support individual efforts.

Medical doctors were among the thousands who trekked northwards to participate in the gold rush and whaling at the turn of the twentieth century. Some used their medical expertise to make money while en route, finding work on whaling ships or in treating local people for injuries, infectious diseases, and chronic illness.[115] Dr George McDonald established a practice at Dawson at the turn of the century, on the third floor of the Hotel McDonald. He appeared first in the mission journal in Fort McPherson in November 1897. There, Dr McDonald was among 'many white men coming down Mackenzie on the way to the Youcon, where rich finds have been made'.[116] That fall, Dr McDonald treated people in McPherson and accompanied the missionary Isaac Stringer to Herschel Island. In March 1898, a Gwich'in woman married

113 The gold fields produced biological and arsenic contamination of waterways. See P. T. Rowe, 'The Yukon Country', *The Chautauquan* (Jan. 1899); L. Piper, 'Chronic Disease in the Yukon River Basin', in *Locating Health: Historical and Anthropological Investigations of Place and Health*, ed. E. Dyck and C. Fletcher (London: Pickering and Chatto, 2011), 131–5; and Yukon Local Ordinance No. 18 of 1899.

114 Yukon College, *Moosehide (Èdhä Dädhëchan Kek'èt): An Oral History* (Dawson City, YT: Yukon College, 1994), interviews with Gerald Isaac p. 39 and Victor Henry p. 92.

115 Walter J. Vanast, '"Arctic Bodies; Frontier Souls": Missionaries and Medical Care in the Canadian North 1896–1926' (PhD diss. University of Wisconsin–Madison, 1996), 134–40.

116 St Matthew's Mission Journal, 5 Oct. 1897.

in the Anglican church reported that she was 'with child, having been seduced by Dr. Geo McDonald, while he was attending her sick child. He denies it, but it is too true.'[117] Seduction was the language of Charles Whittaker, the missionary in charge. The woman's own words have not endured. In the late nineteenth century, 'seduction' was used to describe sexual assault, particularly the assault of poor women, as well as illicit intercourse that resulted in pregnancy.[118] The woman gave birth later that year, and the child died in infancy. The intimacy involved in medical care was one way in which the gendered and racialized violence of colonialism reached Indigenous women.[119] There were other doctors who had intimate relationships with northern Indigenous women.[120] The example of McDonald serves not to characterize all medical practitioners who came north in this period as sexual predators or licentious men but aims rather to counter the sometimes hagiographic depictions of southerners who worked as medical practitioners in the North and to acknowledge instead the power and freedoms that they enjoyed within a colonial context and how this could let them harm, not help, northern people.

By 1909, there was no shortage of trained medical personnel in Dawson, so much so that one doctor from Kansas was discouraged from coming unless he was interested in serving as the city's mayor.[121] Dawson was the only community with too many doctors in the early decades of the twentieth century. By contrast, the Catholic hospital in Fort Simpson had no doctor for its first ten years, from 1916 to 1926. The main obstacle was money. The costs of medical care were shared by the Catholic and Anglican missions and the federal government through the Department of the Interior (which housed the NWT and Yukon Branch) and the Department of Indian Affairs (DIA). The missions provided staff and labour and used their charitable networks to solicit medicines and equipment from organizations such as the Canadian Red Cross.[122] The federal government hired doctors on salary and provided funds to build hospitals, although which departmental budget bore the cost varied with time and circumstance. In general, the DIA paid for medical care for Indigenous peoples who had signed treaty, as well as Inuit, although they occupied a distinct legal category within the racialized administration of colonial

117 St Matthew's Mission Journal, 5 Mar. 1898.

118 Constance Backhouse, *Petticoats and Prejudice: Women and Law in Nineteenth-Century Canada* (Toronto: Women's Press, 1991), 43, 58.

119 For fuller discussion of the gendered and racialized violence of colonialism, see Sarah Carter, *Capturing Women: The Manipulation of Cultural Imagery In Canada's Prairie West* (Montreal: McGill-Queen's University Press, 1997).

120 Vanast, 'Arctic Bodies', 143, 150.

121 Territorial Secretary to F. C. Waldecker, 28 Apr. 1909, GOV 1646, file 25103, YRG 1, Series 1, Central Registry Files, YA.

122 Letter to Colonel Marshall, Canadian Red Cross, 26 Apr. 1920, COR 251 f. 20, Series 1-1a, Anglican Church of Canada, Diocese of Yukon, YA.

government and had not signed treaty. Other branches of government covered the costs for indigent people (including Métis and settlers and sojourners) in the North, while Métis and non-Indigenous northerners with means were responsible for paying their own medical bills.[123] The question, 'who pays?' is the subject of at least a third of the surviving archival correspondence pertaining to northern health and could occupy an entire chapter if not a volume in its own right.[124]

In Dawson, a doctor could find fee-paying patients among the urban population at that place. Elsewhere, doctors sought salaried positions with the police or paid for by the territorial administration or the DIA. Money was always an issue. In the summer of 1920, Dr W. H. Carr was hired from the outside by the territorial administration to work in Whitehorse. Carr was to be paid a monthly salary of $400 supported by the DIA ($100), the territory ($250, of which $50 was for his role as Medical Health Officer), and the RCMP ($50).[125] He also had the opportunity to build a private practice. Carr came, spent a week, and then turned around and left. Writing to his erstwhile employer, Gold Commissioner George Mackenzie, Carr stated that not only was the local (white) population much smaller than he had been led to believe, but also the cost of living was much higher. Inadequate housing and a 'somnolent' attitude in town as to whether he stayed or left further encouraged his quick departure.[126] Doctors who came without advance arrangements could find themselves out of luck. James Rymer arrived from England in Fort Resolution late in 1907 and asked the RNWMP and DIA for a salary and compensation for medicines. Both declined. Rymer stayed on nonetheless, working with the Oblates to provide medical care to the local community until his sudden death in 1911.[127]

With treaty came annual visits by a medical doctor attached to the treaty party.[128] While the annual visits were welcomed, leaders such as Chief Pierre

[123] There were also daily subsidies paid; the flat rate of $1.50 per diem paid by the Department of the Interior for treatment and maintenance of 'indigent whites and halfbreeds' was also applied to Sami (Laplanders) brought to the NWT as reindeer herders. See Memo, 21 Feb. 1934, RG 85, vol. 191, file 554/119-1, part 2, LAC.

[124] The tragic consequences of jurisdictional disputes over responsibility to pay were exemplified in the case of Jordan River Anderson, a Cree child from northern Manitoba, whose experiences prompted the creation of Jordan's Principle. See McCallum and Perry, *Structures of Indifference*, 100–2. See also Walter Vanast, '"Hastening the Day of Extinction": Canada, Québec, and the Medical Care of Ungava's Inuit, 1867–1967', *Études/Inuit/Studies* 15, no. 2 (1991): 55–84.

[125] George Mackenzie to R. E. Tucker, 29 Nov. 1920, Gov 1843 251, YRG 1, Series 2, Central Registry Files, YA.

[126] W. H. Carr to George Mackenzie, 3 Aug. 1920, Gov 1843 251.

[127] See Isidore Edjericon, Albert Fabien, Victor Lafferty, George Sanderson in *That's the Way We Lived*, 71–3; Vanast, 'Arctic Bodies', 106–10; Clermont Bourget, *Douze ans chez les sauvages au Grand-Lac Des Esclaves, comme médecin et agent des Indiens (1923–1935)* (Ste-Anne-de-Beaupré: En vente chez l'auteur, 1938), 35.

[128] Fumoleau, *As Long as This Land Shall Last,* 138.

Squirrel did not consider them sufficient. In the wake of the measles epidemic, Squirrel reportedly said, 'When I made this treaty with your government, I stipulated that we should have here a policemen and a doctor; instead of that you have sent nothing but missionaries.'[129] It took over a decade from when Treaty 8 was signed before Dr Archibald Lawrence MacDonald was hired in 1911 to work in the Mackenzie district. MacDonald was in his fifties when he first came to Fort Smith and stayed on until 1930.[130] He served the local population, including the men who laboured on the Smith portage, worked at the hospital opened in Fort Smith in 1914, and took over travelling with the treaty party. The residential school at Fort Providence lay outside the boundaries of Treaty 8 but was part of MacDonald's responsibilities. He went to the school most years to inspect the health of the children, handing out candies to encourage vaccination. MacDonald travelled only reluctantly by dogsled and so hardly budged from Fort Smith through the long winter months; the police attributed MacDonald's inertia to his age and called for a younger man to be appointed as district physician.

The greater problem though, and one acknowledged by observers at the time, was that a single physician stationed at Fort Smith could hardly provide medical care to communities and people dispersed over hundreds of kilometres of land.[131] People travelled far for medical care, both traditional medicine and the new institutional care. Paul Blondin travelled 300 kilometres to a medicine man who lived near Tłegǫ́htį (Norman Wells) when his son Edward fell ill.[132] In 1921, the hospital at Fort Simpson reported a mother who had travelled 100 kilometres with her three children.[133] But people who were ailing could not be expected to travel long distances to seek help from a physician, especially if they were in need of emergency care. With the signing of Treaty 11, further pressure was applied to the government. It was not just the churches who called on the government to fund doctors and hospitals. In 1922, RCMP Inspector G. L. Jennings emphasized Canada's 'duty' to provide more relief and medical care to people along the Mackenzie River.[134]

To make this more feasible, the government took to employing men in multiple roles: as Indian Agent, Medical Health Officer, coroner, school inspector, and Justice of the Peace all rolled into one. Such was the case with Clermont Bourget, appointed by the DIA to Fort Resolution in 1923. Bourget was French-Canadian and came recommended by the Oblate father Camille

129 As cited in Keith Crowe, *A History of the Original Peoples of Northern Canada*, rev. ed. (Montreal: McGill-Queen's University Press, 1991), 157.
130 McCormack, *Fort Chipewyan*, 262–3.
131 See Conroy as cited in Fumoleau, *As Long as This Land Shall Last,* 139; Vanast, 'Arctic Bodies', 116.
132 Blondin, *When the World Was New*, 140–1.
133 Vanast, 'Arctic Bodies', 125, 293; Okpik, *Survival*, 51.
134 Cited in Vanast, 'Arctic Bodies', 122.

Lefebvre to the government as a good candidate for the post.[135] Bourget travelled with the treaty party down the Mackenzie River, dispensing both medicine and treaty payments in his role as Indian Agent. Like MacDonald, Bourget hardly travelled after freeze-up, making only one winter visit to Providence in 1924 in his twelve years at Resolution. With his wife and daughter, Bourget was comfortably ensconced in the Catholic and francophone settler community on the south shore of Great Slave Lake. As Walter Vanast detailed, Fort Resolution and Fort Smith, at the southern edge of the Northwest Territories and only a day's travel apart, now each had a doctor while Fort Simpson had a hospital but no doctor, and 'huge stretches of terrain' were left unserved, particularly in winter (which lasted for eight months of the year).[136] In 1924, adverse southern publicity about northern healthcare prompted the Minister of the Interior, Charles Stewart, to call a meeting with Minister of Indian Affairs D. C. (Duncan Campbell) Scott, the Director of the Northwest Territories and Yukon Branch O. S. (Oswald Sterling) Finnie, and the Police Commissioner Cortlandt Starnes. They agreed on the need to hire another doctor to serve the Mackenzie district, but Scott stalled – refusing to pay the larger salary for a combined Indian Agent and medical doctor at Fort Simpson or to hire a separate physician outright. In 1926, the wife of the HBC post manager at Fort Chipewyan, Louise Rourke, wrote describing the situation:

> The bi-yearly visit of the doctor is, of course, a farce. Over and over again there are deaths amongst the people which might have been prevented had there been a doctor within reasonable distance: over and over again the cry goes out: 'Send us medical men'. But nothing happens.[137]

That same year a physician named W. A. M. (Arthur) Truesdell replaced T. W. (Flynn) Harris as Indian Agent at Fort Simpson. The shortage of trained doctors remained a feature of medical care in the North through the 1920s and 1930s.

Government-employed doctors inspected the residential schools. The ill health produced by inadequate nourishment and crowded, poorly ventilated indoor environments meant that schools became sites of outbreaks that then spread farther afield, like whooping cough in the 1880s. The regional spread of dysentery in 1900 was shaped by the movement of children to and from school. The same happened again with diphtheria in the 1910s and tuberculosis throughout this period (see Chapter 9). Nevertheless, with the exception of Aklavik, no other community in the Mackenzie district had both a school and a hospital in the 'mission era'. There were those communities with residential schools (Hay River, Fort Providence, Fort Resolution, Fort Chipewyan) and

[135] Bourget, *Douze ans*, 10. [136] Vanast, 'Arctic Bodies', 129.
[137] Cited in Fumoleau, *As Long as This Land Shall Last,* 306.

those with hospitals (Fort Smith, Fort Simpson). The DIA refused to permit schools to incorporate hospitals into their operations because of the potential to spread disease.[138] In practice, schools served as hospices and had sick rooms for children. In 1925, the school at Hay River had a patient who had resided there for twenty-four years. Sick children stayed at the schools and for more serious illnesses than if they had ready access to a hospital. Noel MacKay, a Métis man from Fort Chipewyan born in 1905, described how at the school there, 'I seen there was a little room there was always 2 boys was marched in that room, soon as one of them died there was one to replace them never got out of there alive. [There were] 2 beds there, always filled up especially by the Indians.'[139] Fort Resolution, while it did not have a hospital, did have a doctor. When a child died of tuberculosis and measles at the Fort Resolution residential school in 1935, the death report noted explicitly, 'if we had a hospital handy, we might have saved her life'.[140] When Julius Salu, the Teetł'it Gwich'in leader, lost his daughter to illness at the Hay River school in the early 1930s, he called for both a school and a hospital in Fort McPherson. When Elder Christie Thompson reflected on the importance of establishing these institutions in the village, she noted that now, 'should something happen to the child, the doctor is right there'.[141]

The value of hospitals as outposts of colonial authority was apparent in Aklavik in the late 1920s. There, a dispute broke out between the Anglican and Catholic churches over establishing not one, but two hospitals – one for each denomination. Aklavik also had two residential schools, Anglican and Roman Catholic. This proliferation of institutions did not reflect greater need in the delta, but rather colonial prerogatives. The government depended on the Roman Catholic and Anglican missions in the Mackenzie district to deliver medical care, much as they depended on them to operate day and residential schools.[142] In the 1920s, missionary competition in the Mackenzie district focused on the Arctic Coast, seen as a frontier for Christian proselytizing.[143] Aklavik served as a node connecting Kuukpak with the Arctic Coast and was perceived by both Roman Catholics and Anglicans 'as a crucial stepping stone'. To this end, each established schools and hospitals to 'anchor' their missions.[144] Thus, a few months after providing a $1,250 grant to the Anglican

138 Russell Ferrier Memo to Dr Scott, 29 May 1925, RG 10, vol. 6472, file 905-1, part 1, LAC.
139 Noel MacKay, interview with Jim Parker, 20 Sept. 1978, Fort Chipewyan, AB, James M. Parker Fonds, Acc# 82-46, box 2, file 66, UAA.
140 Memorandum into Cause of Death of ______ of the Fort Resolution Indian Residential School on 27 Nov. 1935, RG 10, vol. 6475, file 916–23, part 1, c-8791, LAC.
141 Christie Thompson, 'A Long Time Ago – Part #1', in 'Gwich'in COPE stories', 651.
142 Chapter 4 in McCarthy, *Great River*; Abel, *Drum Songs*, 114.
143 Usher, *Fur Trade Posts*, 89–92; Jim Edwards, 'Christmas Long Ago', in 'Gwich'in COPE Stories', 182.
144 Vanast, 'Arctic Bodies', 365.

hospital at Aklavik, the Northwest Territories and Yukon branch received a request from Bishop Gabriel Breynat for a grant to the Roman Catholic Hospital, now established at that same site. O. S. Finnie and deputy minister W. W. Cory wanted the Roman Catholics to build a hospital at Fort Good Hope, one of the many places in the Northwest Territories where a hospital was 'urgently needed'.[145] Breynat was not interested in erecting a hospital in Fort Good Hope precisely because he felt the Catholic church already had a strong presence in that community. Hospitals and medical care were tools in the effort to convert souls to Catholicism.[146] This was not the argument that Breynat made to Finnie, however. Instead Breynat claimed that the Anglican hospital had denied treatment to a Roman Catholic man to demonstrate that the competition did not 'satisfactorily [meet] the requirements' of the settlement.[147]

Government officials needed the churches as much, if not more, than the churches needed them. Cory (on Finnie's advice) asked Breynat and Anglican bishop Isaac Stringer to work together to 'come to a mutual recognition of their respective spheres of activity',[148] adding that henceforth his department wanted to be asked for approval over where mission posts and, by extension, potential future hospital or school sites were to be established. Cory asserted this authority on the grounds that missions had to secure trading licences in order to access goods for their posts.[149] Through their authority to regulate trade, the government hoped to exercise greater control over the missionary activity now advancing along the Arctic Coast. Breynat denied the government this authority and rebuffed Cory's 'friendly advice', pointing out that he was bound 'by the directions imparted to me by our ecclesiastical Superior in Rome'.[150]

In the end, the department issued a grant to the Roman Catholic hospital in Aklavik in addition to the Anglican hospital. Breynat had not let up in his advocacy. Then J. A. (Fred) Urquhart, shortly after his arrival in Aklavik as Medical Health Officer, argued for both institutions: demand had increased starkly with the devastating flu epidemic that year. Finnie justified the decision to Cory in October 1929 along racial lines, writing that in the Roman Catholic hospital most of the patients 'are Indians from up the Mackenzie River. There are comparatively few Eskimos treated in that hospital.'[151] This had been the argument made by the Anglicans as well, that their hospital was meant to primarily serve Inuit patients. For Finnie, this distinction opened up the

[145] O. S. Finnie to W. W. Cory, 5 Jun. 1928, RG 85, vol. 191, file 554/119–1, part 1, LAC.
[146] McCarthy, *Great River*, 120.
[147] G. Breynat to W. W. Cory, 25 May 1928, RG 85, vol. 191, file 554/119–1, part 1, LAC.
[148] W. W. Cory to G. Breynat and to I. O. Stringer, 30 Apr. 1928, RG 85, vol. 191, file 554/119–1, part 1, LAC.
[149] Finnie to Cory, 5 Jun. 1928. [150] Breynat to Cory, 25 May 1928.
[151] O. S. Finnie to W. W. Cory, 3 Oct. 1929, RG 85, vol. 191, file 554/119–1, part 1, LAC.

possibility that the DIA could be pressed to contribute funds for equipment in the Roman Catholic hospital, while the Department of the Interior paid for Inuit medical care. But Finnie's embrace of this rationale also reflected the persistent racial logic of the colonial system. The 1920s and 1930s were the period in which interest in the question of whether Inuit were 'Indians' peaked among anthropologists and bureaucrats, with racial differences generally emphasized and Inuit located as closer to 'white' than their Dene, Gwich'in, Tagish, or Tłı̨chǫ counterparts.[152] The provision of healthcare in the Mackenzie was subject to the priorities of colonial authorities, including state and religious officials whose internecine disputes weighed more heavily in decision-making than the needs or desires of the peoples whose health was to be cared for.

Healthcare in the North was more accessible to settlers and sojourners working for the government and engaged in resource exploitation than it was for the original people of the land. Even as Indian Affairs and the Interior dithered over hiring a physician who could provide a minimum of care to those who had signed treaty north of Great Slave Lake, the RCMP employed physicians (at the rank of surgeon or assistant surgeon) at their Yukon posts and in Fort McPherson beginning in 1911. When the government did not find it feasible to construct hospitals or station medical personnel, resource operators hired doctors to serve their sojourning male workers. The federal government celebrated the provision of medical care as an essential element of industrial resource operations.[153] Doctors employed at police posts and work camps did treat local peoples (and were paid to do so by the DIA and the Interior), but there were limits to their willingness and ability to serve larger populations.[154] At Norman Wells, Imperial Oil hired Dr W. A. Richardson in July 1921 'primarily to look after their staff but [he] has the privilege of general practice'.[155] Richardson treated any men, women, or children who needed assistance when he passed through their communities or if they travelled to him.[156] Finnie soon recruited Richardson to work as the Medical Health Officer responsible for the region from Fort Simpson to Fort Good Hope. To secure the funds for this appointment, Finnie assured the Minister of the Interior, W. W. Cory, that it was unnecessary to pay Richardson the normal MHO salary, which started at $200 a month, and that $50 a month would suffice.[157] Finnie did not share with Richardson that his pay was discounted, but money soon became an issue, coupled with the enormous responsibilities that attended his

[152] Constance Backhouse, chapter 2 in *Colour-Coded: A Legal History of Racism in Canada, 1900–1950* (Toronto: Osgood Society for Canadian Legal History, 1999).

[153] See 'Canada Guards Natives' Health in Far North', *Natural Resources Canada*, 10, no. 2 (February 1931), 1.

[154] Joseph P. Dunne to W. W. Cory, 12 Aug. 1921, RG 85, series C-1-a, vol. 585, file 578, reel T-13213, LAC.

[155] O. S. Finnie to W. W. Cory, 3 Jan. 1922, series C-1-a, vol. 585, file 578, reel T-13213, LAC.

[156] Vanast, 'Arctic Bodies', 125. [157] Finnie to Cory, 3 Jan. 1922.

work as MHO. Within two years, Richardson abruptly left his northern post, overwhelmed by the responsibility combined with the government's unwillingness to support the medical care so clearly required.[158] Clermont Bourget, as a government doctor, was expected to fill some of the gap left by Richardson. It is hard to fault individuals for their unwillingness or inability to provide medical care given the disconnect between the needs on the ground and the thinnest of support from the state.

To the west in the Yukon, the expectation that medical services intended for a white, labouring population should extend to the local community encountered obstacles of a different kind. Mayo was a mining town, birthed in the gold rush, which grew up around rich silver deposits. In the summer of 1922, as Dawson settled into prolonged decline, the town's Good Samaritan Hospital was dismantled and shipped to Mayo, along with 'sufficient other second hand material to erect a building of the same size'.[159] From these recycled materials, a two-storey hospital was built to accommodate twelve to fifteen patients. The hospital was supported by a grant from the territorial government and by the Keno Hill and Treadwell Yukon companies, the principal employers in Mayo. Mine employees had $2.50 deducted monthly from their wages to support the hospital.[160]

Within a year of opening, the Mayo hospital was a busy place. So much so that the chairman of the hospital board wrote to the Gold Commissioner calling for the construction of a new wing and additional staff, including at least one more nurse.[161] A 1923 sketch showing the proposed wing outlined new patient, storage, and common rooms. On the upper floor, a larger space was marked out and labelled 'place for extra beds, Indians etc.'.[162] The desire to create a segregated, peripheral space for Indigenous patients was common to hospital care in the Yukon. In the hospitals in Dawson and Whitehorse, 'the Indians are treated in separate wards', a manifestation of the segregated society that had emerged at the insistence of settlers and sojourners in the Yukon in the wake of the gold rush.[163] Segregated space to treat Indigenous patients had not motivated the request for a new hospital wing, but discomfort with sharing a hospital soon emerged as a critical operational issue for Mayo General Hospital.

In April 1924, a power struggle erupted when the matron, Elizabeth McDougall, refused to 'admit Indians to hospital' without a separate ward

158 Vanast, 'Arctic Bodies', 129.

159 Gold Commissioner to J. H. McNeill, 10 Aug. 1922, Gov 1678, file 9, folder 4, YRG 1, Series 1, Central Registry Files, YA.

160 W. J. D. Dempster to G. P. McKenzie, 13 Apr. 1923, Gov 1678, file 9, folder 2, YRG 1, Series 1, Central Registry Files, YA.

161 Gold Commissioner to J. H. McNeill, 7 Aug. 1923, Gov 1678, file 9, folder 2.

162 Sketch showing upper and lower floors proposed new wing Mayo General Hospital, Gov 1678, file 9, folder 2.

163 See Coates, *Best Left as Indians*, 92–6.

where they could be treated.[164] McDougall fired off a telegram off to the Gold Commissioner, demanding to know whether she was in charge of the hospital, to which Commissioner George Mackenzie replied, 'You are in charge of Hospital under direction of Hospital Board.' He continued, 'While I appreciate your objection to treating Indians without special Indian Ward also appreciate awkward position in which Board is placed.'[165] McDougall left for the south, taking another nurse with her. Matron McDougall's defenders included the doctor at the hospital, McClennan, who described her wartime service, including 'honorable mention in despatches' and a 'letter of recommendation from King George'.[166] That McDougall was skilled and highly recommended would have made her an asset in the North, where reports often surfaced of novice personnel saddled with enormous responsibility and unable to rise to the occasion.[167] However, with McDougall's experience came pronounced racism towards Indigenous patients. In his assessment of the situation, Mackenzie wrote that the hospital was not busy at the time, the staff was not overworked, and the revenue was welcome. Moreover, the patient in question was 'free from a contagious or infectious disease'. 'Frankly', he concluded, 'I cannot understand the state of mind of any person who would object.'[168] Mackenzie had the capacity to see the humanity of Indigenous patients and considered them entitled to treatment, even if McDougall did not.

Although McDougall did not return to the Mayo General Hospital and relations between staff and the hospital board improved, the issue of a separate ward lingered. McDougall's opinions about segregation were those of the dominant society – even Mackenzie acknowledged them as valid, although he would not go so far as to argue that they warranted the denial of medical care. Because the employees of the mining companies paid out of their wages to support the hospital, their desire for segregated care carried weight in the cash-strapped Yukon of the 1920s. In 1925, the DIA declined a request for funds to build an 'Indian ward' put forth by John Hawksley. By 1928, the compromise was that Indigenous patients 'were kept in a tent on the Hospital grounds adjacent to the main building'.[169] This was described as a 'temporary arrangement', but it appears to have been the practice for several years at that point. Again Hawksley sent a request to his superiors at Indian Affairs asking

[164] Elizabeth McDougall telegram to G. P. Mackenzie, 31 Mar. 1924, Gov 1678, file 9, folder 3, YRG 1, Series 1, Central Registry Files, YA.
[165] G. P. Mackenzie to Elizabeth McDougall, 1 Apr. 1924, Gov 1678, file 9, folder 3.
[166] Dr McLennan telegram to Gold Commissioner, 3 Apr. 1924, Gov 1678, file 9, folder 3.
[167] W. A. Geddes to Bishop Stringer, 7 Jan. 1927, COR 251 f.22, Series 1-1a, Anglican Church of Canada, Diocese of Yukon, YA.
[168] Gold Commissioner to J. E. Ferrell, 24 Apr. 1924, and Gold Commissioner to W. J. D. Dempster, 24 Apr. 1924, Gov 1678, file 9, folder 3.
[169] G. I. MacLean to O. S. Finnie, 18 Aug. 1928, Gov 1929 file 403–2 parts 1, YRG, Series 4, YA.

the department to cover the costs of a new ward and this time his request was granted with the new segregated ward complete by May 1930.[170]

The infrastructure of care erected and supported in this period can be generally characterized as insufficient. Underfunded and racially contingent, the system prioritized the needs of settlers and sojourners engaged in resource exploitation and, insofar as it focused on the needs of Indigenous northerners, was designed around the objectives of the Christian missions upon whom the government depended to deliver its treaty promises. The missions, the medical practitioners, and the state grappled with material limitations imposed by climate and distance from sites of supply in securing drugs, medical supplies, and equipment. Pathogens could travel northwards more smoothly in this period than the technologies that might dispatch them. While preventive and curative therapies, such as vaccines and antitoxin, were sometimes available through these supply networks, government and medical officials relied heavily on other tools to control the spread of infectious pathogens. New sanitary infrastructures appeared at the beginning of the twentieth century and made disease reporting, quarantine, disinfection, and isolation important tools for disease control across the Yukon and Mackenzie. This is the subject of Chapter 6, which looks at health regulations imported as part of the legal frameworks imposed to control what were now Canada's northern territories. Measures to address the spread of infectious pathogens served multiple objectives in the colonial context.

[170] J. Hawksley to A. F. Mackenzie, Mar. 17, 1930, Gov 1619 1490 J file 2, YRG 1, Series 1, vol. 9, Central Registry Files, YA.

6 Race, Gender, and Control

In the spring of 1921, colonial authorities in Ottawa planned a 'show trial'.[1] A young Deh Cho Dene man, Albert LeBeau, was sitting in a southern jail cell charged with the murder of his wife and child. Previously his trial would have been held in Edmonton, far from LeBeau's home. But in 1921, a treaty party was scheduled to come to Fort Providence, where LeBeau worked at the Roman Catholic mission. Justice officials and territorial administrators decided that LeBeau's trial offered an opportunity to assert the Dominion's control over northern lands and peoples. The trial would be held immediately after the signing of Treaty 11, with signatories invited to attend, although the judge and jury would be all white. LeBeau's would be the first trial held 'in the far north', with the aim to impress 'the natives with a sense of British justice', according to the *Edmonton Bulletin*.[2] The jury found LeBeau guilty, and he was sentenced to hang. Albert LeBeau spent his last months imprisoned at Fort Fitzgerald. In October, he contracted smallpox and was very ill.[3] The executioner, already en route, turned around at Fort McMurray and returned home to Edmonton, prompting rumours that a reprieve would be granted. No reprieve came, and Albert LeBeau recovered from smallpox only to be hanged in Fort Smith on 1 November, as scheduled.

Show trials relied on the enforcement of criminal law to further Canada's control over the lands it claimed as its northern territories. This chapter examines a different show: the performance of germ theory as manifested through public health measures that aimed to control infectious diseases and

[1] For other northern show trials, see Julie Cruikshank, 'Oral Traditions and Written Accounts: An Incident from the Klondike Gold Rush', *Culture* 9, no. 2 (1989): 25–34; P. Whitney Lackenbauer and Kristopher Kinsinger, eds., *Arctic Show Trial: The Trial of Alikomiak and Tatamigana*, introd. Ken Coates and William R. Morrison (Calgary: Documents on Canadian Arctic Sovereignty and Security, 2017), http://pubs.aina.ucalgary.ca/dcass/83260.pdf; Shelagh D. Grant, *Arctic Justice: On Trial for Murder, Pond Inlet, 1923* (Montreal: McGill-Queen's University Press, 2002).

[2] 'Indian Murder Trial at Fort Providence Impressed Natives with British Law', *Edmonton Bulletin*, 19 July 1921, 7.

[3] Bourget, *Douze ans*, 34.

specifically smallpox.[4] Diseases as negotiated social phenomena take on their own character when refracted through the power relations of settler colonialism in the North.[5] The belief that smallpox was particularly deadly to Indigenous peoples shaped how the emergent settler colonial state reacted to the threat of Indigenous smallpox cases. Urban disease anxiety and technologies of surveillance and control were imported to the Yukon and the Mackenzie after 1900. Colonial authorities initially created highly restrictive and intrusive measures to control smallpox that constrained Indigenous mobility and regulated contact with whites.[6] These measures had to be moderated in the face of economic disruption, cost, and effectiveness as well as in response to the inadequate infrastructures of care erected in the North. Examples from the Yukon and the Mackenzie district were alternatively excessive and inadequate, revealing how colonial control over northern bodies and lands was still in-the-making in these years.

Smallpox Control in the Yukon

The smallpox outbreak in the summer of 1900 established the foundation for public health responses in the Yukon that relied on isolation, quarantine, and vaccination. The first cases that appeared in Dawson in June were sent to an isolation hospital 'about two and half miles from town'.[7] The hospital consisted of bell tents used in the Crimean War and after as field hospitals. Erected on Dog Island, directly across from Moosehide, officials described this as 'an isolated spot in the River Yukon'.[8] Dog Island would be used again in 1902 to isolate smallpox patients and to quarantine a steamship. There is no indication that the Tr'ondëk Hwëch'in were asked about the location of the isolation hospital, although they would have seen the tents from shore. Another 'temporary pest house' was set up at Spring Gulch.[9] A handful of cases appeared in Dawson that summer, then more cases appeared at Grand Forks and up the creeks in September. The outbreak ended before winter set in.

In mid-November, James Murphy in Whitehorse fell ill with what appeared to be a severe cold. When blotches broke out on his face, he was reported as a smallpox case to the police, as required under the public health ordinance.

[4] Graham Mooney, *Intrusive Interventions: Public Health, Domestic Space, and Infectious Disease Surveillance in England, 1840–1914* (Rochester: University of Rochester Press, 2015).

[5] Jones, *Rationalizing Epidemics*, 5.

[6] Arnold, *Colonizing the Body*, 7–9; Bashford, *Imperial Hygiene*, 22; Adele Perry, *On the Edge of Empire: Gender, Race, and the Making of British Columbia, 1849–1871* (Toronto: University of Toronto Press, 2001), 111.

[7] William Ogilvie to J. A. Smart, 12 Jul. 1900, GOV 1677, vol. 67, file 7, YRG 1, Series 1, Central Registry Files, YA.

[8] F. Montizambert, Memo for the Minister of Agriculture, 27 Oct. 1902, RG 29, vol. 2, file 937013, part 2, LAC.

[9] Z. T. Wood to NWMP Comptroller, 10 Oct. 1900, RG 18, series A-1, vol. 194, file 587–00, LAC; 'Notice', [Oct. 1900], GOV 1677, vol. 67, file 7, YA.

The NWMP hired Joseph Cardinal to nurse Murphy. According to NWMP doctor L. A. Paré, Cardinal 'had some experience in nursing, having nursed two small pox patients before', and 'he had had small pox himself'. His immune experience established, Paré also noted that Cardinal was reliable, a good cook, and a 'very good worker'. Cardinal had to cut and split all the wood needed for heating, he had to haul water, and he had to cook meals; as Paré put it, Cardinal had to do '*everything*'.[10] Isolation requirements and fear of the disease intensified the work of nursing smallpox patients. A Dawson nurse, Barbara Ross, requested more pay on the grounds that she had to work as 'laundress in addition to nursing because no one else would do it for fear of infection. Also that I had no relief from duty and any rest I got was by sleeping in the ward with my patients.'[11]

Cardinal cared for Murphy in a tent, visited by Paré three times a day 'on foot in the deep snow and the rough ice, there was no beaten trail, my own footsteps were always covered over the next morning, besides each day I made it a point to inspect the surroundings to make sure that nobody was lurking round the premises'.[12] With the appearance of Murphy's case in November and anticipating more, officials built an isolation hospital, 'a good substantial building, quite warm and comfortable'.[13] Murphy's house was disinfected and his clothing burned. As an indigent patient, the Yukon Council compensated Murphy for these losses.[14]

Two white hunters had identified and reported Murphy's sickness. When Murphy went into isolation, they had to quarantine in their tent, which they did, according to Paré, 'without a murmur, their only remark: "It is a bit hard on one, but we see the wisdom and necessity of the measure."' Paré did not have much faith in the hunters and set up 'a picket of our men watching that the quarantine is respected'.[15] This picket reflected a widely held belief in the 'dense ignorance of the multitude', a sentiment expressed by Dr Good (Dawson's first Medical Health Officer (MHO)) and echoed by government officials, physicians, and police.[16] Only after they had respected the quarantine did Paré judge the two hunters as 'men of great common sense'. The assumption that people would not respect quarantines reflected the disorder, from a state-control

[10] L. A. Paré to Officer Commanding, 20 Dec. 1900, GOV 1677, vol. 67, file 7, YA. Emphasis in original.

[11] Barbara Ross to William Ogilvie, 24 Oct. 1900, GOV 1677, file 8, part 1, folder 1, YRG 1, Series 1, Central Registry Files, YA; Ross was paid about $6.50 a day, Cardinal had been paid $8.00 per day.

[12] Paré to Office Commanding, 20 Dec. 1900; L. A. Paré to F. Montizambert, 14 Nov. 1900, RG 29, vol. 2, file 937013, part 1, LAC.

[13] Paré to Office Commanding, 20 Dec. 1900.

[14] See, for example, correspondence between Anna Allen and Territorial Administrator, Oct. 1911 and Jul. 1912, GOV 1677, file 8, part 2, folder 1, YRG 1, Series 1, Central Registry Files, YA.

[15] Paré to Montizambert, 14 Nov. 1900.

[16] Dr Good to W. Ogilvie, 3 Jul. 1900, GOV 1677, vol. 67, file 7, YA.

perspective, of the Klondike gold rush.[17] Controlling the movement of people along the creeks and in the boom town of Dawson was a challenge. Archille Filion was symptomatic when he slipped through the police guard to travel 'about on all the Creeks' before police caught up to him.[18]

There were also the economic costs of quarantine to consider. These ranged from the disruption of individual life to large-scale curtailment of travel and transport, as ships were tied up and people prohibited from moving freely. Quarantines disrupted hunts, and people could go hungry. Along the trails between Dawson and the Forks, which men and women travelled to register claims, to get grub and equipment, and to work their mines, police were now on guard, preventing people 'from doing business'.[19] To mitigate economic hardship and to facilitate surveillance, the commissioner and council eventually replaced the general quarantine with strict controls on houses or cabins or people who were direct contacts of infected cases. A public notice advertised their names and threatened that if they were found outside of quarantine, they would be sent to the isolation hospital (Figure 6.1).

As Alison Bashford wrote in *Imperial Hygiene*, public health as it developed over the nineteenth century was a 'spatial form of governance'.[20] In a colonial context, quarantine regulations defined state control over lands and waters. The appearance of smallpox cases at Grand Forks led the Board of Health to grant the MHO powers that extended outside the city of Dawson.[21] But quarantine measures went far beyond Dawson and the creeks. Border control created pinch-points in transportation networks. Most outsiders arriving in the nineteenth century had travelled from St Michael, Alaska on the southern shore of Norton Sound, east along the lower Yukon River to Dawson. At the head of the Inside Passage, Skagway provided a closer landing point for those headed to the gold fields. By 1900, the White Pass and Yukon Railway connected Skagway to Whitehorse and from there to the river steamers that proliferated during the gold rush, carrying people and goods along the upper Yukon River (Map 6.1).[22] New overland routes also appeared. After 1902, a winter trail connected Whitehorse with Dawson. Beginning in 1904, the RCMP patrolled annually from Dawson over to Fort McPherson in the Northwest Territories.

[17] Allan Patenaude, 'The Administration of Justice in Canada's Northwest Territories, 1870–1990: A Case Study in Colonialism and Social Change' (MA thesis, Simon Fraser University, 1990), 114.

[18] C. Starnes to Z. T. Wood, 30 Oct. 1900, GOV 1677, vol. 67, file 7, YA.

[19] Z. T. Wood to the Comptroller, 10 Oct. 1900, RG 18, series A-1, vol. 194, file 587–00, LAC; C. C. Raven to Officer Commanding, 2 Oct. 1900, GOV 1677, vol. 67, file 7, YA.

[20] Bashford, *Imperial Hygiene*, 1.

[21] William Ogilvie to Z. T. Wood, 25 Oct. 1900, GOV 1677, vol. 67, file 7, YA.

[22] Yukon Archives, 'Sternwheelers of the Yukon / Les Bateaux à aubes du Yukon', https://archives-ftp.gov.yk.ca/exhibits/sternwheelers/en/river.html.

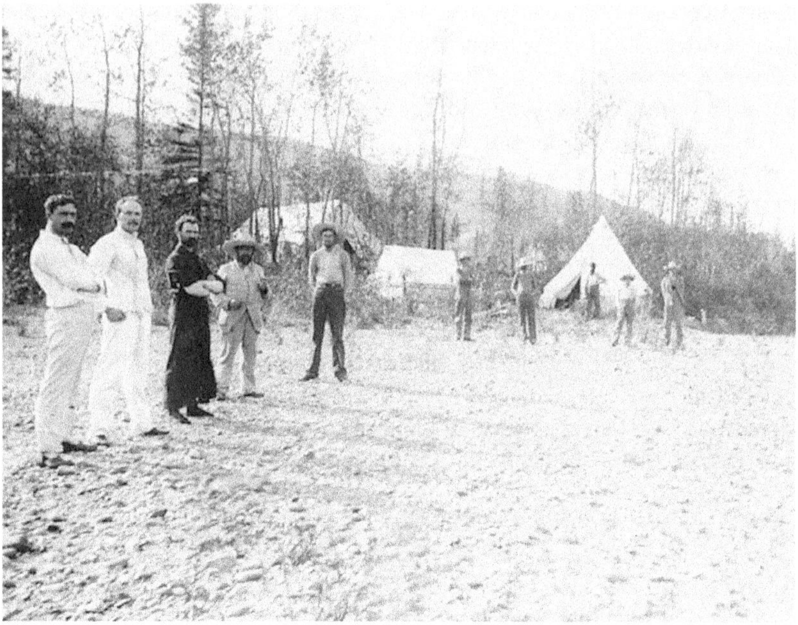

Figure 6.1 Smallpox quarantine station, Yukon, c. 1900. PA-022500/Library and Archives Canada.

When the first reports of smallpox came in the summer of 1900, Yukon Commissioner William Ogilvie directed NWMP Superintendent Zachary Taylor Wood to 'inaugurate a quarantine system at the summit of White Pass and adjacent entries to the country'.[23] Wood sent NWMP assistant surgeon Paré to the detachment at Caribou, just east of Bennett Lake, while assistant surgeon S. M. (Samuel Martin) Fraser was stationed at Dalton Trail. These were both within the Yukon's borders. Paré and Fraser were to examine everyone who entered the territory, 'quarantining suspicious cases or persons from infective districts'.[24] The newly appointed Dominion Director General of Public Health, Frederick Montizambert, was responsible for administering quarantine stations throughout Canadian territory. He sought to coordinate quarantine measures across provincial and territorial borders. Officials on either side of the Canada–United States border cooperated in controlling outbreaks – they shared supplies of vaccine and antitoxin and information about cases and their spread – but such coordination could only go so far.

23 Z. T. Wood to William Ogilvie, 7 Jul. 1900, GOV 1677, vol. 67, file 7, YA.

24 Z. T. Wood to Comptroller, NWMP Ottawa, 6 Jul. 1900, RG 18, series A-1, vol. 194, file 587–00, LAC.

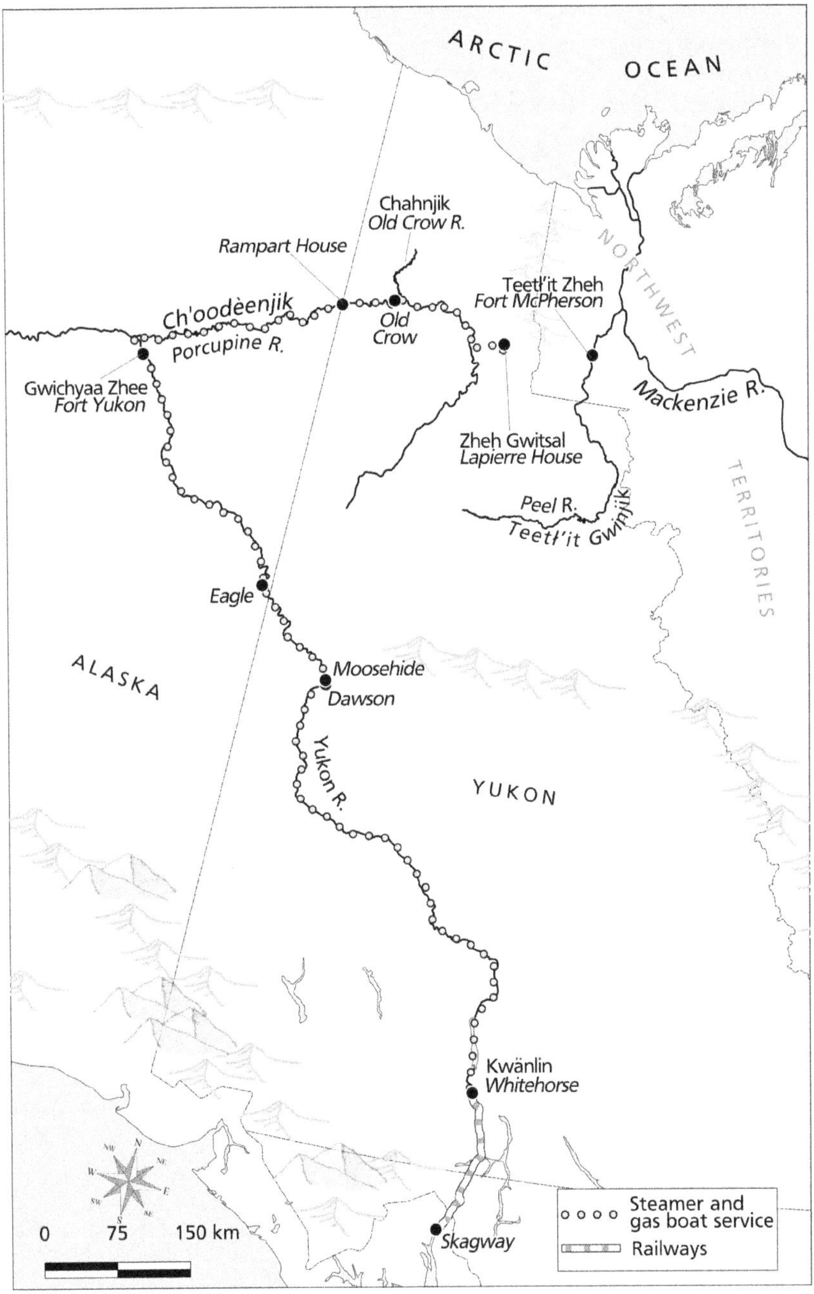

Map 6.1 Yukon and Alaska borderlands around 1911.

Clifford Sifton, Minister for the Interior, did not trust the United States and the transportation companies at Skagway to protect Canada's interests and asked Montizambert to station 'an officer at the frontier directly responsible to this Government'.[25] Samuel Cameron was appointed in July 1901 and lived in Skagway, where he could inspect the outgoing train to protect not only Dawson and the gold fields, but also the British Columbia–Yukon borderlands.[26]

In the summer of 1902, smallpox appeared on the *White Horse*, a mail steamer travelling the busy river corridor between Whitehorse and Dawson. The *White Horse* was made to tie up at Dog Island, with its ninety-three passengers and crew strictly confined, a situation they strenuously protested.[27] The SS *Zealandian*, operated by the White Pass and Yukon, was then also forced into quarantine for a week, as two crew members had transferred mid-river between the ships. When the smallpox case was reported on the *White Horse*, the police came and led the two men off the *Zealandian*, 'no reason given'. During the week the *Zealandian* was in quarantine, the company pressed hard to have the restrictions lifted during what was the 'busiest time of the season', indicative of the pressures applied to officials to limit quarantine.[28] Steamboats on the Yukon River served as vectors for the spread of pathogens, not just because of the speed with which they travelled but also because of the mobility of crew and passengers.

Quarantine measures and placarding were regularly deployed to control the spread of diphtheria, smallpox, and scarlet fever in the Yukon territory. Sometimes measles prompted a quarantine, as did the anticipated arrival of the 1918–19 influenza pandemic.[29] Where quarantine served as an assertion of control over the land, coercive or compulsory vaccination was an assertion of control over bodies.

By 1900, it was well established that a single vaccination against smallpox did not confer lifelong immunity, and revaccination was commonplace. Nurse Cardinal 'had been vaccinated, had the small pox, but I also vaccinated him', according to Dr Paré.[30] Police could expect to be revaccinated multiple times,

[25] F. Montizambert memo 4 Jul. 1901, RG 29, vol. 2, file 937013, part 2, LAC.

[26] F. Montizambert to S. D. Cameron, 31 Oct. 1901, RG 29, vol. 2, file 937013, part 2, LAC; see Andrea Geiger, *Converging Empires: Citizens and Subjects in the North Pacific Borderlands, 1867–1945* (Chapel Hill: University of North Carolina Press, 2022), for broader borderlands history.

[27] [Passengers and Crew of *S.S. White Horse*] to J. H. Ross, 13 Jun. 1902, GOV 1677, vol. 67, file 7, YA.

[28] P. F. Scharschmidt to A. B. Newell, 12 Jun. 1903, GOV 1677, vol. 67, file 7, YA.

[29] 'Smallpox Outbreak of, in Dawson', RG 18, A-1, vol. 194, file 587–00, LAC; 'White Horse, Outbreak of measles amongst Indians at', RG 18, A-1, vol. 514, file 530–16, LAC; 'Scarlet Fever – Whitehorse', GOV 1926 376 (510), YA; Yukon Health Ordinance No. 20 of 1902; Michael Gates, 'How the Yukon Was Spared the Influenza Pandemic of 1918', *Yukon News*, 26 Mar. 2020, www.yukon-news.com/opinion/history-hunter-how-the-yukon-was-spared-the-influenza-pandemic-of-1918/.

[30] Paré to Officer Commanding, 20 Dec. 1900.

and they were among the first to receive vaccines in 1900.[31] When smallpox appeared that summer, officials initially found themselves with only enough lymph material 'to vaccinate one tenth of the population'.[32] This was not through negligence. Commissioner Ogilvie had ordered lymph and points the previous fall. They had yet to arrive, reflecting the challenges of securing medical supplies in a place situated thousands of kilometres from centres of biomedical manufacturing. Vaccine lymph had an expiry date, and shipping took two to three months at least. To ensure stocks were always on hand required regular shipments.[33] Widespread smallpox outbreaks in 1900 intensified demand throughout supply chains, creating further delays.[34] When they arrived from Vancouver in August, Montizambert and his son carried vaccine lymph and points with them. There were otherwise few challenges in terms of transportation in a cold climate when it came to smallpox vaccine. Some therapies, notably diphtheria antitoxin, were much more fragile.[35]

In the autumn, Paré vaccinated or revaccinated over a quarter of the local population at Whitehorse, after offering vaccination to anybody without asking any fee.[36] Paré's efforts came about in direct response to James Murphy's diagnosis. Similar vaccination measures targeted all those in proximity to any identified case. When smallpox was diagnosed on the No. 16 claim by Gold Run, five men were isolated in a cabin, the cabin they had been living in was 'fumigated with sulphur, old clothing burnt, and every person on the claim vaccinated'.[37] But in 1900, the Yukon also implemented a large-scale vaccination campaign supported by a precise and forceful vaccination ordinance, No. 39 of 1900, which stayed in place until repealed by the comprehensive 1902 health statute.

This ordinance, described by Superintendent Wood as 'enforcing compulsory vaccination', was the framework within which a vaccination campaign proceeded in the southern and central Yukon in the fall and winter of 1900.[38] This campaign was a concerted effort from the territorial government and the NWMP, who hired private physicians to vaccinate 15,000 settlers and sojourners in the Yukon where they lived and travelled after freeze-up.[39] As described by MHO MacArthur in late October, the campaign established two vaccine stations on 'the main

[31] P. C. H. Primrose to Officer Commanding, 19 Jul. 1900, GOV 1677, vol. 67, file 7, YA.
[32] Wood to Comptroller, 6 Jul. 1900.
[33] W. E. Thompson to Acting Commissioner, 14 Feb. 1905, GOV 1677, vol. 67, file 8, part 2, folder 1, YA.
[34] Henderson Bros. to William Ogilvie, Oct. 12 1900, GOV 1677, vol. 67, file 8, part 1, YA.
[35] See L. Piper, 'Diphtheria Antitoxin and Tales of Mercy in Northern Health Care', *CBMH/BCHM* 38, no. 2 (2021): 285–319 (pp. 296–7).
[36] Paré to Officer Commanding, 20 Dec. 1900.
[37] F. Candle to Z. T. Wood, 18 Oct. 1900, GOV 1677, vol. 67, file 7, YA.
[38] Z. T. Wood to Commissioner 31 Oct. 1900, GOV 1677, vol. 67, file 8, part 1, YA.
[39] J. H. MacArthur to Yukon Council, 29 Oct. 1900, GOV 1677, vol. 67, file 8, part 1, YA.

thoroughfares through the territory', one at Cooks Roadhouse, and one on the Klondike trail at Upper Ferry. In addition to these stations, there were to be house-to-house visits along the creeks. Physicians were assigned to different locales, with one each at the vaccine stations and another five to work the creeks. Significantly, no Indigenous communities appeared in the list of places to be vaccinated. For instance, while Dr Norquay was assigned to 'West Dawson/Dawson/Klondike City', Moosehide was not included. The archival record is silent on the subject of vaccinating Indigenous peoples during the 1900 campaign.

There was some initial confusion about the role of the police in enforcing the ordinance. Ogilvie wrote Wood, noting 'If the vaccination ordinance does not provide for the punishment of culprits through the direct intervention of your force I think it should be made to do so.'[40] At least one physician expected the police to round people up for vaccination. A plan had to be negotiated by physicians, territorial officials, and the NWMP. There was to be a general call for people to come forward voluntarily to be vaccinated. This would be followed by house-to-house visits by the public vaccinator (for which he was paid $25 per day), accompanied by a police officer. At each house, residents would have to provide evidence of vaccination, and the policeman 'would take the names of all those who refused to be operated on', information that could be used to prosecute people under the ordinance.[41]

After the winter 1900–1 campaign, systematic smallpox vaccination did not occur again in the territory for several years. Cases appeared, such as those that led to the quarantine of the SS *White Horse* and SS *Zealandian* in 1902, but they were effectively isolated. In April 1906, MHO W. T. Barrett called on the commissioner to implement another vaccination campaign targeted at children and adults who had not been vaccinated in the last six years. Barrett recommended that adults 'be compelled to submit to vaccination', and that children be required to show a certificate before returning to school in the autumn. The public notice advertising the vaccination campaign used gentler language, advising adults 'to take advantage of this general vaccination', while effort focused on public-school children. The territory ordered 1,500 vaccine points, which arrived with an expiry date of 15 August 1906, which then determined the last day of the campaign. Public vaccinators were hired and paid per vaccine administered. Based on their accounts, 134 people were vaccinated in Whitehorse, Dawson, and along the creeks over six weeks.[42]

The appearance of smallpox in 1900, 'this loathsome disease', had been met with fear.[43] Letters between territorial officials communicated a sense of

[40] W. Ogilvie to Z. T. Wood, 30 Jan. 1901, GOV 1677, vol. 67, file 7, YA.

[41] MacArthur to Yukon Council, 29 Oct. 1900; Z. T. Wood to Commissioner, 1 Feb. 1901, GOV 1677, vol. 67, file 7, YA.

[42] GOV 1677, vol. 67, file 8, part 1, folder 2, part 2, YA.

[43] Wade and Aikman to William Ogilvie, 30 Aug. 1900, GOV 1677, vol. 67, file 7, YA.

urgency and anxiety. As Dr Good wrote to commissioner Ogilvie, the first case 'is a severe case of smallpox. There is no mistake about this . . . There will be other cases.'[44] Ogilvie immediately called an emergency public meeting 'with the leading citizens and Medical men', to put together a collective response and 'to stamp it [the smallpox] out'.[45] The territorial government then reacted with strict measures: isolation, quarantine, and compulsory vaccination targeted at the entire settler and sojourner population. Then there came a recalibration, apparent first in the reassessment of the seriousness of the cases, which by mid-July had gone from 'severe' to 'mild'; then, when Ogilvie replaced the general quarantine at the Forks with a more limited quarantine.[46]

We see the most significant shifts after the 1900 outbreak and vaccination campaign ended. As early as May 1901, smallpox cases appeared at Sitka in the Alaskan panhandle, and a steamer en route to Skagway was quarantined by American officials. Wood wrote to the commissioner about how to proceed, should cases appear in Skagway. He endorsed a plan put forth by Inspector Snyder as 'a more economical mode of procedure than that adopted last year'.[47] A similar refrain appeared in correspondence and reports in the aftermath of the 1900 outbreak and in the years to come, with commentators emphasizing the cost of smallpox control measures. MHO MacArthur called for more vaccination and inspection stations, the expense of which 'would be infinitesimal in comparison with the cost of last summer's epidemic'.[48] The smallpox outbreak in 1900 had been enormously expensive, including the cost of disrupted business, securing vaccines, paying nurses and physicians to work or visit isolation hospitals, and paying public vaccinators a daily rate. Police officers had their expenses covered too when they accompanied the vaccinators or otherwise enforced public health measures. Subsequent outbreaks also carried significant costs. The steamer quarantine in 1902 was exceptionally costly, as the crew was compensated for lost wages, on top of supplying provisions to everyone on board.

The territorial government asserted considerable authority, exemplified in the compulsory vaccination ordinance, and expended enormous resources in reaction to the smallpox outbreak in 1900–1. These decisions were rooted in a fear of smallpox as part of a culture of anxiety in the Yukon that was an extension of broader Western cultural fear of infectious disease shaped in the urban environments of the nineteenth century. The thousands of outsiders who poured into the territory from urban places brought diseases, ideas about

[44] Dr Good to W. Ogilvie, 3 Jul. 1900, GOV 1677, vol. 67, file 7, YA.

[45] W. Ogilvie to Z. T. Wood, 6 Jul. 1900, GOV 1677, vol. 67, file 7, YA.

[46] Telegrams from Commissioner to R. P. Peel and Commissioner to D. Menzies, both 14 Jul. 1900, GOV 1677, vol. 67, file 7, YA; Mooney, *Intrusive Interventions*, ch. 5.

[47] A. E. Snyder to Officer Commanding 14 May 1901, GOV 1677, vol. 67, file 7, YA.

[48] MacArthur, 'Sanitary Report', 10.

disease, and ideas about differential racial susceptibility to disease with them. The exceptional circumstances of the gold rush made it difficult for the commissioner, physicians, and NWMP to know the best response. They recognized how the Yukon was at risk from disease outbreaks in distant urban centres: reports of 'smallpox in Seattle and of the Bubonic Plague in San Francisco' prompted calls for 'earnest watchfulness' and intensified control measures in 1903; reports of smallpox in Eastern Canada in 1904 spurred the territory to stock up on vaccines and diphtheria antitoxin.[49] But the government lacked the resources to mount a response to each outbreak equivalent to the measures taken in 1900–1. Moreover, some measures were deemed unnecessary. Compulsory vaccination was not needed annually, particularly as the population stabilized and declined, and so the vaccination ordinance was superseded by the broader 1902 public health ordinance.[50] Subsequent vaccination campaigns, like the one in 1906, were limited in scope. Targeted isolation, surveillance, and control measures were used in later outbreaks in Dawson and Whitehorse. Then in 1911, the Yukon government confronted its first smallpox outbreak in a Gwich'in community, and the response was telling.

Rampart House 1911–12

On 2 April 1911, two men arrived from California to work on a dredge up Hunker Creek. They were sick with smallpox, but their illness went unnoticed until two co-workers ended up in Dawson's St Mary's Hospital in late May. Shortly thereafter, a barber in the city fell ill and went to the Good Samaritan Hospital. All three men developed smallpox rashes, and with both hospitals 'infected', fumigation, isolation, and control measures were put in place.[51] A 'pest house' was opened, this time at Jackson Gulch three miles outside town.[52] Schools and movie theatres in Dawson were closed as more cases appeared, with nine men and women admitted to hospital in June. On 29 June, the MHO Alfred Thompson got smallpox and had to be replaced by William E. Thompson for the duration of the outbreak.[53]

The territorial administration stopped short of a general quarantine and only required isolation for direct contacts and patients. Anyone passing through or leaving Dawson had to secure a certificate from health authorities 'that they

[49] J. A. Fraser to F. Montizambert, 17 Feb. 1903, RG 29, vol. 2, file 937013, part 2, LAC; Medical Health Officer to Commissioner, 30 Mar. 1904, GOV 1677, vol. 67, file 8, part 1, folder 2, YA.

[50] Territorial Secretary to I. W. Burke, 20 Jun. 1902, GOV 1677, vol. 67, file 8, part 1, folder 2, YA.

[51] Arthur Wilson to W. W. Cory, 19 Jul. 1911, GOV 1677, vol. 67, file 8, part 2, folder 1, YA.

[52] Supt. Commanding to Territorial Treasurer, 21 Jun. 1911; W. E. Thompson to Arthur Wilson, 12 Jul. 1911, both in GOV 1677, vol. 67, file 8, part 2, folder 1, YA.

[53] Alexander Henderson to Ben Levy, 10 Jun. 1911; A. Henderson to Alfred Thompson, 18 Jun. 1911, both in GOV 1677, vol. 67, file 8, part 2, folder 1, YA.

have not been in contact with smallpox or its contagion'.[54] But people and freight continued to come and go. This prompted great concern from Whitehorse. City officials and businesspeople begged the territorial commissioner for a quarantine of Dawson: 'If not done Skagway threatens quarantine against ####All Yukon####', wrote Whitehorse's elected council representatives.[55] The White Pass and Yukon Railway said they were willing to stop passenger traffic, so long as they could continue to freight goods. There were reports of mining operators closing down operations rather than face an international quarantine.[56] But commissioner Alexander Henderson, on Thompson's advice, refused to quarantine Dawson.[57] Instead, they chose compulsory vaccination. US authorities promptly closed the border from the Yukon through Eagle and Summit.

The vaccination ordinance was passed on 7 July 1911.[58] With fewer doctors living in the district, local druggists were hired as vaccinators and paid $1 per vaccination. The ordinance directed that anyone who had not been vaccinated in the last year 'shall procure the vaccination', under penalty of a $400 fine, although there was provision for medical exemptions. The standard of proof was 'marks upon the body' along with 'the person alleging himself, or herself, to have been so vaccinated'.[59] In this campaign, physicians and territorial officials had to contend with significant anti-vaccinationist sentiment.[60] MHO Alfred Thompson, who contracted smallpox in June, did not 'believe in vaccination' according to Ida May Burkholder, matron of the Good Samaritan Hospital. Two nurses also fell ill after being recruited to work at the isolation hospital. According to Burkholder, one of these nurses had lied when she was examined before admission to the smallpox ward.[61] Thompson went on to be elected in September as the Yukon's representative in the federal parliament. His opposition to vaccination, and similar sentiments among nurses, reflected more

54 Tr'ondëk Hwëch'in were prohibited from using the ferry between West Dawson and Dawson; see Memo to Charles Heinrich and A. D. McKeen, 20 Jun. 1911, GOV 1677, vol. 67, file 8, part 2, folder 1, YA.

55 Robt. Lowe and W. L. Phelps to Commissioner, 24 Jun. 1911, GOV 1677, vol. 67, file 8, part 2, folder 1, YA.

56 Telegram to Arthur Wilson, 28 Jun. 1911, GOV 1677, vol. 67, file 8, part 2, folder 1, YA.

57 A. Henderson to R. Lowe, 26 Jun. 1911, GOV 1677, vol. 67, file 8, part 2, folder 1, YA. Similar telegrams were sent to the mayor of Skagway, the governor of Alaska, and the deputy minister of the Interior.

58 Thompson to Wilson, 12 Jul. 1911; A. R. MacFarlane to National Drug and Chemical Co., 26 Aug. 1911, L. A. Paré to A. Henderson, 16 Jun. 1911, all in GOV 1677, vol. 67, file 8, part 2, folder 1, YA.

59 W. E. Thompson, 'Compulsory Vaccination: An Ordinance Respecting the Public Health', 7 Jul. 1911, GOV 1677, vol. 67, file 8 part 2, folder 1, YA.

60 Anne Hardy, '"Straight Back to Barbarism": Antityphoid Inoculation and the Great War, 1914', *Bulletin of the History of Medicine* 74, no. 2 (Summer 2000): 265–90 (pp. 268–9).

61 Thora McIlroy Mills, 'Gold Rush Nurse', *north/nord* 20, no. 5 (1973): 10–13; 'Small pox cases treated in the Isolation Hospital June to August 1911', GOV 1677, vol. 67, file 8, part 2, folder 1, YA.

widespread vaccine hesitancy and helped these sentiments to proliferate.[62] Commissioner George Black wrote to MHO H. C. Davis in early 1912 to encourage him to vaccinate as many people as possible, while minimizing conflict: 'Very often the exercize of a little tact will bring about the desired result when a peremptory order would excite indignation and antagonism.' Black further told Davis to get advice 'as to the law defining your authority', signalling broader opposition to public health measures within Yukon's settler population.[63]

By mid-July, territorial authorities believed that the outbreak was on the wane. The US quarantine was to be lifted 1 August, although with a vaccination certificate required to cross the international border.[64] The territorial administrator wrote to the federal deputy minister of the interior, emphasizing that 'unless a new outbreak occurs, of which I think there is little or no danger, the expense in connection [to the outbreak] will cease in about 4 or 5 weeks'.[65] By mid-July, eight patients had been released from the isolation hospital in Jackson Gulch, and W. E. Thompson anticipated that the hospital would soon close. Thompson was more circumspect in his assessment than the territorial administrator. No new cases had appeared for two weeks and, 'as far as the outbreak is concerned, it is at an end', he wrote, 'but our vigilance cannot be relaxed because an isolated case might occur at any time from latent germs'.[66] Ten days later, a case appeared at Rampart House.

Rampart House was situated along Ch'oodèenjik, or the Porcupine River. Gwich'in had long travelled through the area and harvested fish in the shallow waters near that place. When the HBC left Fort Yukon, they moved first to a site near Howling Dog Canyon, then to Old Rampart House (still on the US side of the border), then finally to what they initially called New Rampart House, just on the Canadian side of the line. The HBC did not last long at Rampart House. They left after three years, closing their LaPierre's House post at the same time.[67] Independent traders soon proliferated in the Yukon. One of them, Dan Cadzow, born in Ontario of Scottish ancestry, built a store at Rampart House in 1904. For the first two to three decades of the twentieth century, the community around Rampart House thrived, with people gathering there in the spring, before ratting season, from Van Tat (Crow Flats), Fort Yukon, and Arctic

62 Bashford described stronger opposition in the Australian colonies compared to England, in part because smallpox was not endemic in the former, *Imperial Hygiene*, 51–2; see also Nadja Durbach, '"They Might as Well Brand Us": Working-Class Resistance to Compulsory Vaccination in Victorian England', *Social History of Medicine* 13 (2000): 45–62; Paré to Henderson, 16 Jun. 1911.

63 George Black to H. C. Davis, 3 Apr. 1912, GOV 1677, vol. 67, file 8, part 2, folder 1, YA.

64 W. E. Clark to Arthur Wilson, 23–4 Jul. 1911, GOV 1677, vol. 67, file 8, part 2, folder 1, YA.

65 Arthur Wilson to W. W. Cory, 10 Jul. 1911, GOV 1677, vol. 67, file 8, part 2, folder 1, YA.

66 Thompson to Wilson, 12 Jul. 1911.

67 Ken Coates, *The Northern Yukon: A History* (Parks Canada Manuscript Report Number 403, 1979), 27–8.

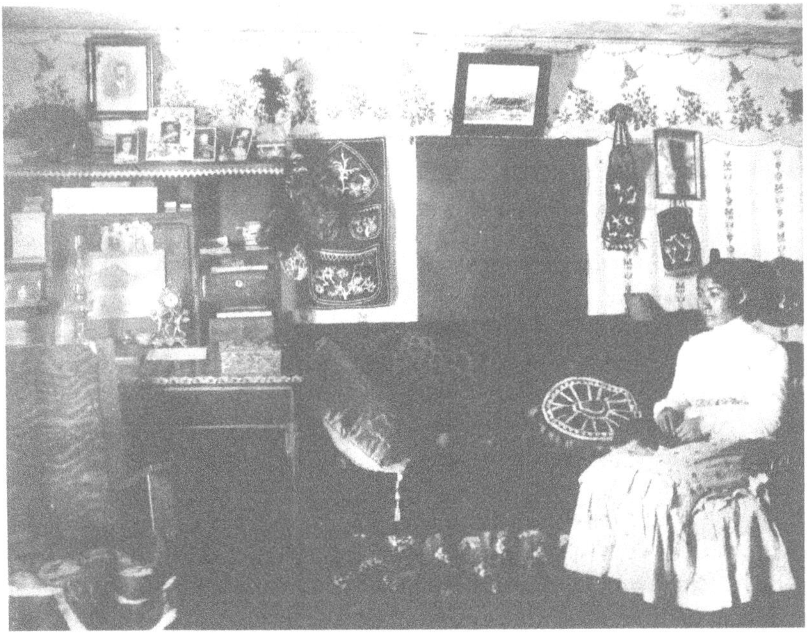

Figure 6.2 Monica (Njootli) Cadzow at home, Rampart House. Dan Cadzow Papers, UAF-1965–31–37, Alaska and Polar Regions Collections and Archives, University of Alaska Fairbanks.

Village. 'Everybody used to travel together', according to Alice Frost.[68] There would be big feasts at Rampart House, and people would come from as far as Fort McPherson. Charlie Thomas told how his family spent a lot of time in Crow Flats in summer and winter; when the caribou came, they went to the mountains and came into Rampart House to trade, get supplies, and visit.[69] Cadzow and his family were important within the village. Cadzow married twice, both times to Gwich'in women. His first wife was Monica Njootli, a Teetł'it Gwich'in woman (Figure 6.2). In 1911, she was twenty-seven and Cadzow was forty-five.[70] Archie Linklater was also prominent in the community at Rampart House. He married a Van Tat Gwich'in woman, Catherine Netro. Born into a fur-trade family in Moose Factory, Linklater arrived in the Yukon around 1898 when he was in his mid-forties. Linklater appears first in

[68] Hannah Netro in *People of the Lakes*, 217; Alice Frost interviewed by Shelagh Beairsto, in *Rampart House*, 66.

[69] Charlie Thomas interviewed by Louise Profeit-Leblanc, in *Rampart House*, 27.

[70] Her name also given as Veronica. See Hannah Netro interviewed by Shelagh Beairsto, in *Rampart House*, 15.

the archival record as a Special Constable with the NWMP in the Yukon in 1900. By 1905, Linklater was living in the northern Yukon, trapping, hunting, and fishing with his wife Catherine and raising a large family; they had at least nine children born between 1905 and 1926. Linklater kept a daily diary from 1906 until his death in April 1941 that gives prosaic but remarkable detail into his family's daily life through those decades.

Isaac Stringer, Bishop of Selkirk in the Yukon, served as census enumerator in 1911. He recorded 206 people at Rampart House (and LaPierre's House), most of whom were Gwich'in. Stringer was a more precise enumerator than most, differentiating Van Tat, Neets'ąįį, Teetł'it, Gwichaa, Dagoo, and Draanjik Gwich'in, and including also ten Inuvialuit who lived in the area of the census. Many of the Gwich'in had their birthplace recorded as Alaska, indicative of the ongoing strong relationships and regular movement across what was now being redefined as an international boundary.[71] There were a handful of non-Gwich'in men, seven of whom (including Cadzow and Linklater) were married to Gwich'in women and who were part of the Gwich'in community. There were another five or six men 'scattered around the country prospecting'.[72] In the hierarchical logic of the colonial census, Dan and Monica Cadzow were the first household enumerated.

On 1 June 1911, an international survey party arrived in Rampart House from Fort Yukon. The first smallpox case appeared six weeks later. According to a RNWMP report, the disease appeared first in the cabin of 'preacher John ... and it is thought that smallpox probably was brought into the country by means of infected cast off clothing brought from Dawson'.[73] Alternatively, the virus may have travelled in someone with only mild symptoms. After all, the first two cases of the disease that year had passed unnoticed because 'they were mild cases and not diagnosed as smallpox'.[74] An asymptomatic carrier was no more likely a member of the survey party (who came via Fort Yukon) than one of many others who were on the land or travelling on the river with the normal comings and goings of summer.

This was the first time since the gold rush that smallpox had been identified in a Yukon Indigenous community. The reaction by territorial officials drew on the same tools – isolation, quarantine, vaccination – that were the foundation of smallpox control elsewhere in the territory. There were, however, marked differences between efforts used to control the disease in Rampart House as

71 Geiger, *Converging Empires*, 51.

72 A. E. Acland to Officer Commanding, 27 Jun. 1912, RG 18, series A-1, vol. 532, file 206–17, LAC.

73 J. F. Fyfe to Officer Commanding, Dawson, 15 Sept. 1911, RG 18, series A-1, vol. 532, file 206–17, LAC.

74 Thompson to Wilson, 12 Jul. 1911.

compared to Dawson, and in the experience of the disease for the Gwich'in and their families living in this place.

Neil McDonald, now in his early twenties, worked for Dan Cadzow for two years. He recalled how the first police had come to Rampart House 'during the smallpox ... There was a nurse and the first policeman, Jimmy Five [James Fyfe].'[75] Earlier that year, Constable Fyfe had served on the party that found and recovered the bodies of the Lost Patrol.[76] Fyfe and nurse Arthur Lee arrived in the evening of 5 August, on board the *Midnight Sun* from Fort Yukon and bringing 300 vaccine points with them. By this time, the head of the US survey party, Thomas Riggs, had 'taken command' along with Dr Gilbert T. Smith. Smith, the survey physician, remained in charge of the response to the outbreak for the duration. Fyfe reported on the quarantine that had been swiftly imposed: 'No person is allowed here unless they are going to stay and no one is allowed to leave. Everyone here has been vaccinated and two men are out in the hills vaccinating all the natives and surveyors they can find.' All outgoing mail was being 'well fumigated', as well as the buildings and tents in town.[77]

Hannah Netro was born in 1919, eight years after the epidemic. She was told a story about the smallpox by her father, Joe Kaye (or Kyikavichik, older brother of Johnny Kyikavichik who signed Treaty 11). At the time, Hannah's stepmother Myra was nineteen years old and married to Jacob Tizya, aged twenty-one. Myra and Jacob had a baby girl named Anna, who was about a year old. 'One morning she got up and she got sick – she had spots all over her. Somehow they contacted the doctor and he arrived here', according to Netro.[78] It was unusual that there was a doctor in the community; Dr Smith was there only because of the survey. Little Anna was the first case of smallpox. Where Fyfe referred to the case appearing in the home of 'preacher John', he was referring to Anna's grandfather, John Tizya, an important Anglican leader. Linklater recorded the case in his diary as well.[79] Linklater had been hired to feed the survey-party dogs. Essential in winter, the surveyors had little use for dogs in summer, but they still needed to be looked after. Linklater took the dogs to his fish camp and by the last week of July had fifteen in his care. But then, when he travelled back to Rampart House on 5 August, Linklater noted that he 'could not go in, it being in quarantine', so

[75] Neil McDonald in *People of the Lakes*, 133.

[76] See Dick North, *The Lost Patrol* (Anchorage: Alaska Northwest Pub. Co., 1978). James Falconer Fyfe was born in 1888 in Arbroath, Scotland and died in Seattle, WA on 29 Aug. 1919. See his obituary, 'Well Known Man Found Dead', *Douglas Island News*, 12 Sept. 1919.

[77] J. F. Fyfe to Officer Commanding, 6 Aug. 1911, RG 18, series A-1, vol. 532, file 206–17, LAC.

[78] Netro in *Rampart House*, 14.

[79] 23 Jul. 1911, Diary, Archibald (Archie) Linklater Fonds, MSS O/S 6 (95/30), YA [hereafter Linklater Diary].

he returned home to the fish camp.[80] In those early weeks of August, Linklater described the *Aurora* and the *Midnight Sun*, with Fyfe and Harry Anthony as guide, going up and down the river vaccinating people in all the fish camps. Then, on 17 August, Linklater's two-month-old boy, Archie Jr, got very sick. Archie and Catherine took the baby to Rampart House where he was diagnosed with smallpox. Two days later, Archie left the fish camp with the dogs, 'bound for quarantine island'. Another of his 'little ones got small pox', he noted.[81]

Archie Linklater spent the next two months on the quarantine island with his wife and four children. During all that time, he fed eight government dogs, as well as the dogs of all the families quarantined with him on the island, a number that grew from 65 on 20 August to a peak of 155 dogs and 11 pups in the first week of October. Thereafter, the numbers in quarantine subsided. For the most part, Linklater fished and fed the dogs. In late September, as the number of dogs on the island rose and the weather grew colder, Linklater had to shoot one of the survey-party horses 'for dog feed'.[82]

James Fyfe took photographs during the epidemic, including of the quarantine tents and hospital on a low-lying island in the river (Figure 6.3). Elder Stephen Frost Sr knew stories of the epidemic but expressed disbelief at the location of the hospital, 'you can see for yourself that island floods every year. I can't imagine a hospital there.'[83] Carpenters were brought in from Fort Yukon and began construction on the hospital on 21 September. Three weeks later, everyone was moved into the hospital, tents were set up for washing, and a dog yard built for the dogs and pups that Linklater was feeding.[84] As Hannah Netro shared, 'There was hardly any willows on that island and they built that hospital there. That's where they moved everybody and took care of them.'[85]

Families quarantined together on the island. Those who were healthy fished, snared rabbits, and packed firewood, work that kept them busy. There were at least four babies on the island, one of whom, Moses, died of smallpox on 7 September and was buried the same day. It was a source of criticism from the Gwich'in at the time and after that they were not permitted to gather for religious services on the island. Amos Njootli (John Ttssietla's son-in-law) had come from Fort McPherson to minister to the people at Rampart House during the epidemic.[86] As Sarah Abel recalled, 'While everyone was still staying on the island, the minister got there. The surveyors didn't want the minister to land at Rampart, so he was told to go [to]

80 Linklater Diary, 5 Aug. 1911. 81 Linklater Diary, 17–19 Aug. 1911.
82 Linklater Diary, 27 Sept.1911.
83 Stephen Frost Sr, interviewed by Shelagh Beairsto, in *Rampart House*, 21.
84 Linklater Diary, 21 Sept.–13 Oct. 1911; J. F. Fyfe to Officer Commanding, 6 Nov. 1911, RG 18, series A-1, vol. 532, file 206–17, LAC.
85 Netro in *Rampart House*, 14; significant growth of willows is a product of climate change and was also remarked on by Frost, p. 21.
86 Sarah Abel Chitzi, interviewed by Adeline Charlie, in *Rampart House*, 8.

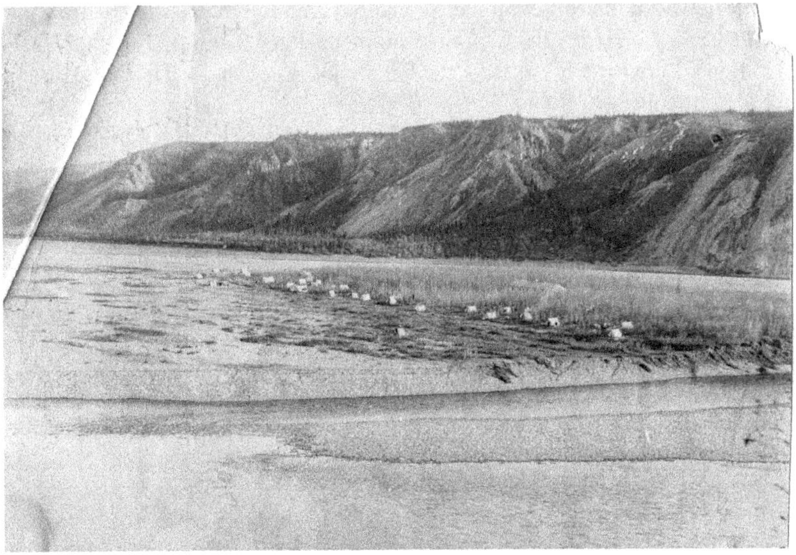

Figure 6.3 Quarantine island in the Porcupine River at Rampart House. The hospital is the long building visible behind the tents. Yukon Archives, James Fyfe fonds, 86/42, #64.

the island'. After the epidemic, Njootli complained to the DIA investigator about not being permitted to hold services. The death of baby Moses would have made religious services an urgent desire for the devout members of the community; three other babies were baptized three days later. Another baby, Ellen Bruce, was born in December 1911.[87] Hannah Netro noted that after the hospital was built, 'the doctor kept the mom and the baby separate (from the other patients), way at the other end of hospital somewhere. That way, the baby and mom didn't get sick.' Ellen Bruce went on to live a long, rich life, passing away in 2010 at the age of ninety-eight.

In addition to the quarantine island and hospital, Fyfe, Smith, and the survey party also established an isolation camp down the river, where those who wished to leave Rampart House would stay for two weeks before travelling on. Constable Fyfe with Dr Smith patrolled along the river to the Inuvialuit fish camps, where everyone was found to be healthy. Charles Whittaker at McPherson cancelled visits to Rampart House in October and again at Christmas on account of the outbreak.[88] Through the autumn and winter and

[87] Yukon Tourism and Culture, *Rampart House* (Whitehorse: Yukon Historic Sites, 2010), 6. See also Diocese of Yukon, Anglican Church of Canada, 'Ellen Bruce – Saint of the Month', https://anglican.yukon.net/ellen-bruce.html.

[88] St Matthew's Mission Journal, 2 Oct. 1911.

into the new year, patrols continued along the river. In December, a patrol went to Old Crow, to 'warn them against going to Peel River and to note their condition'. Fyfe posted bulletins 'in Indian and English on the various trails to notify travellers of the condition prevalent here and warning them to keep away from the infected district'.[89] While this work aimed to communicate to people, dispersed along the rivers and in camps, about the dangers of the outbreak at Rampart House, the level of surveillance of the Gwich'in and Inuvialuit was remarkable.

In August, Fyfe had reported to his commander that 'the Indians' who had been out hunting, 'are being sent in from the hills to be vaccinated, and so that they can be watched'.[90] In addition to the quarantine on the island and the isolation camp downriver to hold those who wished to leave, Fyfe also established 'detention camps back of the Indian village' to keep all of those who were not sick. With the assistance of Harry Anthony, 'I have seen that the camps are kept clean and that the natives give themselves frequent baths'.[91] Everyone in the camps was examined daily by the doctor. By early November, the last five people had been released from the detention camp, with no signs of disease. People released from detention or quarantine were first examined and then 'disinfected' with formaldehyde or bichloride of lime.[92] Linklater and Gwich'in men left the quarantine island in late October to hunt to feed the families who stayed behind. Even after leaving the island, Linklater remained subject to controls on his movement. He quarantined for two weeks over Christmas so that he could travel to Fort Yukon in the new year. He spent Christmas away from his family and celebrated with 'a dog salmon boiled' for dinner. On 1 January, he wrote 'this has been the dullest New Year's day I ever spent in my time'. But the next day, the doctor 'disinfected myself, clothing, bedding, dog harness, toboggan wrapper and dogs. Then I left, going to Fort Yukon at dark.'[93]

Those diagnosed with smallpox in the Yukon commonly had belongings destroyed, but in Rampart House this destruction was far more aggressive. Three days after the first case was diagnosed, Linklater noted 'they had the small pox tent and clothing burned'.[94] Because of the fear of fomite transmission, and the assumption that this was the source of the epidemic in Rampart House, Constable Fyfe went up to the confluence of the Porcupine and Old Crow rivers, the site of Old Crow, 'for the purpose of destroying infected camp sites and fumigating cabins', including John Tizya's cabin.[95] Fumigation (and what Linklater referred to as 'disinfecting' people) created health hazards and could

[89] F. T. Horrigan to Commissioner, 4 Mar. 1912, RG 18, series A-1, vol. 532, file 206–17, LAC.
[90] J. F. Fyfe to Officer Commanding, 11 Aug. 1911, RG 18, series A-1, vol. 532, file 206–17, LAC.
[91] J. F. Fyfe to Officer Commanding, 27 Aug. 1911, RG 18, series A-1, vol. 532, file 206–17, LAC.
[92] Fyfe to Officer Commanding, 6 Nov. 1911. [93] Linklater Diary, 25 Dec. 1911, 1–2 Jan. 1912.
[94] Linklater Diary, 25 Jul. 1911. [95] Fyfe to Officer Commanding, 15 Sept. 1911.

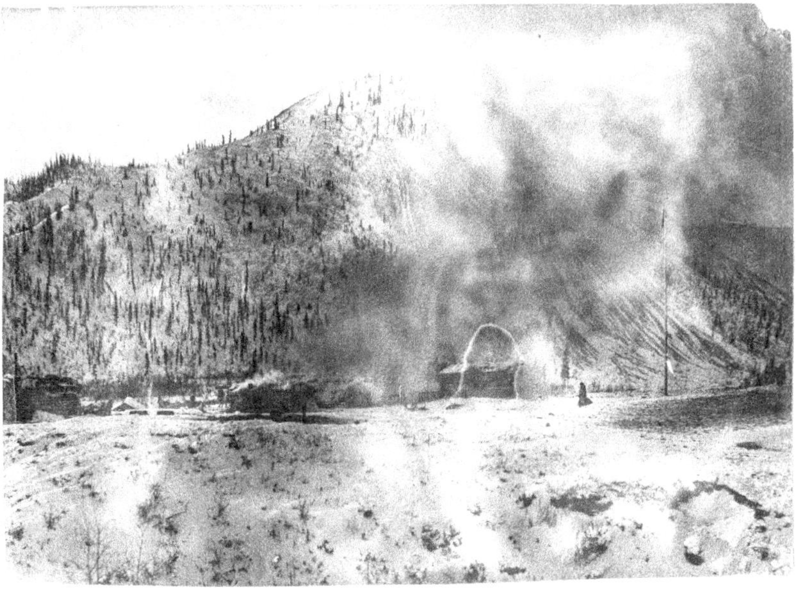

Figure 6.4 Two cabins burning at Rampart House, February 1912. Yukon Archives, James Fyfe fonds, 86/42, #60.

damage property. Chloride of lime, also called bleaching powder, could burn skin, was harmful if ingested or inhaled, and was not to be used as a powder in unvented areas (like a poorly ventilated cabin). Formaldehyde is a carcinogen that can cause death if ingested, while low-level exposure over long periods can cause respiratory problems and skin irritation. Sulphur was the least toxic to human bodies, although when burned it created an acrid smoke that irritated the eyes, mucous membranes, and skin and could cause permanent damage. It also stained belongings.

On the morning of February 5th, Archie Linklater spent the day at Rampart House before returning to his winter camp. While there he 'saw the cabins being burned' (Figure 6.4). In addition to what was destroyed at the outset of the epidemic, and then at the mouth of the Old Crow River in early September, this last measure was the most significant. As Constable Fyfe wrote to his superior, using the passive voice common to police reports, 'There have been twelve Indian cabins destroyed by fire.' Of course, this destruction was no accident. Rather, as Fyfe continued, this 'was the only possible method on account of their unsanitary condition and their danger of infection'.[96] As Charlie Peter Charlie remembered hearing from his mother, 'And then, they

[96] J. F. Fyfe to Officer Commanding, 1 Mar. 1912, RG 18, series A-1, vol. 532, file 206–17, LAC.

even burn people's houses. Too much of sickness in there so they burn it, I guess.'[97] Although there was no overt resistance to fumigation and property destruction by the state, the burning of homes in particular was a loss remembered for decades thereafter. Sarah Abel recalled how at the time of the outbreak, 'They (the people of Rampart House) now had log houses, and nice caches with everything that they needed like dog harnesses and toboggans. The surveyors burnt everything down; no one was allowed near the full caches of meat and they were all moved to the island.'[98] Abel emphasized the value and importance of this property, while Fyfe and the surveyors deemed Indigenous homes less sanitary and less valuable, which in turn made them targets for destruction. Fyfe captured the burning of the cabins at Rampart House in two photographs. One was captioned, 'Fire in Indian Camp in far north of Canada', as though that fire was not set by Fyfe himself. The framing might suggest that Fyfe wanted to distance himself from the decision to burn people's homes were it not for a second image, of a man posed in front of a burned-out building. The man in front of the building is not identified, but it may have been Fyfe or a member of the survey crew (Figure 6.5). The way the man is posed does not suggest any shame or ambivalence, rather the photograph is a souvenir. Although the image is blurred, the man is clearly smiling.

Once the snow was off the ground, Fyfe reported 'in Indian town the whole surface will be burned over. The disenfectant [*sic*] ordered by the doctor will be used on this place as an additional safeguard to prevent the spread of the disease.'[99] The hospital was burned down after all the patients were discharged and the epidemic had passed. Alice Frost, who heard stories about the epidemic from her grandmother Rachel Cadzow (Dan Cadzow's second wife), shared 'They said a big hospital was built on the island. They quarantined everything and everybody. Everybody was put on the island. They stayed there for a while, and then when everyone was okay, they moved everybody back. They burnt down the hospital after that.'[100] Hannah Netro also ended her story by noting that 'after everybody got well again, they burned the hospital down'.[101] The ephemerality of the hospital had meant that the poor choice of location did not matter. Its construction was about infection control (like the 'pest house' in Jackson Gulch) rather than the ongoing provision of medical care to the people of the northern Yukon.

In the end, there were ninety-eight cases of smallpox identified in Rampart House in the summer and autumn of 1911, and one death: Rachel's three-week-old

[97] Charlie Peter Charlie, interview by Veronica Germaine and Georgina Griffith, in *Rampart House*, 47.

[98] Abel in *Rampart House*, 8. [99] Fyfe to Officer Commanding, 1 Mar. 1912.

[100] Alice Frost, interview by Shelagh Beairsto, in *Rampart House*, 68.

[101] Netro in *Rampart House*, 14.

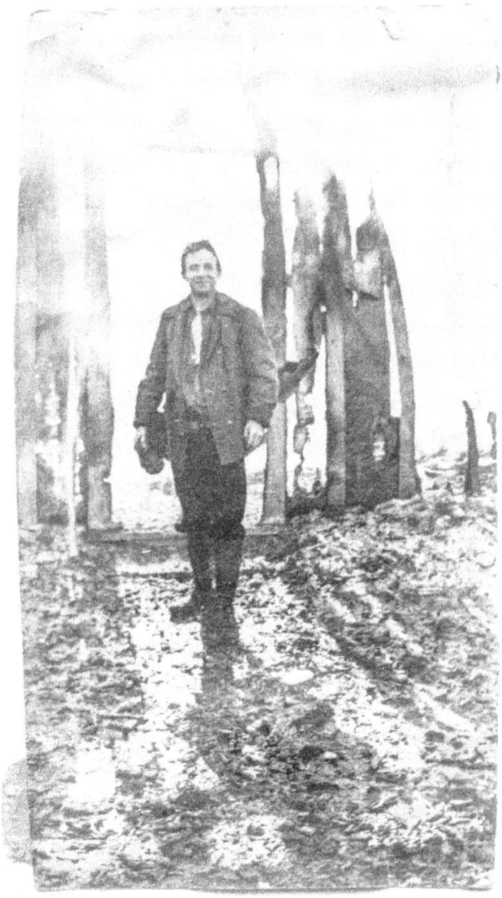

Figure 6.5 Man, possibly James Fyfe, posed in front of burned-out building. Yukon Archives, James Fyfe fonds, 86/42, #8.

baby, Moses. The initial outbreak in Dawson saw nineteen cases, no deaths, and far less restrictive measures than in Rampart House when it came to quarantine, surveillance, and detention. It would seem the significant disparity in cases between the two outbreaks was the degree to which the Dawson population was vaccinated, or otherwise previously exposed to smallpox, compared to the Rampart House population. Certainly, Dawsonites had been subject to general and even compulsory vaccination campaigns in 1900, 1906, and 1911. Many would have been vaccinated because of their occupation (not only police but transportation employees were vaccinated for preventive reasons) or previously exposed to smallpox in distant urban centres.[102] By 1908, immigrants from England to Canada were required to show proof by vaccination or previous infection.[103] Indigenous peoples in the Yukon, by comparison, were rarely targeted for smallpox vaccination. The general vaccination campaigns in 1900 and 1906 had paid no attention to Indigenous communities.[104] This changed in 1911. In addition to the sustained efforts to vaccinate Gwich'in, Inuvialuit, and others in the immediate vicinity of Rampart House, the outbreak prompted concern with vaccinating other Indigenous communities. In September 1911, Seymour Rowlinson in Carmacks wrote to the Commissioner about his (relatively unsuccessful) efforts to vaccinate the 'Big Lake Indians'.[105] In February 1912, the Dawson patrol carried vaccine supplies to Fort McPherson, and the local doctor proceeded to vaccinate everyone there as well.[106]

After they were released from the quarantine island, most Gwich'in families went back out on the land, where many caribou were now to be found. Fyfe did not expect their return until the river opened up in spring. The spring also saw RNWMP inspector Arthur E. Acland travel to the Yukon to assess Gilbert Smith's management of the epidemic on behalf of the DIA. Acland travelled up the Old Crow River with Charles Whittaker and D'Arcy Arden. 'Most of the Indians speak some English', wrote Acland, 'and I got all the information I could interviewing them as I found them along the Rivers.'[107] Acland asserted that from these interviews, the Gwich'in felt 'they had been well used and taken care of', although this ignored the complaints made by Njootli and others about restrictions on religious services. The course of the epidemic otherwise suggests that there was not strong resistance among the Gwich'in to the quarantine measures. The only people charged with disregard for the quarantine were two members of the survey party who failed to isolate before travelling to Fort Yukon, and who were convicted with $5,000 fines. The focus of Acland's investigation lay with Dr Smith and his 'general business management of the epidemic', which Acland concluded was 'very poor'. Acland found that Smith was apparently not well liked and demonstrated poor judgement. Specifically, 'he has kept no track of the goods received', and 'there were no written requisition for supplies'.[108] This meant that Gwich'in at Rampart House were not reimbursed for the destruction of their property, as they may have otherwise been (and as indigent

[102] N. E. Culbertson to Percy Reid, 17 May 1926, GOV 1677, file 6, YRG 1, Series 1, Central Registry Files, YA.
[103] Bashford, *Imperial Hygiene*, 38.
[104] Z. T. Wood to J. H. Ross, 20 May 1901, GOV 1677, vol. 67, file 7, YA.
[105] Seymour Rowlinson to Arthur Wilson, 30 Sept. 1911, GOV 1677, vol. 67, file 8 part 2, folder 1, YA.
[106] St Matthew's Mission Journal, 3 Feb. 1912.
[107] Acland to Officer Commanding, 27 Jun. 1912.
[108] Acland to Officer Commanding, 27 Jun. 1912.

patients elsewhere in the Yukon were).[109] Dan Cadzow did provide some replacement goods, and Elders were divided on whether Cadzow had profited or lost out financially in the epidemic.[110] The final criticism levied against Smith, and used to protect the Crown from having to pay him more money for his services, was that 'he continued the quarantine for an unjustifiable length of time'.[111] This conclusion was not used as a foundation to compensate the Gwich'in who had been subject to the quarantine measures. But it is telling that the government itself recognized that what amounted to over six months of quarantine was 'unjustifiable'.

The Gwich'in criticism of the handling of the epidemic came in a different form. For those who remembered the epidemic or who had heard stories from their family about their experiences in 1911–12, the outbreak was not smallpox. Neil McDonald said, 'It was chickenpox, not smallpox'.[112] Charlie Peter Charlie who heard about the epidemic from his mother, said, 'Yeah, smallpox, but not really, not strong one, I don't know. Maybe it's not even smallpox.'[113] Robert Bruce Sr (husband of Ellen Bruce) said, 'They say smallpox, but I don't know what they got now after I hear all the B.S.! They made all that up, most of it.'[114] Other histories, rooted in this evidence, call the diagnosis of smallpox into question.[115] We see here the distrust of government officials, rooted in this epidemic experience. In arguing that the disease was *not* smallpox, Gwich'in historical memory asserts that the measures taken were disproportionate to the threat the community faced. That assessment illuminates smallpox more clearly in colonial context.

As historians have long asserted, 'diseases exist as negotiated social phenomena that patients, doctors, and societies use to assign value and meaning to bodily phenomena'.[116] We see this negotiation at work in the histories of Rampart House in 1911. Gilbert Smith, an American physician placed in charge of managing the epidemic, appears to have viewed smallpox with the fear shared by many American and Canadian observers at this time: that the disease would spread viciously, that Indigenous people were disproportionately vulnerable to the pathogen, and that many would die. Smith

[109] J. D. Craig to W. F. King, 6 Aug. 1911, RG 18, series A-1, vol. 532, file 206–17, LAC.

[110] Sarah Abel maintained that Cadzow 'went broke, because of what the surveyors did to the people', p. 9, Charlie Peter Charlie said that Cadzow profited, p. 47, both in *Rampart House*.

[111] W. D. Hogg to A. E. Acland, 24 Mar. 1917, RG 18, series A-1, vol. 532, file 206–17, LAC.

[112] Neil McDonald in *People of the Lakes*, 133.

[113] Charlie Peter Charlie in *Rampart House*, 47.

[114] Robert Bruce Sr, interview by Lawrence Charlie, p. 52, see also Mary Kassi, interview by Angela Nukon, p. 58 both in *Rampart House*.

[115] Yukon Tourism and Culture, *Rampart House*, 6.

[116] Jones, *Rationalizing Epidemics*, 5; see also Andrew Cunningham, 'Transforming Plague: The Laboratory and the Identity of Infectious Disease', in Andrew Cunningham and Perry Williams, eds., *The Laboratory Revolution in Medicine* (Cambridge: University of Cambridge Press, 1992), 209–44.

originally described the disease as 'virulent, two [cases] being of the confluent type'.[117] After the death of baby Moses in September, Fyfe reported that 'as the cold weather will set in soon the Doctor expects to see more deaths'.[118] Northern Indigenous bodies in winter were assumed to be particularly vulnerable. But that was not what happened. Instead, while many people were infected, only one infant passed away. And Gwich'in Elders often emphasized the birth of Ellen Bruce during the epidemic, reinforcing how this episode was marked by life, survival, and endurance. Another account of smallpox that year, found in *I, Nuligak*, emphasized Indigenous resilience and expertise in a northern environment. Nuligak described how he and his Uncle Nuyaviak got sick with sores, 'all over our hips thighs and feet'. For relief from the sores they sat in the snow, which turned red with their blood. Nuligak concluded, 'We very nearly died. I believe that we had what the white men call smallpox. This frequent sitting in the snow cured us, healing our sores.'[119]

By the 1940s, most Van Tat Gwich'in and Dagoo had moved from Rampart House to Old Crow at the mouth of the Old Crow River, where John Tizya had his cabin in 1911.[120] Some families moved back across the border to Fort Yukon.[121] Old Crow had advantages. It had long been an important fishing site and was close to Crow Flats and good muskrat trapping. Rampart House and Old Crow both had access to good moose and caribou hunting, but at Rampart House there were steep banks that were 'hard to climb'.[122] By 1926, a church had been built at Old Crow. Then, in 1929, Dan Cadzow got sick and went to Dawson for treatment, dying there in St Mary's Hospital. 'Nobody took over' the store at Rampart House, according to Neil McDonald.[123] There were other trade posts at Old Crow, Whitestone Village, Johnson Creek, Lapierre House, and Fort Yukon where people could get what they needed. So there were a variety of reasons why people left Rampart House that speak to the fluid geographies of this period. But the epidemic of 1911 had its own role to play. Some Elders spoke of the enforcement of the international border and the presence of the police as a reason why they left Rampart House. Although game wardens did not arrive in the community right away, by the

117 Fyfe to Officer Commanding, 11 Aug. 1911.
118 J. F. Fyfe to Officer Commanding, 7 Sept. 1911, RG 18, series A-1, vol. 532, file 206–17, LAC.
119 Nuligak, *I, Nuligak*, 84–7, quotation p. 87.
120 Bruce Sr in *Rampart House*, 53; Vuntut Gwitchin First Nation and Smith, *People of the Lakes*, 154–5.
121 Kassi in *Rampart House*, 57–8; also J. J. Hillard to G. A. Jeckell, 26 Aug. 1939, Gov 1619 1490J file 3, YRG 1, Series 1, Vol. 9, YA.
122 Frost Sr in *Rampart House,* 22.
123 Cadzow's death is recorded online in the 'Dawson City Mortuary Records 1898–1938', www.alaskaweb.org/dawmort/c_d.html; Neil McDonald in *People of the Lakes*, 134–5.

late 1920s they patrolled the area to keep Gwich'in hunters from crossing the border freely.[124] As Hannah Netro put it:

> the surveyors . . . made a border line with the horses. That's another reason for us to move to Old Crow. The people, they had difficulties hunting and trapping. They shoot caribou on this side, but really they were on the American side. . . . They move to Old Crow where it's easier. There's more freedom (in Old Crow) for them to do whatever they need to do to survive.[125]

In Rampart House, Ben Kassi's home was twenty-five metres from the boundary monument, Archie Linklater's about seventy-five. The history of the boundary and the survey was also the history of the smallpox epidemic, when the police first came to Rampart House and closely watched everyone's movements, controlling their actions, and destroying their valuable property. If narratives of the mild epidemic at Rampart House, the birth of Ellen Bruce, and the survival of Nuligak and his uncle are smallpox counter-narratives, so too is the way that the epidemic served to realize police and state control on the ground.

You Have No Brains!

In late June 1921, after watching Albert LeBeau's trial for murder at Fort Providence, RCMP inspector George Frederick Fletcher continued on his patrol through the southern Mackenzie. In addition to the treaty party, Fletcher noted, 'there has been a great deal of travel into the country this year, that is for the North'. There were people working with Imperial Oil and headed to the finds at Norman Wells, there were geologists, oilstakers, prospectors for gold, and a large party of Dominion surveyors.[126] Among those who came north was acting secretary of the NWT, O. S. Finnie, based at Fort Smith that summer to attend to government business. In mid-July, anticipating that Fort Smith would become the administrative headquarters of the NWT, Finnie spent a few days selecting lots overlooking the Slave River, 'for the future requirements of the Department'. They were, he noted, 'excellent sites'.[127] Amid the bustle and excitement of opportunity in the North, there were reports of sickness. Fletcher observed that, 'the Indians have been suffering from a very severe form of cold all down the River'; only the community of Fort Liard appeared in good health. Moreover, 'a

[124] Clara Tizya in *People of the Lakes*, 241; J. Hawksley to J. D. McLean, 28 Mar. 1927, Gov 1619 1490J, file 3, YA; J. Hawksley to H. Reed, 24 Jan. 1931, Gov 1619 1490J, file 2, YRG 1, Series 1, vol. 9, YA; J. J. Van Bibber, *I Was Born under a Spruce Tree*, comp. Niall Fink (Vancouver: Talus Publishing, 2012), ch. 10.

[125] Netro in *Rampart House*, 15.

[126] G. F. Fletcher to Officer Commanding, 19 Sept. 1921, June Helm Fonds, N-2002–021, box 3, file 'RCMP Patrol Reports 1919–21', NWTA.

[127] O. S. Finnie to W. W. Cory, 26 Jul. 1921, RG 85, series C-1-a, vol. 585, file 578, reel T-13213, LAC.

light form of smallpox, or chicken pox' had broken out at Fort Smith, Fort Fitzgerald, and Fort Resolution.[128]

Smallpox had been on the increase in southern and central Alberta since 1918.[129] In early February 1921, the Anglican missionary reported 'news of smallpox at [Fort] MacKay'. A 'mild case' appeared in Fort Chipewyan on 28 March, and by late April there were ten cases in the village.[130] Smallpox spread through the spring. By June, Isabel Gibson, the missionary's wife and a nurse in her own right, was vaccinating people in Fort Chipewyan.[131] Around that time, the SS *MacMurray* arrived and was prohibited from landing. With the arrival of the treaty party at the end of the month, Rev. William Gibson noted in the mission diary, 'the doctor investigates Smallpox'. On 28 June 1921, 'smallpox found to be very bad Chipewyan quarantined for 15 days'.[132] As it was, the outbreak in Fort Chipewyan was nearing its end, and the new restrictions were akin to closing the barn door after the horse had bolted. Most of the community had been vaccinated, but the day school closed for the rest of the summer, while the Roman Catholics quarantined the residential-school children on Goose Island, nineteen kilometres from the mission.[133] Two RCMP officers arrived to maintain the village quarantine. The province sent a nurse to Fort Chipewyan in early June, and in mid-July they sent a doctor. Gibson's last record of a smallpox case came on 14 July.

What made the smallpox 'mild' in April but 'very bad' in June? The virulence of the pathogen did not shift over the course of the outbreak, and there was no increase in mortality. What changed was that the scale of the outbreak became clear when Dr George Ings, with the Treaty 11 party, confirmed that the disease was smallpox. MacDonald, the government physician at Fort Smith, had diagnosed the first cases as chicken pox and let a sick riverboat pilot travel on from Hay River.[134] The misdiagnosis allowed smallpox to spread widely through the southern Mackenzie, from Fort Chipewyan to Fort Resolution, Fort Smith, and to smaller communities like Fort Fitzgerald, Hay River, and Jackfish Lake, before significant control measures were taken.[135]

Finnie appointed Ings as temporary MHO for the southern Mackenzie. Ings rushed through Fort Smith on his way back home to Fort McMurray, visiting 'only a few of the smallpox patients in the Settlement. He was at the hospital only about

[128] Fletcher to Officer Commanding, 19 Sept. 1921. [129] McCormack, *Fort Chipewyan*, 269.

[130] 28 Apr. 1921, Daily Journal of Activities – St Paul's – Fort Chipewyan, Anglican Diocese of Athabasca, Acc. A. 13, item 11, box 14, PAA [hereafter St Paul's Daily Journal].

[131] Rutherdale, *Women and the White Man's God*, 114–15.

[132] St Paul's Daily Journal, 27 Jun. 1921; 'River Boats Making Good Time North', *Edmonton Bulletin*, 21 July 1921.

[133] Bishop Grouard to Charles Stewart, 10 Aug. 1922, RG 15, vol. 1123, reel T-14684, file 3460900, LAC.

[134] This was not the only questionable diagnosis that MacDonald made. See Piper, 'Diphtheria Antitoxin', 303.

[135] L. M. Lloyd-Walters to Officer Commanding, 31 Aug. 1921, RG 85, series C-1-a, vol. 585, file 578, reel T-13213, LAC.

five minutes', wrote Finnie. Perhaps Ings's greatest omission was that he failed to vaccinate any government officials during his stopover. The nursing sisters at the hospital and the RCMP officer criticized Ings's handling of the outbreak in Smith. Finnie wrote describing his disappointment: 'Had I not already recommended him for Health Officer, I would not do so now.'[136] And in a separate letter, Finnie concluded, 'if Dr. Ings's duty is to look after the epidemic at Fort Smith, he has failed absolutely'.[137] The problem was not just Ings, but that MacDonald – the physician normally stationed at Fort Smith – spent the summer travelling with the Treaty 8 party, 'so we have been entirely without medical assistance', observed Finnie. This was common in the Mackenzie. That summer, there were actually more doctors in the district than usual. In addition to MacDonald and Ings, there was Richardson at Norman Wells (MHO for the area between Fort Simpson and Good Hope) and Philip Doyle, a police surgeon in the delta. Before leaving Fort Smith in early September, Finnie got a taste for the failures of care in the territory that he helped to administer.

Infection-control measures were similar in 1921 as compared to a decade earlier in the Yukon: isolation, quarantine, and vaccination. By mid-July, with twenty cases in the community, the hospital at Fort Smith was full, treating women and 'the more serious cases'.[138] Men convalesced in tents on the hospital grounds. In Fort Chipewyan, Jenny Flett remembered five to six people to a tent and three tents in total.[139] At Fort Resolution, the sick were removed to a camp on a nearby island. Less serious cases, who did not require medical attention, quarantined in their own homes. Everywhere, food was an issue.[140] Initially, there was hope that everyone in the district could be vaccinated to prevent the epidemic from spreading. But there was a shortage of vaccines. Finnie placed an order in mid-July that did not arrive until early September, after he had left for the south. Adolph Mercredi remembered that his family had been vaccinated, except him (and he fell ill).[141] Moreover, during the outbreak, vaccines went first to people in the posts and only after to people who lived on the land. When Ings returned to Fort Smith in late August, he vaccinated the nursing sisters at the hospital and 'whatever Indians and halfbreeds that were in the settlement'.[142]

In total, there were around 100 cases in the southern Mackenzie, with forty-three at Fort Smith and thirty-seven in Fort Chipewyan. The other communities

136 Finnie to Cory, 26 Jul. 1921.

137 O. S. Finnie to J. P. Dunne, 10 Aug. 1921, RG 85, series C-1-a, vol. 585, file 578, reel T-13213, LAC.

138 Lloyd-Walters to Officer Commanding, 31 Aug. 1921.

139 McCormack, *Fort Chipewyan,* 270.

140 See food lists 15 July, 21 July, and 31 September 1921, and Lloyd-Walters to Officer Commanding, 31 Aug. 1921 in RG 85, series C-1-a, vol. 585, file 578, reel T-13213, LAC.

141 Adolph Mercredi, interview with J. Overvold, 4 Feb. 1977, Yellowknife, N-1992–084, Metis Heritage Association Fonds, NWTA [hereafter MHAF].

142 Lloyd-Walters to Officer Commanding, 31 Aug. 1921.

had fewer than ten cases each. Six deaths were attributed to the epidemic.[143] The deaths included two elderly Indigenous women in Fort Smith who, like baby Moses at Rampart House, were the people most vulnerable to infectious disease. Adolph Mercredi, at Fond du Lac and Fort Chipewyan in 1921–2, remembered 'old timers' died from smallpox and a subsequent flu outbreak discussed in Chapter 7.[144] Jenny Flett remembered that those who died of smallpox in Fort Chipewyan were wrapped in grey blankets and buried in the lakeshore cemetery.[145] The Oblate missionary at Fort Resolution wrote in November that he had tallied thirty-two deaths in the community since January, more than in recent years. He attributed the excess deaths to smallpox and diphtheria.[146] That both diseases appeared that summer can be tied to the increase in visitor traffic described by Inspector Fletcher. Nevertheless, in the words of one RCMP officer, 'the percentage of deaths has been amazingly low'.[147] The disparity between expectations about the severity of smallpox and the course of the epidemic reflect the persistent cultural assumptions about the vulnerability of Indigenous bodies to smallpox.

After 1921, smallpox rarely appeared again in the Yukon or the Mackenzie district. In 1932, reports from Vancouver and the Pacific Coast prompted the MHO to require all passengers arriving in Whitehorse by train or otherwise to 'submit to vaccination for smallpox, unless they can produce a certificate of recent vaccination'. These measures were in place for less than two weeks, and fourteen people were vaccinated before the provisions were cancelled.[148] Possibly the last archival record of a smallpox outbreak comes from Great Bear Lake in 1936. In the Codex Historicus kept at Tulita, the Oblate missionary noted that the police had declared that a sickness among the Sahtu Dene was smallpox and placed them in quarantine for fifteen days. During that time, the Dene went hungry, 'because that police officer had them locked up in Franklin'. One Dene man who spoke out in protest of the restrictions told the police constable, 'You have no brains!'[149] The Oblate missionary also felt the police response was disproportionate to the threat posed by smallpox, given his description of the event. This again showed the gulf between the response of the colonial state to smallpox and the lived experience of

[143] O. S. Finnie to W. W. Cory, 18 Jul. 1921, RG 85, series C-1-a, vol. 585, file 578, reel T-13213, LAC; Indian Agent Card's Diary, Annuity Payments, 1921 as cited in Fumoleau, *As Long as This Land Shall Last*, 139.

[144] Mercredi interview, MHAF. [145] McCormack, *Fort Chipewyan*, 269–70.

[146] A. Duport to G. Breynat, 26 Nov. 1921, PR1997.0109/1582, reel #14, PAA.

[147] R. Field to Commissioner, 13 Sept. 1921, RG 85, series C-1-a, vol. 585, file 578, reel T-13213, LAC.

[148] Re: Yukon Health Ordinance, 26 Mar. 1932, GOV 1843 251, part 2, YRG 1, Series 2 Central Registry Files, YA.

[149] Codex Historicus, Fort Norman, Mar. 1936 (1935–40), pg. 6, PR1997.0109/2022, box 91, OMI, PAA.

Indigenous northerners with that disease, one of the least fatal that they had encountered since the arrival of Euro-Canadians on their lands.

Chasing Out Catherine

Public health regulations give the force of law to intrusions in people's private lives. Concern about smallpox, combined with the role of the RCMP as the arm of colonial power in the North, meant that hunters could be locked up or families quarantined for months on an island and their possessions burned, all justified in the interests of public health. Ideas about race contoured public health responses and the ways in which smallpox outbreaks realized police and state control over the daily lives of people living in the Yukon and Mackenzie district. In a patriarchal colonial state, gender also has a significant role to play. Nowhere was this more apparent than in the control of sexually transmitted infections. A case study from the southern Mackenzie district, involving a Métis woman and her sister, whom I refer to as Catherine and Eliza, offers insight into gender dynamics as part of the history of health, care, and colonization of the Northwest Territories.[150] Catherine's experience with Clermont Bourget in Fort Resolution further illustrates the character of colonialism in the small hamlets and posts of the North, where a handful of men held enormous power over the legal, medical, and educational institutions under construction by the state. Some used the implementation of public health measures and the surveillance and control of intimate lives to advance their own interests and pursue their own vendettas. That race and gender shaped experiences with these nascent institutions in these tiny communities is readily apparent not only in Catherine's case, but also in the experiences of Peter Baker, a Christian from Lebanon who came to the Northwest Territories in 1907. Baker, like Catherine, found himself at odds with those who wielded colonial power in the southern Mackenzie and was threatened with deportation. Baker ended up before 'a kangaroo court' that found him guilty 'on a trumped-up charge of knowingly receiving stolen property' and received a six-month suspended sentence.[151] These experiences deepen our understanding of the kind of communities that many colonizers endeavoured to construct in the North.

Born at Nishì (Old Fort Rae) in the 1890s, Catherine attended residential school at Fort Resolution then married an HBC trader. The couple had no children and, by the early 1920s, Catherine had left her husband and was 'maintaining herself' in Fort Resolution. In January 1924, Catherine was convicted of vagrancy – a charge used to arrest a person for prostitution – and sentenced to three months' hard labour. After she arrived at the RCMP guard

[150] 'Catherine' and 'Eliza' are pseudonyms. I have excluded details that could be used to identify the women.

[151] Peter Baker, *Memoirs of an Arctic Arab: A Free Trader in the Canadian North: The Years 1907–1927* (Yellowknife: Yellowknife Pub. Co., 1976), 65–6; Ray, *Industrial Age*, 163–6.

room in Resolution, Dr Bourget examined her, and 'she was found to be suffering from Venereal disease'.[152] During her sentence, Catherine worked for the RCMP doing general housework and sewing dog shoes to protect their paws when they pulled sleds across the ice. She was also taken regularly to Bourget at the mission hospital for treatment for gonorrhea.[153] Bourget's bill for $95 came due after she was released from the Fort Resolution guardroom in April, and her estranged husband agreed to pay it a few months later.[154] In February 1930, Catherine and her husband were again living apart when she was convicted a second time, now under section 307 of the Criminal Code for knowingly communicating a venereal disease. Two Métis men gave evidence against her.[155] With Bourget as Justice of the Peace, Catherine was sentenced to six months' imprisonment with hard labour, the maximum penalty. In delivering his sentence, Bourget emphasized that 'he would use every endeavour to have the accused sent to some institution outside where she could receive proper treatment for gonorrhea'.[156]

Although Bourget presented this as an issue of 'proper treatment', the idea of removing Catherine from the Northwest Territories stemmed foremost from a desire to see her deported (much like HBC manager Willy Lyall wanted Baker deported). As a sexually active woman living apart from her husband, Catherine was perceived as immoral, a bad influence, and a threat to community health.[157] In 1924, Inspector H. L. Fraser had said as much in his report on Catherine and her sister Eliza.[158] Fraser raised concerns about the spread of venereal disease 'in a country where Doctors are scarce, and where so many people are already suffering from Tuberculosis'. He recognized the failures of healthcare in the Mackenzie district. But his next comment was that 'the influence of these women is having a very detrimental effect on the morals, not only of the men, but also of the young Indian girls in the District'. Eliza, 'has no visible means of subsistence', reported Fraser, 'is an equally dissolute character, and should be charged under the same section, but she has seven children – all illegitimate, and is about to be confined again'. He concluded with a strong recommendation that 'if possible, steps be taken to remove both of these women from this neighbourhood to some place where proper supervision can be kept over their action as they are a menace to the life and health of the community here'.[159] In their surveillance of two women, 'not men in the circulation of the disease and the regulation of sex',

152 H. L. Fraser to Officer Commanding, 16 Jul. 1924, RG 85, vol. 751, file 4535, LAC.

153 Jan.–Apr. 1924, 'G' Division, Fort Resolution Journals, RG 18-C-6, vol. 3470, LAC.

154 G. F. Fletcher to Officer Commanding, 12 Aug. 1924, RG 85, vol. 751, file 4535, LAC.

155 J. Clifford, Crime Report, 3 Feb. 1930, RG 85, vol. 751, file 4535, LAC.

156 Clifford, 3 Feb. 1930.

157 See Sarah Carter, *The Importance of Being Monogamous: Marriage and Nation-Building in Western Canada to 1915* (Edmonton: University of Alberta Press, 2008), 15, *passim*.

158 Fraser to Officer Commanding, 16 Jul. 1924. In that year, communicating venereal disease was a crime under Section 316A of the Criminal Code.

159 Fraser to Officer Commanding, 16 Jul. 1924.

state officials in the NWT acted consistently in policing female sexuality as elsewhere in imperial context.[160]

Catherine and Eliza were both 'natives of the Territories, and could not, therefore, be deported to wherever they came from', in the opinion of the department solicitor.[161] Officials investigated whether they could remove Eliza's children.[162] O. S. Finnie thought the best solution was that the children 'might be looked after by the Salvation Army, or placed in charge of a nunnery at Government expense'. Such action required legislation for the NWT to address 'deserted wives' and 'illegitimate children', and Finnie directed that ordinances to this effect be prepared.[163] Eliza fades from the archival record after 1924. It appears that her children were not apprehended in the absence of existing legislation that provided for their removal. We see in this brief moment the ways that public health could trigger the desire for greater state control over northern lives and bodies, as well as its failures to follow through.

When Catherine came before the court again in 1930, Bourget was determined to have her removed. His efforts made little headway. Finnie considered 'the expense of bringing this woman to Edmonton would no doubt be quite high'.[164] Moreover, notwithstanding Bourget's claim that Catherine needed 'hospital treatment for venereal disease until rendered harmless', the treatment available in Edmonton was the same that she had access to in Resolution, specifically, regular administration of urotropine (a urinary antiseptic) and liquor sedans (a 'utero-ovarian sedative' and painkiller).[165] While liquor sedans was an older therapy derived from various plants indigenous to the Americas (Black Haw, Jamaica Dogwood, and Hydrastis or Goldenseal), urotropine was a more recently formulated chemical therapy combining ammonia and formaldehyde. In a wire to Bourget declining to remove Catherine, Finnie observed that 'if as you state there is an epidemic of venereal disease in your district the sending of one case out of the country will obviously not be of much effect'.[166]

In the year that followed, Bourget used health and expense (he argued that it was cheaper 'in the long run' to have Catherine sent to Edmonton) as cover

[160] Bashford, *Imperial Hygiene*, 167.
[161] K. R. Daly to O. S. Finnie, 12 Sept. 1924, RG 85, vol. 751, file 4535, LAC.
[162] Daly to Finnie, 12 Sept. 1924.
[163] O. S. Finnie to W. W. Cory, 1 Oct. 1924, RG 85, vol. 751, file 4535, LAC. The correspondence ends here, no ordinance was passed; see H. H. Rowatt, *Ordinances of the Northwest Territories Passed by the Northwest Territories Council from 1905 to 1930* (Ottawa: F.A. Acland, 1931).
[164] O. S. Finnie to D. C. Scott, 10 Feb. 1930, RG 85, vol. 751, file 4535, LAC.
[165] Bills for payment, March–August 1930, RG 85, vol. 751, file 4535, LAC; Hannah Landecker, 'Antimicrobials before Antibiotics: War, Peace, and Disinfectants', *Palgrave Communications* 5, no. 45 (2019), https://doi.org/10.1057/s41599-019-0251-8; also advertisement for liquor sedans in *British Medical Journal* no. 3314 (5 Jul. 1924); n.a., *Manual of Therapeutics* (Detroit: Parke, Davis, and Company, 1909), 405.
[166] O. S. Finnie, telegram to C. Bourget, 19 Feb. 1930, RG 85, vol. 751, file 4535, LAC.

for what was a moral argument. Treating Catherine in 1930 was more expensive than in 1924 because, in the first instance, Bourget's decision to sentence her to six not three months' imprisonment had doubled the cost of her care. Moreover, in 1930, in addition to medicine and doctor's visits, a matron – the wife of RCMP Sergeant J. Clifford – was tasked with looking after Catherine. A 'white woman' had been deemed necessary to cook, clean, and provide nursing care.[167] A. E. Acland (the same official who investigated the epidemic at Rampart House) forwarded Clifford's report on his wife's work, noting, 'This is just another of those cases where members of the Force and their families have to step in and take over very unpleasant duties that no one else wishes to perform.'[168] The treatment and care for people sick with sexually transmitted infections had long been compromised by the intimate nature of these infections, and the context in which they are transmitted, as well as the prevailing moral ideologies that can outweigh concern for health.[169] In Catherine's case, Bourget – like Fraser before him – made explicitly moral arguments about the need to remove her from the territory. In a long letter to Finnie written in February 1931, Bourget repeatedly argued about the moral value of removing Catherine in deterring others 'who were more or less following her path'.[170]

In 1931, faced with the bills for the matron, the medicine, and the doctor's care, Finnie looked into the possibilities for removing Catherine from the NWT. In writing to Dr J. J. Heagerty with the Department of National Health about the matter, Finnie noted that his branch 'wishes to control the spread of communicable diseases so far as it is possible to do so, not forgetting, however, that this must be done without incurring a large expenditure of public funds'. In this letter, Finnie noted that at a provincial institution, a patient like Catherine, 'will receive proper care and treatment under more favourable conditions than those prevailing in the North West Territories'.[171] In writing to the Alberta Attorney General's office, Finnie further noted the precedent whereby people from the Mackenzie district 'adjudged insane, are treated in the Provincial Mental Hospital at Ponoka, Alta'.[172] Through this correspondence, Finnie was able to ascertain that Catherine could be sent to the provincial jail at Fort Saskatchewan, which had 'excellent facilities' for treating venereal disease.[173]

167 J. Clifford to Officer Commanding, 13 Jan. 1931 and C. Bourget to O. S. Finnie, 9 Feb. 1931, RG 85, vol. 751, file 4535, LAC.

168 A. E. Acland to the Commissioner, 17 Jan. 1931, RG 85, vol. 751, file 4535, LAC.

169 Jay Cassel, *The Secret Plague: Venereal Disease in Canada 1838–1939* (Toronto: University of Toronto Press, 1987), 8–9.

170 Bourget to Finnie, 9 Feb. 1931.

171 O. S. Finnie to J. J. Heagerty, 6 Mar. 1931, RG 85, vol. 751, file 4535, LAC.

172 O. S. Finnie to G. B. Henwood, 10 Apr. 1931, RG 85, vol. 751, file 4535, LAC.

173 M. R. Bow to J. J. Heagerty, 13 Mar. 1931; Finnie to Henwood, 10 Apr. 1931, both RG 85, vol. 751, file 4535, LAC.

Catherine avoided relocation to Fort Saskatchewan because she completed her sentence before Finnie finished his inquiries. But the last document in her file is chilling. In December 1932, over a year after Finnie had determined that she could be sent out of the territory on the grounds of disease treatment, and over two years after her release from prison, the MHO at Fort Smith, Dr J. M. Morrow, sent a police patrol to Salt River to bring her to the Fort Smith hospital for examination. Catherine had been living at Salt River for over a year.[174] What prompted the patrol at this moment in time is not explained in the documents. There is no record of a complaint. When Dr Morrow examined her, he 'cannot say at present whether this woman has the disease, and we cannot up to the date of reporting obtain any evidence of her having communicated this disease'.[175] Catherine's file ends there.

We should not take Clifford's, or Fraser's, or Bourget's characterizations of Catherine and Eliza as gospel. In addition to the racism so blatant in all of these communications, Bourget was also a fervent Catholic. Catherine, a young French-speaking Métis woman educated in the Catholic residential school, drew his particular ire. Bourget considered himself as the pinnacle of Fort Resolution society. He wrote as much in his self-published memoirs (titled *Douze ans chez les sauvages*), contrasting life among the 'official class' in Fort Smith (where 'everyone thought they were called to administer, and as a result, social life was extremely strained') to Fort Resolution, where 'I at least had the pleasure of being alone and, after putting (in the figurative sense) my boot in the right place to whoever deserved it, I was king and master'.[176] Bourget, after all, was Indian Agent, Medical Officer of Health, coroner, school inspector, and Justice of the Peace.[177] The nuns and priests at the Oblate mission and school considered his family 'exemplary', favoured his daughter Yvette (the only white child at the school), called him 'the good doctor', and went out of their way to support him in his work.[178] And Bourget did not like Catherine.

There is other evidence in the archival record about Catherine and her sister that can bring these women and their experiences further into the light. Notwithstanding Fraser's hostile description of Eliza and her purportedly large, illegitimate family, others felt differently. In 1921, H. A. Conroy signed a note in Eliza's scrip file strongly recommending 'that the grant be allowed for both the applicant and her child, as she is a hardworking woman, not living the Indian mode of life'.[179] The application was paid in 1924 with Dr Bourget, now in his

174 C. Bourget to O. S. Finnie, 9 Feb. 1931, RG 85, vol. 751, file 4535, LAC.
175 RCMP report, 6 Dec. 1932, RG 85, vol. 751, file 4535, LAC.
176 Bourget, *Douze ans*, 32–3.
177 Bourget, *Douze ans*, 34; Fumoleau, *As Long as This Land Shall Last*, 172 – Gerald Card at Fort Smith in 1920 had a similarly long list of responsibilities.
178 See Vanast, 'Arctic Bodies', 117–21.
179 H.A. Conroy, 31 Dec. 1921, RG 15, series D-II-8-d, vol. 1372, reel C-15011, file ******, ******, LAC.

role as Indian Agent, signing the receipts. Catherine also received her scrip payment from Bourget, just months after her release from the guardroom at Fort Resolution. In spite of himself, Bourget's descriptions give us greater insight into Catherine as well. In a 1931 letter to Finnie, Bourget observed that Catherine had 'at times . . . enough money by alleged genuine work that vagrancy could not even be a charge against her'.[180] In that same letter, he also made grand claims about the disorder that would invariably come to pass, should she not be controlled.[181] Had Catherine returned to Resolution in the summer of 1931, Bourget would have done something about it, given how closely he kept an eye on Catherine and sought to control her. It is telling that none of this came to pass.

There is a photograph of Catherine, taken in 1920, of a beautiful, well-dressed young woman with a gentle smile and a shawl over her head and dress. We know that she worked hard and supported herself. She had no children, possibly because of the effects of the gonorrhea or its treatment. The combination of urotropine and liquor sedans that she received in 1930 was very painful; Catherine had to stay in bed for a week each time she received these therapies.[182] And we know that Catherine had relationships with men, mostly Métis, some of which were longer than others, before moving to Salt River in 1931. Her decision to move to Salt River was possibly to put distance between herself and Bourget without being forced to leave the lands where she was born. Catherine knew, because Bourget said as much when he delivered his sentence, that he wanted her removed to the south. For both Catherine and Eliza, their status as Métis women, neither 'Indian' nor white, and in Catherine's case, her education at the residential school, made them more vulnerable in Fort Resolution. This status shaped expectations that they were supposed to represent what southern 'civilization' could bring to the North. Bourget did not want Catherine making Resolution – where he was 'king and master' – her home. Bourget wielded enormous power in the colonial society created in the Mackenzie district and, in the case of Catherine, and in the context of her illness, Bourget used this power against her.

Conclusions

The history of smallpox in the Yukon and Mackenzie district is a history of control: the effective control of an infectious pathogen and intensifying colonial control over northern lands and bodies. Northerners were fortunate that, by the time smallpox found its way to their communities, carried in the flood of people who came in search of gold, oil, and furs, the pathogens that arrived were markedly less virulent than in the past. That was by chance. But from that

[180] Bourget to Finnie, 9 Feb. 1931. [181] Bourget to Finnie, 9 Feb. 1931.
[182] Bourget to Finnie, 9 Feb. 1931.

circumstance flowed a very different history of smallpox in the North, one where the very identity of the disease was called into question. Smallpox deaths hardly appear in burial registers and other sources. There were a handful of deaths attributed to that disease, in 1900, 1911, and 1921–2, but fewer than diphtheria, dysentery, or whooping cough at this time (not to mention the far more serious infectious diseases: influenza, tuberculosis, or pneumonia). Meghan Highet in her analysis of the Yukon territorial death register made a similar observation: she found no deaths attributed to smallpox in the Yukon between 1898 and 1904, in contrast to the significant newspaper coverage of the disease and official correspondence about it in that same period.[183] We have to account, then, for the discrepancy between seriousness of the disease (as measured by mortality), compared to the degree of concern and intervention.

Pathogens scare us because they appear as actors beyond our control, driven by their own needs, and wholly indifferent to our pain. Colonial narratives of smallpox married this viral indifference to what were perceived as vulnerable Indigenous bodies and thence came the supposed unintentional devastation of contact-era epidemics, disproportionately borne by the colonized. As smallpox changed, these colonial narratives and anxieties did not. This dissonance produced the smallpox that was not in Rampart House: an outbreak, six months of quarantine, detention camps, an isolation hospital, cabins and caches burned to the ground, and yet only one death of a little baby. Not to diminish that loss, which was surely deeply felt, but community memories emphasized instead a birth (of Ellen Bruce). And the response at Rampart House was, in the words of the government itself, 'unjustifiable'.

The smallpox epidemic at Rampart House was a product of a hastily constructed, reactionary public health infrastructure: governed by a remote state, implemented by police, missionaries, and local officials, which focused on isolation, quarantine, surveillance, sanitation, and vaccination to bring the threat of smallpox under control. This health infrastructure was, as Finnie himself experienced in 1921, inadequate to the task. Again, northerners were fortunate that smallpox arrived when it did – weak and unable to wreak the anticipated havoc. This infrastructure, hastily erected as it was, still served a valuable purpose. Vaccination especially helped to keep smallpox in check. These public health measures also helped community members deal with the other infectious pathogens – diphtheria, typhoid, and scarlet fever – that now appeared more frequently at their doorstep. But this infrastructure was also a tool of settler colonial power that could be deployed unevenly depending on race and gender. There is no better example of the arbitrary exercise of power, drawing on tools intended to control infectious disease, then the experience of Catherine.

[183] Highet, 'Gold Fever', 114–15.

7 Experiences of Influenza

Northern Elders often spoke of sickness as 'flu', referring in a general way to what we might also identify as infectious respiratory illness. Yet the use of 'flu' in oral histories contained within it other elements: of change over time in the experience of sickness, of severity, and of the role of trade posts in the spread of disease. Julienne Andre, in Chapter 3, recalled her childhood, when 'we travelled all year from spring through the fall and nobody got the flu or cold'.[1] George Vittrekwa also shared stories from a time 'before the flu disease came to this country'.[2] Michel Grandjambe, who grew up on the land by Fort Good Hope, testified at the Berger Inquiry how 'the men used to go to the settlement for groceries at Christmas time and Easter. We had no worries, no flu or even common cold. We would all come to settlement only sometimes about mid-June.'[3] If smallpox was not a defining colonial disease in northern Canada, then the 'flu' was. A narrower interpretation of 'flu' as 'influenza' shows this in the burial registers as well. Tuberculosis was the single most common cause of death (n=541), followed closely by accidents (n=539), then influenza and pneumonia (n=347 and n=338, respectively). Influenza moved through the Yukon and Mackenzie district in outbreaks and epidemics that ranged from moderate to world-changing.

A world-changing flu came to Dehcho in 1928, ten years after the pandemic that swept most of the globe but whose flames had only burned the edges of Canada's northern territories. This chapter opens by looking at the 1918–19 influenza pandemic and the reactions it elicited in the Yukon and Mackenzie district, even where it was largely kept out. This pandemic was part of a history of relatively frequent influenza outbreaks and epidemics in the North which gave people experience in identifying this sickness, in caring for those who fell ill, and in staying away from posts when disease was circulating. Colonial authorities in both territories drew on tools used in recent years to deal with smallpox. But where the threat of smallpox was exaggerated in these decades,

[1] Julienne Andre in *Gwichya Gwich'in Googwandak*, 262, 269.

[2] George Vittrekwa, interview 27 Feb. 1974, GSCI, GLC files, tape 68.

[3] *MVPI Fort Good Hope, NWT* (7 August 1975), vol. 20 (testimony of Michel Grandjambe), 1991–2.

the threat of influenza would be underestimated in 1928, with devastating consequences. This chapter details the experience of 1928, primarily by moving along the path of the SS *Distributor* as it delivered influenza down the length of the Mackenzie River. While this was an epidemic that reached across the Mackenzie district almost all at once, there were also divergent experiences at each village, camp, and trade post, which serve to illuminate important parts of the larger story.

Before 1928: The 1918–1919 Pandemic and Seasonal Flus

Influenza viruses were among the earliest pathogens introduced and described by colonizers in the Yukon and Mackenzie district. Although the worst epidemics came in the twentieth century, influenza travelled frequently in the North well before then. Influenza acted syndemically with other pathogens – scarlet fever in the 1860s, measles around 1900 – to produce the devastating epidemics in those years. In the late nineteenth century, numerous influenza outbreaks occurred, with deaths from influenza or 'grippe' recorded in every decade before 1900. Severe outbreaks in 1891 and 1892 were part of a Russian pandemic that spread swiftly, initially along rail routes. In 2005, researchers presented evidence that this pandemic involved a coronavirus that had spread from cattle, acting in combination with influenza to shape the pandemic's three waves.[4] In the North, the frequency of influenza outbreaks and deaths intensified after 1892.[5] The cause of death database has deaths from influenza in each *year* from 1895 through 1902. Between 1891 and 1902, cases and deaths from influenza were recorded all along the Mackenzie River – from Fort Smith to Kitigaaryuit on the Arctic Coast. This pattern of recurrent epidemics of 'influenza-like illness' between 1890 and 1901 occurred in other parts of the world as well.[6]

The frequency of influenza outbreaks slowed in the years that followed, but continued to cause serious illness and death. In 1907 and again in 1913, the residential school at Providence had outbreaks of influenza that 'laid almost everyone low'.[7] At Behchokǫ̀, there was influenza at Christmastime in 1910. In

4 L. Vijgen, E. Keyaerts, E. Moës, et al., 'Complete Genomic Sequence of Human Coronavirus OC43: Molecular Clock Analysis Suggests a Relatively Recent Zoonotic Coronavirus Transmission Event', *Journal of Virology* 79, no. 3 (2005): 1595–604, http://doi.org/10.1128/JVI.79.3.1595-1604.2005; Harald Brüssow and Lutz Brüssow, 'Clinical Evidence That the Pandemic from 1889 to 1891 Commonly Called the Russian Flu might have been an Earlier Coronavirus Pandemic', *Microbial Biotechnology* 14, no. 5 (2021): 1860–70, https://doi.org/10.1111/1751-7915.13889; George Dehner, *Influenza: A Century of Science and Public Health Response* (Pittsburgh: University of Pittsburgh Press, 2012), 39–41.

5 Heine et al., *Gwichya Gwich'in Googwandak*, 200.

6 G. Dennis Shanks and John F. Brundage, 'Pathogenic Responses Among Young Adults during the 1918 Influenza Pandemic', *Emerging Infectious Diseases*, 18, no. 2 (2012): 201–7 (p. 202).

7 Vanast, 'Arctic Bodies', 231; McCarthy, *Great River*, 206.

July 1916, the Anglican missionary at McPherson reported, 'An epidemic of Le Grippe going. Fry and I have it. Several Indians quite ill.'[8] Similarly there was influenza at Fort Chipewyan in January 1917 with 'some one or more sick in every home', although no deaths were reported.[9] Influenza was a frequent visitor to communities along Dehcho well before the 1918 influenza pandemic. It appeared both in winter (the season when influenza viruses flourish) and in the summer, with the open-water transportation that allowed more fluid relationships between the Mackenzie and Yukon rivers and distant places. It was at times fatal, particularly when it appeared alongside other pathogens. More often, it brought sickness and recovery – an experience which would have conferred some immunity to survivors.

With that in mind, previous encounters with influenza did not, for the most part, protect people during the 1918–19 influenza pandemic. That influenza pandemic, also known as the 'Spanish flu', spread in three waves between March 1918 and May 1919. About one-third of the world's population, approximately 1.8 billion before the pandemic hit, were infected, and an estimated 50 million people died. The influenza pandemic that year killed more people in a short period of time than any other pandemic, famine, or war in history.[10] The second wave between September and November 1918 was the most fatal, and both the second and third waves were characterized by a high frequency of 'complicated, severe, and fatal cases'.[11] One of the defining features of the 1918–19 pandemic were the W-shaped mortality graphs. Normally, deaths from influenza are among the very young (under five) and very old (over sixty-five), producing a U-shape when graphed. But in 1918–19, in many parts of the world, healthy young adults aged twenty to thirty-five died at disproportionate rates for reasons that remain only partially understood but have been linked to shared immunological histories of that age cohort.[12] Cause aside, the effect of disproportionate mortality among this age cohort meant that in some communities the effects of influenza in 1918–19 were much greater because of the loss of young adults who were also parents, workers, and providers.

[8] St Matthew's Mission Journal, 10 Jul. 1916. [9] St Paul's Daily Journal, 21 Jan. 1917.

[10] Alfred W. Crosby, *America's Forgotten Pandemic: The Influenza of 1918* (New York: Cambridge University Press, 1989), 311.

[11] Jeffery K. Taubenberger and David M. Morens, '1918 Influenza: The Mother of All Pandemics', *Emerging Infectious Diseases* 12, no. 1 (2006): 15–22 (p. 17); K. J. Bolton, J. M. McCaw, J. McVernon, J. D. Mathews, 'The Influence of Changing Host Immunity on 1918–19 Pandemic Dynamics', *Epidemics* 8 (2014): 18–27.

[12] Alain Gagnon, Matthew S. Miller, Stacey A. Hallman, et al., 'Age-Specific Mortality During the 1918 Influenza Pandemic: Unravelling the Mystery of High Young Adult Mortality', *PLoS ONE* 8, no. 8 (2013), http://doi.org/10.1371/journal.pone.0069586; Shanks and Brundage, 'Pathogenic Responses', 204–6.

In Canada, the estimated death toll from the 1918–19 pandemic was 50,000 people, fewer than the estimated 61,000 killed in the First World War. Historians have assessed the pandemic's role in shaping post-war labour activism and state involvement in public health.[13] Popular awareness of the experience of the 1918–19 pandemic in the North has emphasized the devastating effects of influenza in a number of small, predominantly Indigenous northern communities. In 1985, Anne Budgell and Nigel Markham made a documentary for the National Film Board that looked at the experience of Okak, a Moravian mission post in Labrador where 204 of 263 Inuit residents perished from influenza in 1919. Okak was subsequently abandoned. Brevig Mission in Alaska, similarly, is well known because of the effects of the pandemic (seventy-two of eighty adults in the village died), and more so because it was from an Inupiat gravesite in Brevig Mission that samples of the 1918 virus were recovered in 1951, with the permission of village Elders.[14] These samples later provided the basis for detailed genetic research into the virus. Svenn-Erik Mamelund, Lisa Sattenspiel, and Jessica Dimka examined influenza mortality in Alaska and Labrador in 1918–19 and emphasized the degree of regional variation, although overall mortality, they noted, at 2.5 to 5 percent was 'substantially higher than the worldwide average'.[15]

In the autumn of 1918, influenza reached Juneau, Anchorage, St Michael, Nome, and many other points between.[16] Thomas Riggs was governor of Alaska. This was the same Thomas Riggs who headed up the US survey party in Rampart House during the smallpox epidemic of 1911. That experience influenced his approach to the appearance of influenza, including his efforts both to secure an influenza vaccine and more importantly to establish quarantines prohibiting travel to Alaska's interior and at Skagway, the southern entrance to the Yukon. The principal of the residential school at Carcross wrote that 'every precaution is being taken in Skagway the stevedores even being obliged to wear medicated veils over their faces when unloading the boats'.[17] By this point, establishing a quarantine at Skagway was well-worn practice and, as in the past, Canadian and US officials cooperated in sharing

[13] Esyllt W. Jones, *Influenza 1918: Disease, Death and Struggle in Winnipeg* (Toronto: University of Toronto Press, 2007); Mark Osborne Humphries, *The Last Plague: Spanish Influenza and the Politics of Public Health in Canada* (Toronto: University of Toronto Press, 2013).

[14] Douglas Jordan, 'The Deadliest Flu: The Complete Story of the Discovery and Reconstruction of the 1918 Pandemic Virus', *Centers for Disease Control and Prevention,* www.cdc.gov/flu/pandemic-resources/reconstruction-1918-virus.html.

[15] Svenn-Erik Mamelund, Lisa Sattenspiel, and Jessica Dimka, 'Influenza-Associated Mortality during the 1918–1919 Influenza Pandemic in Alaska and Labrador: A Comparison', *Social Science History* 37, no. 2 (2013): 177–229 (p. 177); see also Svenn-Erik Mamelund, 'Geography May Explain Adult Mortality from the 1918–20 Influenza Pandemic', *Epidemics* 3 (2011): 46–60; Crosby, *Forgotten Pandemic*, 245.

[16] Mamelund et al., 'Influenza-Associated Mortality', figure 1.

[17] Charles F. Johnson to Bishop Stringer, 12 Nov. 1918, COR 252 File 11 A, Anglican Church, YA.

information and costs.[18] This quarantine alongside the prohibitions on travel to the interior also protected Dawson; as Mamelund, Sattenspiel, and Dimka showed, none of the communities along the Yukon River in Alaska's interior were affected by influenza in 1918–19.[19] The geography of vulnerability in 1918–19 saw communities on the eastern and western edges of northern North America (Labrador and Alaska) hit first by the pandemic, while other communities in the interior and along the harder-to-access Arctic Coast were better protected.

One of the key protections afforded communities in 1918 was that news of the deadly pandemic travelled faster than the virus. Vilhjalmur Stefansson sent a letter from Victoria, BC on November 18, 1918 that reached Aylesworth Bowen Perry, the RNWMP Commissioner in Regina, and from him, federal officials in Ottawa. Stefansson had heard by telegram from Nome, 'that six out of the seven Esquimeaux that used to work for us have just died there of the Influenza'. He went on to speculate about Indigenous mortality ('about 75%') but spent most of his letter offering practical advice for how to best check the epidemic, whether from the west along the Arctic Coast or from the south via the Mackenzie River.[20] RCMP comptroller A. A. McLean promptly sent a telegram to Riggs in Alaska asking for more information. D. C. Scott in Ottawa sought information from John Hawksley in Dawson and from Fort McMurray. From these points, federal officials learned that no cases had been reported north of Jackfish Lake in Alberta. Riggs advised strict quarantine measures along the Arctic Coast and at Herschel Island.[21] The Alberta Board of Health took measures to prohibit travel north of Fort McMurray.[22]

At Fort Chipewyan, on 2 December 1918, the Reverend Gibson received word from McMurray 'that the War had come to an end', and of 'a terrible epidemic – Spanish influenza – otherwise known as the "Flu". People becoming a little scared. It seems to be affecting the whole of the North American continent.'[23] The same dual report arrived at Fort McPherson a few weeks later.[24] Ronny Pascal (Gwich'in) remembered these events well.[25] 'It was in 1918, the Dawson patrol came over to Ft. McPherson', said Pascal. 'The police from Herschel Island all gathered in Ft. McPherson. The mail came in and said the war was over. So we came, five teams, over to McPherson with the Dawson patrol.' Pascal and two other men got some dog food from the police, who asked that they head back to Dawson first, 'and they would follow us later'.

18 Crosby, *Forgotten Pandemic*, 251–2.
19 See also Lux, 'Disease and Dawson City'; Gates, 'Spared the Influenza'.
20 V. Stefansson to A. Bowen Perry, 18 Nov. 1918, RG 18, A-1, vol. 567, file G6 [hereafter file G6], LAC.
21 T. Riggs to A. A. McLean, 25 Nov. 1918, file G6, LAC.
22 J. Thomson to Comptroller, 16 Nov. 1918, RG 18, A-1, vol. 565, file 560, LAC.
23 St Paul's Daily Journal, 2 Dec. 1918.
24 St Matthew's Mission Journal, 20 Dec. 1918.
25 Ronny Pascal, 'Trip to Dawson', in 'Gwich'in COPE stories', 445–8.

After they left, Pascal and the others met up with Gwich'in who had had successful caribou hunts. Pascal and the others continued on.[26] 'Somehow or other, we heard there was the epidemic flu in Dawson City', recalled Pascal, 'and we weren't sure we should continue on to Dawson or not.' Staying away from the trade posts when there were reports of sickness was a critical means by which people stayed safe during outbreaks and epidemics. Soon thereafter, not far from Dawson, Pascal and the others met 'two white men . . . and we asked them if there was some kind of sickness going around Dawson. The white men told us they had just left Dawson two days ago everything was fine; no sickness in Dawson.' The group continued on, reaching Mitchell Creek. People who had moved on from there had left a letter behind asking people 'not to return to McPherson this year because of the epidemic flu'.[27] Pascal's story tells not just of that trip but of going back and forth between Dawson and McPherson through the next year as well. He spoke of meat and food, of hunting, and of travelling – the focus of many oral histories of this time that provide the framework within which an episode like the 1918 influenza was situated. The other element apparent from Pascal's account was that the northern interior was not isolated at this time. People were coming and going. News, while in one sense slow to arrive, also circulated widely by word of mouth and notes left on trails, including big news about the end of the war and about the pandemic, and local news about sickness in communities. We see how information travelled, and how people and families made decisions about whether to go into a post or stay out on the land.

Meanwhile, officials in Ottawa made plans. RCMP commissioner Perry had asked McLean whether a doctor could be sent in.[28] The request was put to Scott with the DIA. But as was often the case with Scott, he 'decided not to'.[29] At the time, the only doctor in the Yukon who could be sent elsewhere in case of an outbreak was D. R. McLennan, 'who is reported to be at Mayo engaged in mining'.[30] To the east, in the Mackenzie district in 1918, the only doctor was A. L. MacDonald at Fort Smith. Inspector K. F. Anderson expressed his opinion that MacDonald 'would have his hands full at Fort Smith alone, if the sickness got there, this would leave Fort Resolution, and Hay river, without any Doctors assistance, and at Fort Resolution there is about 75 Indian children and at hay River [*sic*] about 60.' Anderson advised that doctors be sent 'to each of these places by first boat in the Spring'.[31] No doctors came, but medicines and other supplies, including masks, were sent in. Even then, there was concern

26 S. G. Clay to Officer Commanding, Dawson, 26 Dec. 1918, file G6, LAC.
27 All quotations Pascal, 'Trip to Dawson', 447.
28 A. B. Perry to Comptroller, Ottawa, 22 Nov. 1918, file G6, LAC.
29 D. C. Scott to A. A. McLean, 3 Dec. 1918, file G6, LAC.
30 Memo to the Deputy Minister of the Interior, 6 Dec. 1918, file G6, LAC.
31 K. F. Anderson to 'N' Division, Peace River, 8 Mar. 1919, file G6, LAC.

from some quarters about the DIA's parsimony: 'I understand that there are over 1000 Eskimos in those regions', McLean wrote, 'and I am not satisfied that a small quantity of medicine as Mr. Scott in the accompanying letter says he is sending in will meet the requirement in case the Influenza should spread.'[32] There was further debate among federal officials about the potential efficacy of the available medicines. A serum sent north froze in transport, notwithstanding Sergeant Dempster's best efforts to protect the bottles, including sleeping 'with them inside the robe'.[33] This was not the first time that weather and cold curtailed the availability of medicines in the North. Eventually vaccine made its way to the Yukon. When Ronny Pascal got to Dawson in the summertime, 'the doctor told us there was a very bad cold going around and everyone had to get vaccinated – men, women and children. After everything was over, and everyone was well enough, we all went back to the mountains again.'[34]

By the end of 1918, travel to the north-west interior was blocked from northern Alberta, at Skagway in the panhandle, prohibiting travel in the Alaskan interior, and along the Arctic Coast. Only access overland from the east was and would remain unprotected. In January 1919, Anderson met with Corporal Walters at Fort Resolution and the Indian Agent Gerald Card at Fort Smith. Their plan, should the virus appear, included measures for distributing provisions and fishing nets. Procedures to curtail social interaction were devised: if the flu appeared at Fort Smith, word would be sent to stop any dances from being held.[35] On 29 January, Anderson travelled to Hay River and met there with Dene, holding a long conference with them 'in our Indian Room', wrote Reverend A. J. Vale. The policy that emerged from this long meeting was most certainly shaped by Dene leadership and insight into how best to control the spread of disease. The plan was for people to go out on the land and stay there. Vale described that 'Red Flags to be put on the trails a safe distance out of village if sickness is prevailing. No Indian is allowed to pass the Red Flag.'[36] While Vale and Anderson described the plan using a language of force and prohibition, communicating to people with notes (or flags) out on the trails was how news travelled in the North at this time. It was how Ronny Pascal heard about sickness at Dawson. There is no doubt that this plan arose from Dene and colonial leadership and was embraced as an effective tool to check the spread of disease.

In the end, the 1918–19 influenza pandemic never reached the Mackenzie district. There were isolated reports of sickness, but nothing unusual compared

[32] A. A. McLean to Newton Rowell, 4 Dec. 1918, file G6, LAC.

[33] W. J. D. Dempster to Officer Commanding, Dawson, 11 Mar. 1919, file G6, LAC.

[34] Pascal, 'Trip to Dawson', 447. [35] Anderson to 'N' Division, 8 Mar. 1919.

[36] 29 Jan. 1919, St Peter's Hay River, Anglican Diocese MacKenzie River, MR 4/5, box 1, PAA [hereafter St Peter's Daily Journal].

to other years.[37] On Herschel Island, there was widespread sickness in the fall 1918, 'almost all of the people on the Island were sick'.[38] One child, reported as Albert, son of Joseph, died. But this was not thought to be influenza at the time.

Across the border, in the Yukon, they were, for the most part, similarly able to keep influenza out. The exception was in the south, between Champagne Landing and Whitehorse, where at least eleven people died in the spring of 1919. Riggs lifted the quarantine at Skagway in March, even after the flu appeared at that place, and Yukon officials and police scrambled to contain the disease. The Medical Health Officer W. B. Clarke was sick with typhoid in hospital when cases were diagnosed at Skagway and missed the initial reports, delaying an official response. Soon enough, the Gold Commissioner and Dr N. E. Culbertson in conjunction with the RNWMP quarantined all arrivals destined for Yukon or Atlin.[39] They also established quarantine stations at Carcross and Whitehorse. Train passengers were inspected, and suspected cases quarantined immediately. But there were problems with communication across the border, as information was relayed and details lost.[40] There was pressure to lift the quarantines, particularly as the weather warmed and businesses (the transport companies especially) did not want to miss out on the usual spring rush. Scheduled excursions were to bring Americans to Whitehorse to celebrate Victoria Day in mid-May. 'Our idea', wrote A. W. Bell, 'is to have the citizens call it off themselves, so that no official action will be necessary.'[41] Only if necessary would the government intervene to prohibit the celebrations. State officials and the police hesitated to coerce settler communities.

Flu spread in the southern Yukon in the spring of 1919 to Champagne Landing, Canyon, Lake Mendenhall, and Hutshi Lake, with a handful of cases in Whitehorse. Champagne Landing was the hardest hit. Influenza appeared there in late May, and by early June there were sixty-nine cases and two deaths. At Hutshi Lake, everyone fell ill – four families that numbered eighteen people in all. Two died from the flu. There were also deaths reported at Lake Mendenhall and Canyon. At Whitehorse, five cases appeared, and families were quarantined. The only death was of a baby girl, born prematurely when her mother fell sick. The parents both recovered. In total, while influenza was widespread (Bell described it as a 'wholesale epidemic among the Indians in all directions'), there were eleven deaths attributed to the flu that spring.[42]

[37] Report of Constable Smyth, 22 Jul. 1919, RG 18, F1, vol. 12, file G-1316, LAC.

[38] W. H. Fry to Bishop Stringer, 12 Jan. 1919, COR 251 16, Anglican Church, YA.

[39] R. S. Knight to Commissioner, Regina, 22 Apr. 1919, file G6, LAC.

[40] A. W. Bell to Officer Commanding, Dawson, 23 Apr. 1919, file G6, LAC.

[41] A. W. Bell to Officer Commanding, Dawson, 14 May 1919, file G6, LAC.

[42] A. W. Bell to Officer Commanding, Dawson, 3 Jun. 1919; H. Salkeld to Officer Commanding, Whitehorse, 8 Jun. 1919, file G6, LAC; COD Database.

The RNWMP supplied provisions to the sick. They also disinfected 'all the Indian shacks' and burned two cabins, following a logic similar to that which had prevailed at Rampart House earlier in the decade.[43] It was this outbreak which triggered the vaccinations at Dawson that Ronny Pascal remembered. But the disease did not spread farther that spring, and the 1918–19 influenza pandemic did not reach the rest of the Yukon territory.

Pandemic influenza means that the virus spread globally but does not mean that it travelled uniformly everywhere. In 1918, influenza arrived in the North late enough in the year that not only was there time after word of the pandemic's spread to implement controls on travel, but it also did not appear during the busy open-water season.[44] This autumn arrival worked against some Alaskan communities, where the virus was dropped off just before freeze-up, so then help could not get in as easily.[45] But the combination of freeze-up, the slower travel season, and the early implementation of travel restrictions around the delta and the north-west interior kept these places safe. In the Mackenzie district, the red flags never had to be posted on the trails. In the southern Yukon, years of recent experience with smallpox epidemics meant that there were both tools in place to implement quarantine and isolation, and people were familiar with the controls being imposed. Even though the flu appeared in the Yukon in spring, just as things were opening up, it did not spread far. Isolation in the North was a tool used to keep a virus in check; not a pre-existing condition, but a practice.

After 1919, influenza kept returning to the Yukon and Mackenzie district. Between 1919 and 1928, there were repeated outbreaks: at Carcross in 1920, remembered by Johnnie Johns; a 1925 epidemic that affected Mayo, Fort Selkirk, Dawson and Moosehide, and Fort Yukon; a devastating outbreak along the Arctic Coast near Kugluktuk in 1926–7; and significant outbreaks on Lake Athabasca between 1921 and 1924. Table 8.1 in the next chapter presents a summary of these 1920s outbreaks, each of which saw high mortality among elders. Kitty Smith, interviewed in the 1970s, recalled the deaths in Carcross in 1920 as part of a generational change. One of the original prospectors who triggered the Klondike gold rush, Keish (Skookum Jim), had died in 1916, then in 1920 'lots of people die Mrs. Carmack die, Tagish John die and then Mary die his mother'.[46] Smith herself did not fall ill, as she and others were in Little Atlin at the time and stayed away from Carcross because they heard the 'flu was bad' there. Johnnie Johns lost his father in this outbreak; as he put it, 'See a lot of the old timers died with the Spanish Influenza that went through the country here in 1920, killed off a lot of the older people. So we lost

[43] A. W. Bell to Officer Commanding, Dawson, 29 May 1919 and 3 Jun. 1919, file G6, LAC
[44] McCormack, *Fort Chipewyan*, 268. [45] Crosby, *Forgotten Pandemic*, 246.
[46] Kitty Smith interview, Skookum Jim Oral History Project Fonds, COR 1096 (88/58R), YA.

a lot of these old Indian names.'[47] Stories from Lake Athabasca in the 1920s emphasize the speed with which the influenza moved through families, the loss of elders, some of whom died abruptly, and – for those who fell sick but survived – the seriousness of their illness.[48]

Epidemics could affect more than one community in an area and yet still be geographically confined. In 1925, despite severe influenza raging at Fort Yukon and Dawson, there is no evidence that people at Rampart House and Old Crow were affected, nor that the pathogen travelled to or from the Mackenzie district, in spite of important social connections between Dene from the east and the Tutchone at Selkirk.[49] Tommy McGinty remembered how in 1925, people from the Mackenzie had come to Fort Selkirk for gambling but 'bad flu came in' and one 'Mackenzie Joe' died.[50] The deaths along the coast in 1926–7 also involved a gastrointestinal disease and saw high infant, child, and adult mortality. The number of people who passed in a short time made these devastating experiences. They also highlighted the increasing summer activity along the coast. Seasonal movement, the ease and speed of travel, and the timing of major gatherings made a big difference to the movement of pathogens in the North. Moreover, the experience of influenza between 1918 and 1927 influenced the contours of the 1928 epidemic as is discussed in Chapter 8. But the experience of 1928 is valuable historically not just because of the insight it offers to understanding the reverberations of 1918, but most importantly, in its own right.

The 1928 Epidemic

The 1928 influenza epidemic came from the south after spring break-up and with the activity of early summer. From Fort Simpson north, the virus was carried on board the *Distributor*, the HBC's main supply steamship, on its first trip of the year bringing trade goods, food, and visitors to posts along Dehcho, arriving in Aklavik on 5 July 1928. The disease was not confined to the path of the *Distributor*. From treaty gatherings, the pathogen was picked up and carried east around Great Slave Lake, to Great Bear Lake, and south-west from Fort Simpson to Fort Liard (see Map 7.1). A belated quarantine kept the virus from travelling long distances east or west along the Arctic Coast, although people in the delta and nearby – from Herschel Island to Tuktoyaktuk – were affected. The epidemic raged

47 Johnnie Johns interview, Skookum Jim Oral History Project Fonds, COR 1096 (88/58R), YA.

48 St Paul's Daily Journal, 30 Mar.–11 Apr. 1922; MacKay interview Parker, 20 Sept. 1978; 'The diary of Victor Mercredi'; McCormack, *Fort Chipewyan*, 270–1.

49 Linklater Diary, 5 Jul.–1 Aug. 1925.

50 Tommy McGinty, interview with Sharon Sims, 21 Jul. 1985, tape 1, side 2, transcript, in *Fort Selkirk Elders Oral History Project* (1987), 204.

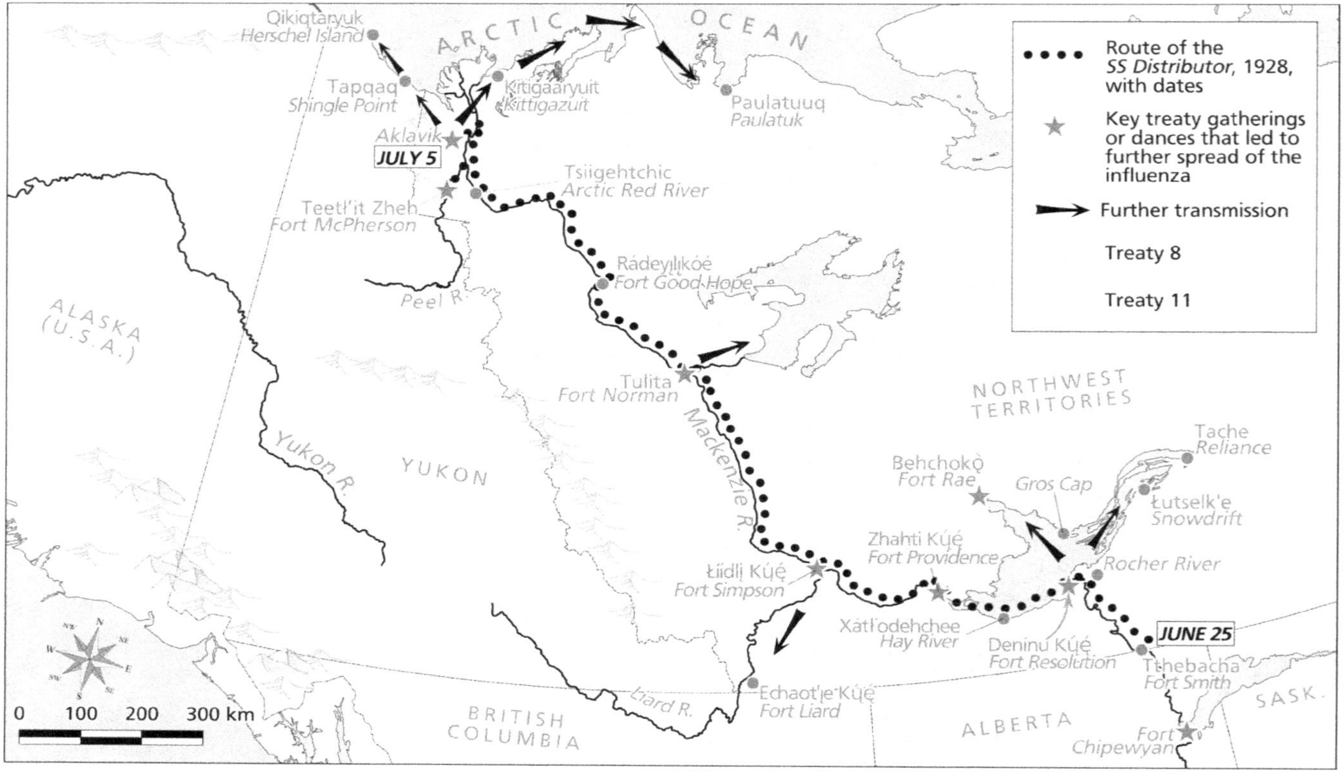

Map 7.1 The 1928 influenza epidemic.

Table 7.1 *Mortality from influenza, 1928*

	Total Population		Deaths in 1928		Percentage of Population	
	1921 Census	Population	Low	High	Low	High
Kitigaaryuit	14	14	2	2	14%	14%
Shingle Point	14	95	10	14	11%	15%
Paulatuk	–	–	6	6	–	–
Aklavik	21	200	17	20	9%	10%
Tsiigehtchic	178	178	7	9	4%	5%
Fort McPherson	283	283	31	35	11%	12%
Fort Good Hope	366	368	17	18	5%	5%
Tulita (incl. Great Bear River)	278	343	26	35	8%	10%
Fort Wrigley	85	85	6	7	7%	8%
Fort Liard	207	217	6	6	3%	3%
Fort Simpson	507	507	37	51	7%	10%
Fort Providence (incl. Trout Lake)	328	328	23	50	7%	15%
Other people and places (NWT), including deaths from Willow River, Gros Cap, Goulet's Camp, Rocher River, Yellowknife River	20	550	59	83	11%	15%
Behchokǫ	779	779	34	80	4%	10%
Hay River	167	167	11	15	7%	9%
Fort Resolution	961	961	25	45	3%	5%
Fort Smith	405	405	2	2	0%	0%
Fort Chipewyan, AB	882	882	9	9	1%	1%
TOTALS	*5,516*	*6,398*	*332*	*494*		
Deaths as Percent of Total Population			*5%*	*8%*		
Average Mortality					*7%*	*9%*

Communities are organized from north (top) to south (bottom). The place names were made consistent with the rest of the text so this is no longer accurate. For people living along the Arctic Coast, the 1921 census estimated the population from the Alaska boundary to Kent Peninsula at 1,515 people. However, the only communities and camps where people caught influenza are those listed here (Herschel Island, Kitigaaryuit, Shingle Point, Paulatuk).

Sources: RG 10 vol. 4042, file 336–877, c-10178, LAC; RG 85 C-1-a, vol. 789, file 6099, LAC; Fleming Diary; Nagy, *Yukon North Slope*; Canada, Sixth Census.

through the month of July. As can be seen in Table 7.1, the total recorded mortality from the influenza was between 332 and 494 people, from a population of around 6,400 – meaning that overall mortality was as much as 8 percent of the total population, and average mortality in those communities affected was between 9 and 10 percent. Multiple observers at the time estimated that the deaths in a given locale represented as much as one-tenth of the local population.[51] Some communities were much harder hit than others: Fort Chipewyan, Fort Smith, and Tsiigehtchic had the lowest numbers of deaths, while Fort McPherson, Fort Providence, and people living on the coast and in camps around Great Slave Lake had the highest death tolls.

The SS *Distributor*

The ice was moving on Lake Athabasca in mid-May, heralding the arrival of spring. Two boats arrived in Fort Chipewyan on 23 May, and then the HBC's paddle-wheeler, SS *Athabasca* arrived from the south on 25 May, bringing back the Anglican missionary family of William and Isabel Gibson and a worker for the residential school in Hay River. As the ice moved out, boats began travelling between communities along the Athabasca, Slave, and Mackenzie rivers through the month of June. A carpenter went north to Tulita for work. There was travel between Tulita and Tsiigehtchic by the river. Trappers and independent traders started coming in to the posts. On 17 June, Dene arrived in Tulita from the mountains in mooseskin boats, with furs and dried meat to trade. Mail and freight were delivered to Fort Chipewyan and Hay River in the south. Seasonal visitors also started to trickle in, like the DIA inspector Charles C. Parker who arrived in Fort Simpson on board a Northern Traders (NT) schooner on 22 June. By later in the month, the NT schooners and the Catholic gas boat the *Immaculata* were going as far as Aklavik, carrying people and floorboards cut at the mill in Fort Resolution. Around this time as well, families starting coming into the posts from the land. The treaty gathering at Fort Chipewyan was held on 23 June. That same day, at Hay River, Rev. William Singleton noted that Dene families were arriving from Buffalo River: 'thus life begins again in the Community'.[52]

In 1928, the role of sick passengers and crew on the SS *Distributor* was to provide speed and range in the transmission of the influenza virus, creating an epidemic that spanned the length of Dehcho in one go. When exactly the virus boarded the ship is not clear. In spite of efforts to trace the origin of the epidemic that year, no conclusive findings were made.[53] The SS *Distributor* left Fort Smith on its first voyage north on Monday 25 June. Sickness was reported at Fort Chipewyan during the treaty gathering.[54] And there was already much coming and going between communities (Figure 7.1). After leaving Fort Smith, the *Distributor* stopped at Fort Resolution on the 26th and at Hay River on the 27th (Figure 7.2). Philip Godsell, with the HBC, was on board and recalled in his 1932 memoirs that the pilot David McPherson was among the first to fall ill: 'by

[51] See, for example, Bourget, *Douze ans*, 205. [52] St Peter's Daily Journal, 23 Jun. 1928.
[53] See, for example, A. W. Duffus to O. S. Finnie, 28 Aug. 1928, file 6099, LAC.
[54] St Paul's Daily Journal, 26 Jun. 1928.

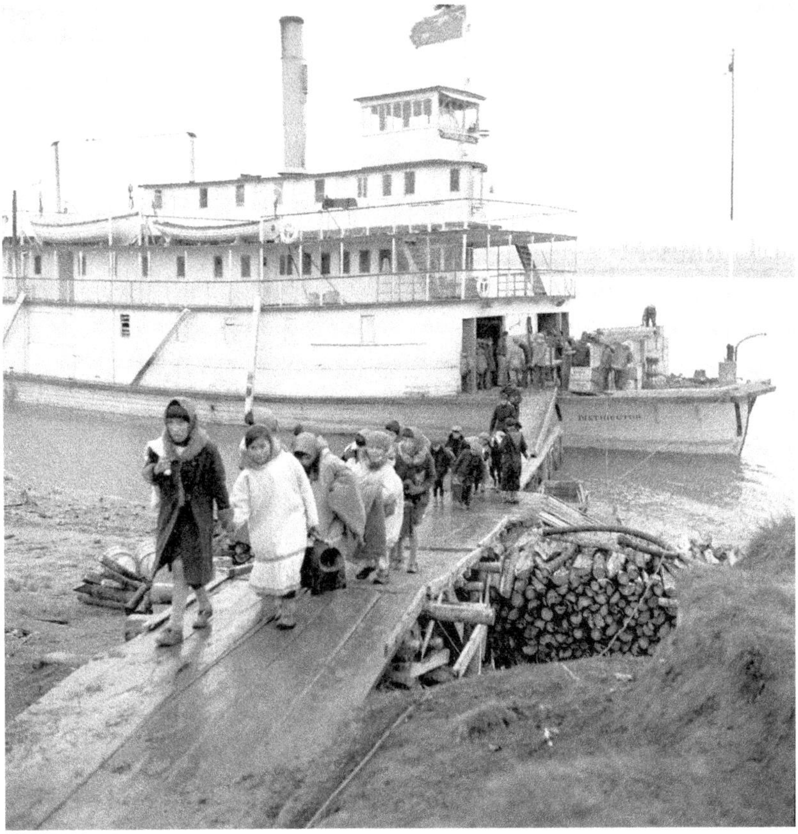

Figure 7.1 Passengers disembarking from the SS *Distributor*, including children either headed to or returning from residential school. Photograph by Richard Hourde while on an assignment for *The Beaver* magazine, HBCA 1987/271/NAA37, Hudson's Bay Company Archives, Archives of Manitoba.

the time I stepped ashore at Hay River', Godsell wrote, 'there was quite a number sick on board'.[55] The steamer went on to Fort Providence. When Dr Arthur Truesdell boarded at Fort Simpson on 29 June, he also noted illness on board but deemed it mild, and so he asked only that people give those who were sick 'a wide berth'.[56] But cases on board kept developing, new ones every 'two

[55] Philip H. Godsell, *Arctic Trader: The Account of Twenty Years with the Hudson's Bay Company*, new ed. (London: Travel Book Club, [1950?]), 304.
[56] W. A. M. Truesdell to O. S. Finnie, 28 Sept. 1928, file 6099, LAC.

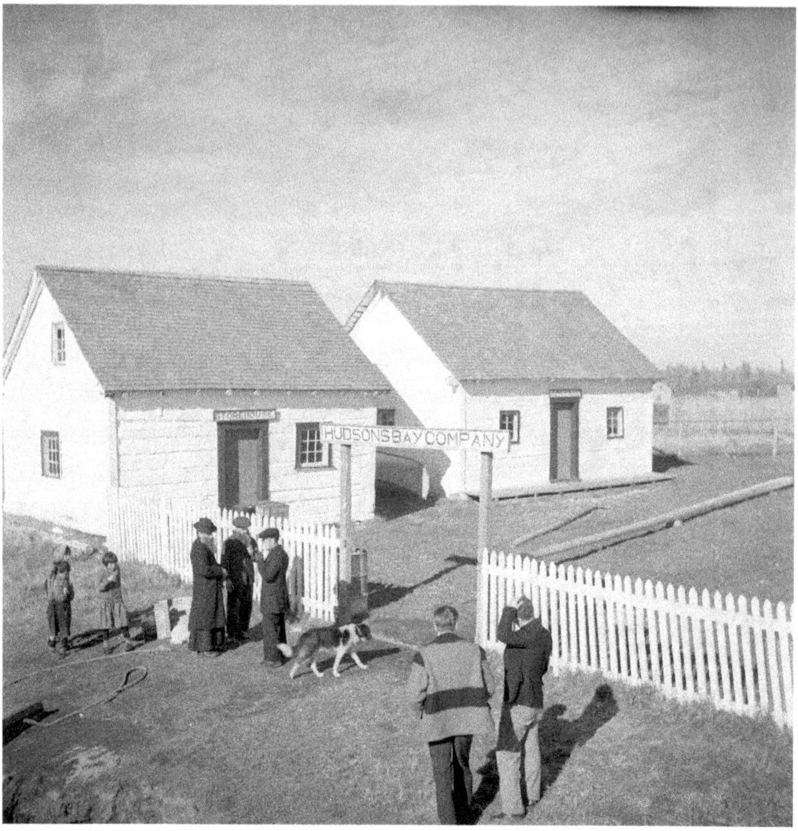

Figure 7.2 Hay River, 1936. Photograph by Richard Hourde while on an assignment for *The Beaver*, HBCA 1987/271/NAA20, Hudson's Bay Company Archives, Archives of Manitoba.

or three hours', such that by Monday 2 July, Archdeacon Fleming observed, 'so many people have colds on board. There seems to be a regular epidemic.'[57]

Fleming had been on board since the steamer's departure, and this was his first mention of illness or colds, suggesting that there was a marked change in the seriousness of the situation north of Fort Simpson. Nevertheless, among those who Fleming said were sick was Gaston Herodier, born in Paris and now the post manager at Fort Good Hope, who promptly disembarked. The *Distributor* then stopped at Tsiigehtchic, where Fleming 'visited the HBC and RCMP. Chatted to

57 Diary of Episcopal Tour, 2 Jul. 1928, Archibald Lang Fleming Fonds, M70-1 Box 1, file 14, GSA [hereafter Fleming Diary].

various trappers and traders.'[58] Two others among the sick were from a Gwich'in family: James Simon and his four-year-old daughter Doris. James, his wife Sarah, and their daughters Susie and Doris had been living at Hay River since 1926, where James studied the bible and Sarah studied music 'so that they could both minister to the people' (Figure 7.3).[59] They were returning home on the *Distributor* when they caught the flu. Sarah Simon remembered how 'my children really was sick on the boat coming back so they got better quick enough. Just my two little girls and I was sick for long time but after I got better.'[60] The boat landed at McPherson on 4 July, and Simon wrote down that by 10 July,

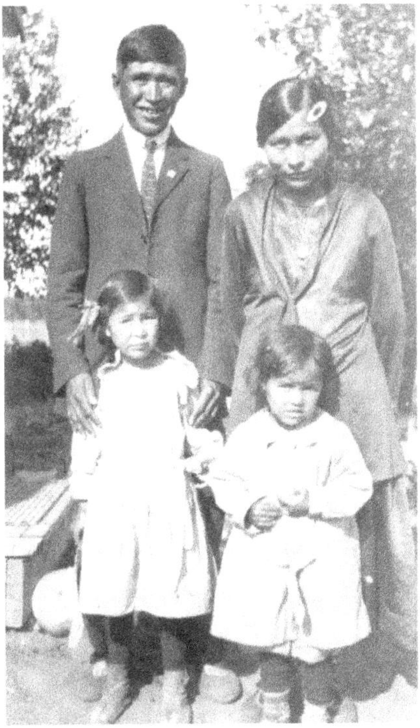

Figure 7.3 James Simon, Sarah Simon, and their daughters Susie and Doris. The General Synod Archives, Anglican Church of Canada.

58 Fleming Diary, 3 Jul. 1928.
59 'Sarah Simon', Life Histories of Elders, GSCI, GTC Department of Culture and Heritage, https://gwichin.ca/elders-biographies; Sarah Simon, *Fort McPherson, N.W.T.: A Pictorial Account of Family, Church, and Community* (Whitehorse: Yukon Native Language Centre, 1982), 5, 15.
60 Sarah Simon, interview 27 Jul. and 4 Aug. 2000, GSCI, Gwich'in Elders' Biographies Research Project, tape 22.

the epidemic was bad in the community.[61] Sarah and James Simon helped the sick in the weeks and months to come.

While the *Distributor* was docked at McPherson, Fleming and William Geddes visited with Edward Sittichinli. In 1903, Sittichinli had been ordained as a Gwich'in minister. By 1928, he was in his seventies. With his wife Annie Sha-Dah Sittichinli, Edward had nine children and was among the most important community leaders at McPherson.[62] Back on board the *Distributor*, nurse Mildred McCabe (originally from Nova Scotia) was 'not feeling well today having contracted the flu from the children', whom she had been helping to look after.[63] And by the time they landed at Aklavik about half past midnight on 5 July, Fleming himself was 'not feeling very fit – seem to have caught the "flu" that has been going the rounds on the boat' (Figure 7.4). He took to bed

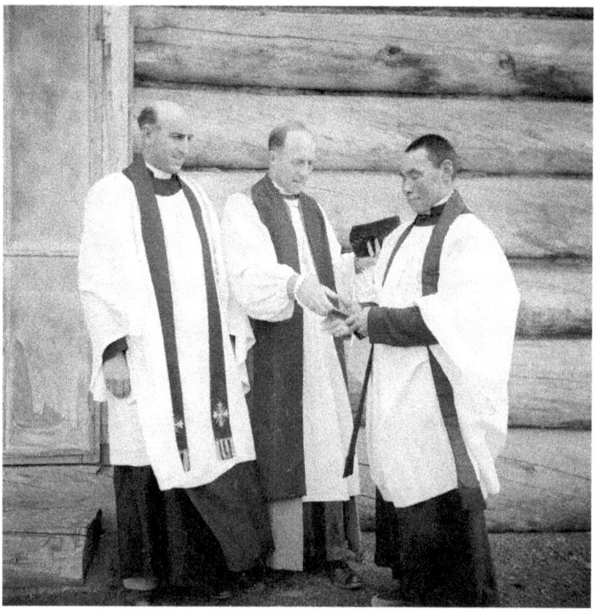

Figure 7.4 A. L. Fleming, Anglican Bishop of the Arctic, speaking with Rev. H. S. Shepherd and Rev. Thomas Umaok, 1936. HBCA 1987/271/NAB3, Hudson's Bay Company Archives, Archives of Manitoba.

[61] Simon interview, Gwich'in Elders' Biographies.

[62] Beaumont, *Jijuu*, 46; his son Jim Edward Sittichinli would also be ordained an Anglican minister, see 'Jim Edward Sittichinli', *Gwadàl' Zheii: Belongings from the Land*, Canadian Museum of History, www.historymuseum.ca/gwichin/storytellers/jim-edward-sittichinli/.

[63] Fleming Diary, 4 Jul. 1928; see McCabe in Rutherdale, *Women and the White Man's God*, 47–8, 113–15.

but not before visiting at the mission and the hospital. 'Eskimos and Indians very friendly', he recorded, as well as receiving visitors while he was ill. The epidemic was in full force in Aklavik by 10 July, when services were cancelled because so many were sick, and by the 11th, 'the whole village is laid up'.[64]

Feasts, Dances, Treaty

The *Distributor* did not just unload cargo and people at each stop, but those travelling on would disembark and visit around the community – as Fleming had done at Tsiigehtchic and McPherson. This was the social season along Dehcho. Federal public health advice from 1920 alerted people to the risk of 'mild cases' or asymptomatic carriers of influenza who play 'a larger part in the spreading of the disease than is realized'.[65] Most people at Fort Resolution – where the *Distributor* stopped before Hay River – directly connected the arrival of the sickness to the steamer. Harold Balsillie, born in 1917, suggested that 'some of the deck hands had the Flu'.[66] Francois King, born in 1902, recalled that 'The boat came in and some people went to visit the people on the boat and after that they got sick'.[67] Others, though, disagreed. Joseph Jerome, born in 1917, remembered everyone arriving for treaty, 'the Slaveys too. Maybe they brought the Flu here.'[68] At the same time as the *Distributor* and other boats were moving through the communities, people came together in big seasonal celebrations, including dances and weddings held at Fort Resolution, Tulita, Fort Simpson, and Tsiigehtchic. As Lucy Vaneltsi recalled, 'People never gathered – only once a year, and that was in the summertime, just waiting for the boat to arrive and the boat didn't come until the first part of July.'[69] While they waited, people held dances, feasts, and games. Dances were the major social events and could last for two or three days.[70] There were drum dances, fiddle dances, and square dances. People played handgames and 'gambled all day long', although as Victor Lafferty pointed out, they didn't gamble for money, 'they played for tobacco or matches or little things like that'.[71] These dances were opportunities to see family and friends and to meet new people.

64 Fleming Diary, 5–11 Jul. 1928.

65 Deputy Minister, Dept. of Heath, 21 Jan. 1920, RG 29, Vol. 1192, File 311-J2-2, Part 1, LAC; Judith Walzer Leavitt, *Typhoid Mary: Captive to the Public's Health* (Boston: Beacon Press, 1996).

66 Harold Balsillie in *That's the Way We Lived*, 75.

67 Francois King in *That's the Way We Lived*, 77.

68 Joseph Jerome in *That's the Way We Lived*, 77.

69 Lucy Vaneltsi, 'Traditional Life #2', in 'Gwich'in COPE stories', 715.

70 Heine et al., *Gwichya Gwich'in Googwandak*, ch. 16; Alphonse Lemoule, 'Power for Dance', in Blondin, *Yamoria*, 185.

71 Harold Balsillie and Victor Lafferty in *That's the Way We Lived*, 79–80.

The dances that were held around treaty gatherings were among the larger ones held during the year, although the dances at Christmas and New Year were also big celebrations. Julienne Andre remembered exactly how a dance at Aklavik preceded the flu epidemic in 1928:

> The Eskimos wanted to dance for us, and then we had to dance for them. They danced all night. That night after mass they all went down to dance. A chant was sung. We really had lots of fun. Everybody danced – some rested and then took the place of the dancer. That's when the flu came. Everybody was sick and lots of people died.[72]

Along with the festivities of dances and feasts, there was also the formal anniversary of treaties that was acknowledged at this time of year. Together, these activities amplified the spread of influenza. By 1928, many of the people who lived along the Mackenzie River were signatories to either Treaty 8 or Treaty 11, the most significant exception being the Inuvialuit along the coast. And so, while the *Distributor* made its way north, Indian Agents, including Flynn Harris and Clermont Bourget, accompanied by RCMP escorts, travelled in smaller boats across the region to pay out money and distribute fishnets, twine, ammunition, axes, flour, tea, sugar, and bacon. Treaty was delayed at Resolution because a late break-up and more hazardous ice conditions had slowed travel.[73] Bourget waited a couple days, 'to give a chance to all the straglers [*sic*] to arrive'. When the time came to pay treaty, influenza was already going around. Bourget described how that day 'all the Indians cough and are sick, they can hardly come to the tent to receive their money'. Because people were 'suffering from bad colds, headaches, fever', there were no speeches made during the treaty ceremonies that year. There was a light rain outside, and 'at times the treaty tent was filled' as people, many of whom clearly felt ill, sought shelter from the weather while they waited.[74]

As Indian Agent for the Great Slave Lake agency, Bourget travelled to Behchokǫ̀ to distribute treaty annuities. In his memoirs and reports, Bourget rationalized his decision to cross the lake as the influenza spread. Bourget sought to justify why he left sick people behind in Resolution and also then helped further transmit the sickness. Bourget travelled with his daughter and sister-in-law, a pilot, an engineer, an RCMP constable, and two nuns. George Sanderson's father (also named George) was the pilot who accompanied Bourget. In previous years, young George had joined the treaty party too, but in 1928, Sanderson recalled, 'I stayed home and my father went travelling with

[72] Julienne Andre in *Gwichya Gwich'in Googwandak*, 272.
[73] C. Bourget, Medical Report, 19 Sept. 1928, file 6099, LAC; Canada, *Historical Climate Data*, Monthly Data for Fort Resolution, 1911–36.
[74] Bourget, Medical Report, 19 Sept. 1928; Bourget, *Douze Ans*, 197.

Dr. Bourget'.[75] Similarly, in other years, children from the Resolution residential school would travel with Bourget to visit their parents during the treaty gatherings. But that year, because of the sickness, Bourget decided they should stay behind. George Sanderson Sr warned Bourget that he felt ill even before they departed. The boat engineer was also sick but thought he was recovering. They both were so ill that the voyage took twice as long as normal. Bourget emphasized that their party was not the first to carry the sickness to Behchokǫ̀ but were preceded by another small boat, 'with her crew already ill'. Bourget felt pressured to go to Behchokǫ̀ because he was already behind schedule: there were 'eight hundred Indians', he wrote, who had been 'waiting for us for a long time, with no big fish to eat; they want to return home, to their hunting and fishing grounds'.[76] When they arrived, Bourget was so sick his legs wobbled and his eyes played tricks on him. Still, he and his sister-in-law distributed the treaty payments. When this job was done, Bourget fell into bed for four days, cared for by the Oblate fathers and Grey Nuns.

Meanwhile, the flu gathered momentum in Behchokǫ̀. Those who were well helped to nurse the sick, but there were limited supplies of southern medicine in the community. Ten cases of medicines had not arrived, and Bourget complained that 'it was ridiculous, we had the whole population sick and all we had left from the previous year were a few pills of quinine'.[77] It was not the first time, either, that the medicines had not come as expected. Bourget insisted that they should arrive with the first boat to be distributed during the treaty meetings. As it was, medicines arrived in August, by which time most Tłı̨chǫ and Dene had left the trade post. 'But', Bourget noted acerbically, 'the liquor permits for the white individuals are delivered on the first boat'.[78] The Tłı̨chǫ spoke to Bourget through an interpreter asking for a permanent nurse. Behchokǫ̀ was distant from the hospitals at Fort Smith and Fort Simpson and would not get its own hospital, Faraud Hospital, until 1940.[79] In the meantime, the Sisters who had accompanied Bourget 'for the recruiting of children' for the residential school at Resolution turned instead to help care for the sick in this moment of crisis. They did not, in the end, bring any children back to the school, 'due to the sickness of all'.[80]

Back in Fort Resolution, many people were sick. The *Distributor* had come and gone, treaty had been paid, and then 'you didn't see anyone walking around town, they were all sick', remembered Judith Giroux.[81] People who had come in for treaty and social gatherings were camped along the lakeshore in tents and tipis. George Sanderson remembered that the weather was hot that summer too.

[75] George Sanderson in *That's the Way We Lived*, 16. [76] Bourget, *Douze ans*, 197.
[77] Bourget, Medical Report, 19 Sept. 1928. [78] Bourget, Medical Report, 19 Sept. 1928.
[79] 'Faraud Hospital Fort Rae', F115 – 47/2, Archives of the Grey Nuns of Montreal.
[80] Bourget, Medical Report, 19 Sept. 1928. [81] Judith Giroux in *That's the Way We Lived*, 77.

Those in town who fell sick could not cook for themselves, if they even wanted to eat. Many people, like Sam Norn, lost their appetite altogether.[82] A café in town, run by Jim Mason, made soup for the sick.[83] Bourget's wife and a Dene girl who lived with the family also made 'soup, Bovril, tea and cocoa'.[84] Pierre Hilaire remembered that 'some people really suffered', lying in bed for as long as ten days.[85] Giroux's mother, who had already been sick for a long time, died during the epidemic. At its peak, people recalled as many as three or four people dying in one day. When interviewing Sam Norn in the early 1990s, Jeanette Mandeville shared how her father's father and stepmother both died on the same day. Norn remembered this too, that one had passed in the morning and the other at night.[86] Victor Lafferty, who was fourteen at the time, helped Willie Norn and Pierre Smith to dig graves, working steadily for more than two weeks. George Sanderson helped out too. Many people recalled William Clawhammer, an older man who stayed healthy and spent every day building coffins to bury the dead.[87] People who were well enough left Fort Resolution to head back to Rocher River. Virginie Calumet, who was fifteen years old at the time and lost her mother in the epidemic, remembered how 'a lot of people died while they were travelling back to Rocher River. A lot of people died when they stopped at Stoney Island. They buried them there.'[88] Fifty-four people died at Fort Resolution and Rocher River in the epidemic, most of whom were adults and elders.[89]

Hay River, Fort Providence, Fort Simpson

The *Distributor* had stopped at Hay River at 5:30 am on 27 June and was stuck there for the day on account of rough water, departing late at 9:30 pm. By 3 July, an 'Epidemic of Influenza quickly spreading throughout the village', wrote Singleton in the mission diary. 'Whole households down with it. School so far free.'[90] The next day, a boy at the Anglican residential school fell ill, and, although they made efforts at isolation, within days all of the boys and most of girls were sick. The matron and nurse also fell ill. As Singleton noted, 'Isolation becoming difficult and apparently useless.'[91] The epidemic lasted about six weeks, with the last death attributed to it on 5 August, and Singleton

[82] Sam Norn, interview with Jeanette G. Mandeville, 19 Mar. 1992, Fort Resolution, N-1997-012, MHAF; Joseph Jerome in *That's the Way We Lived*, 77.

[83] Albert Fabien in *That's the Way We Lived*, 76.

[84] Bourget, *Douze ans*, 200.

[85] Pierre Hilaire in *That's the Way We Lived*, 76.

[86] Norn interview, MHAF.

[87] Beatrice Daniels, interview with Jeanette Mandeville, 25 Mar. 1992, Yellowknife, N-1997-012, MHAF; George Sanderson in *That's the Way We Lived*, 77.

[88] Virginie Calumet in *That's the Way We Lived*, 75; David M. Smith, *Moose-Deer Island House People: A History of the Native People of Fort Resolution* (Ottawa: National Museums of Canada, 1982), 134.

[89] Beatrice Daniels in her 1992 interview said only one young girl was among the dead at Fort Resolution.

[90] St Peter's Daily Journal, 3 Jul. 1928.

[91] St Peter's Daily Journal, 7 Jul. 1928.

complained the weather was hot and close all that time. The children recovered, although some remained weak after their illness. Most of those who passed away were adults and elders, including Old Chief Lamalice, who had been present at the signing of Treaty 8 in 1900.[92] A government nurse, D. M. M. Bradford, visited the sick, bringing medicine. When Bradford fell ill, Minnie Hackett, who had just recovered from the sickness, stepped in. Singleton carried water for families, while a white commercial fisher, E. Demelt, caught fish for the community and their dogs, as well as carrying wood and water.[93]

Jimmy Sabourin was five years old in the spring of 1928 when he travelled with his family to Fort Providence for treaty. He remembered the epidemic in detail, and his account is one of the most widely circulated. The trip started off well, his family had had 'good luck' trapping that year and were able to buy a gramophone with the money they got for their furs. But then, after the treaty with the fields covered with tipis, 'the sickness came so suddenly. What could we do? We couldn't even run away.' Sabourin's grandmother prepared 'powerful medicine' by boiling manure, which helped him to recover.[94] Few who remembered 1928 spoke in detail of the medicines prepared by families, but there were many plant, animal, and other remedies available that eased the suffering of those who were sick and other medicines that could help frighten or send the disease away. Among the Gwich'in, boiled mooseberries, bear root, and northern ground cone were used to increase a sick person's appetite. Juniper berries were used as 'medicine for chest pains, bad colds, coughs, and congestion'.[95] Spruce tea and steam from boiled spruce boughs were used to relieve cold symptoms such as coughing, sore throats, and sore chests. 'Those who are sick with colds can take [spruce tea] three or four times a day for about five days.'[96] Tea made from the white flowers of yarrow could reduce nosebleeds, a symptom that appeared with influenza that year. The great challenge in 1928 was that so many fell sick at the same time that there were few well enough to gather plants or prepare medicines that were not on hand. As Sabourin recalled from Fort Providence, 'Gabriel Denetre's father was drumming to ask the sickness to go back to where it came from. By the next morning hardly anyone could stand.'[97] Sabourin's grandmother died, as did his uncle, bringing grief to the family.

The police report from Fort Providence suggested that it was people from Willow River who had brought the sickness in with them when they arrived for

[92] Fumoleau, *As Long as This Land Shall Last*, 102

[93] Bourget, Medical Report, 19 Sept. 1928; F. Cook to Officer Commanding, Fort Smith, 12 Sept. 1928, file 6099, LAC.

[94] Jimmy Sabourin, 'The Flu Epidemic', in *Nahecho Keh*, 59–60.

[95] Andre and Fehr, *Gwich'in Ethnobotany*, 48.

[96] Andre and Fehr, *Gwich'in Ethnobotany*, 17–18.

[97] Sabourin in *Nahecho Keh*, 59.

treaty.[98] Bourget said that it was Oblate brothers from Providence who travelled to Resolution for lumber, contracted the illness there, and then returned.[99] The *Distributor* had also stopped at Providence on 28 June and docked for about seven hours – enough time for Fleming to disembark and baptize the daughter of the HBC post manager, with James and Sarah Simon acting as godparents.[100] There had been multiple opportunities for the virus to spread.

The Anglican missionary at Fort Simpson, Franklin Clarke, anxiously anticipated the arrival of the *Distributor* on 29 June, delivering supplies and staff for the mission before departing the next morning. Other boats came and went over the next few days. A tea dance was held behind the NT post on 3 July. Then, on 6 July came the first reports of illness. Clarke visited six families, noting that 'many whites also sick with cold, "Grippe" I think'.[101] As the weather warmed, the community was overwhelmed by influenza. People were sick in almost every tent, 'generally the whole family'.[102] The first deaths, of a man and woman in their seventies, came within a week. But Clarke was most taken aback by the death of Harriet Denethlon, a woman in her thirties who, just a couple of weeks earlier, had helped to clean the church for the celebration of St John the Baptist. On 10 July, Clarke recorded in the mission journal that 'Josephine got us up this mg. at 6 a.m., "Harriet is dead! H. is dead!" A shock to us both. I saw her Sat. did not seem seriously ill.'[103] This was but one account of people whose deaths during the epidemic came suddenly without warning.

The government doctor, Truesdell, had departed with the *Distributor* on 30 June. But there was medicine at the post including quinine, mustard plasters, and 'Grip tablets', a commercial preparation of acetanilide that reduced fevers and offered pain relief.[104] By mid-July, Truesdell placed an urgent order for cough medicines, smelling salts, laxatives, quinine and sodium salicylate to ease fevers, stimulants, and sedatives.[105] At Simpson, Clarke used mustard plasters; these were a common treatment relying on the heat of the mustard against the skin to relieve congestion. Fort Simpson had a hospital, where Clarke and his wife recovered when they fell ill. Many others stayed in their tents. By 23 July, thirty-seven people had died in Fort Simpson or nearby. But the comings and goings of the summer season continued. The *Distributor* passed back through the community on 12 July, headed south with nurse Minnie Hackett on board. So too was the government doctor from Aklavik, A. E. Ward, departing the district 'owing to serious

[98] R. E. Parker to Officer Commanding, 31 Aug. 1928, file 6099, LAC.
[99] Bourget, *Douze ans*, 201. [100] Fleming Diary, 28 Jun. 1928.
[101] St David's Mission Journal, 6 Jul. 1928, Fort Simpson, Diocese of Mackenzie River, II 5 a vol. 2, GSA.
[102] St David's Mission Journal, 7 Jul. 1928. [103] St David's Mission Journal, 10 Jul. 1928.
[104] St David's Mission Journal, 7 Jul. 1928; see, for example, 'Foley's Cold and Grippe Tablets', Grand Rapids Public Museum, http://grpmcollections.org/Detail/objects/52385.
[105] J. F. Moran to O. S. Finnie, 20 Jul. 1928, file 6099, LAC.

illness in the family'.[106] The government's failure to replace Ward left Truesdell as the only physician from Fort Simpson to the Arctic Coast that summer. Quite a few people left Simpson on that same boat. The *Edmonton Journal* described the *Distributor* as 'crowded with passengers', fleeing the epidemic.[107]

Even as some people left for the south, others continued to arrive. Jean Godsell, wife of Philip, wrote in her memoirs 'that summer proved to be an extremely busy one indeed, the house being filled with more visitors than usual'.[108] When the *Distributor* landed again at Fort Simpson on 26 July, on board was Dr F. H. Mewburn, a seventy-year-old surgeon from Edmonton. Rev. Clarke asked Mewburn to examine his wife (there was no doctor at Simpson as Truesdell was away), and Mewburn advised that Mrs Clarke had bronchitis and pneumonia and would need careful nursing. Mewburn then went with Clarke 'to see Bella Andrew and the other sick Indians. Ellen Nadiya he said would hardly weather through.'[109] Mewburn was not the only tourist who visited at the post that day, a 'Prof. Gates of London (Eng.)' and his assistant ('a young Cambridge student') were in the North, 'taking blood tests fr. Indians'.[110]

Northern research and tourism continued apace that summer.[111] James Mackintosh Bell, who had previously surveyed the region in 1900 with Charles Camsell for the Geological Survey of Canada, was back prospecting on Great Slave Lake. He was joined by A. Y. Jackson of the Group of Seven and Frederick Banting, who were there for the wilderness experience rather than the geology. Banting offered medical assistance at Fort Resolution on their way out in late July.[112] Early August brought prospectors heading up the Liard River to Fort Simpson who arrived in a seaplane and others who came by more conventional transport, on the *Fort Rae*, a schooner from Resolution. R. H. Patterson was on the Nahanni River at the time. He would go on to fame for his book from his Nahanni adventures in 1927 and 1928. On 5 August, Patterson met up with Fenley Hunter, an American explorer travelling with Albert Dease and another man. Hunter told Patterson that 'flu is killing off the Mackenzie & Liard Indians by scores – &, most important, Sherwood & Poole Field mean to leave South Nahanni for the Flat with their big outfit

[106] D. L. McKeand to Lt. Col. E. Forde, 24 Jul. 1928, file 6099, LAC.
[107] '15 Dead at Resolution in Epidemic', *Edmonton Journal*, 17 July 1928.
[108] Jean Walker Godsell, *I Was No Lady; I Followed the Call of the Wild* (Toronto: Ryerson Press, 1959), 187.
[109] St David's Mission Journal, 26 Jul. 1928. [110] St David's Mission Journal, 26 Jul. 1928.
[111] For broader context, see Tina Adcock, 'The Maximum of Mishap: Adventurous Tourists and the State in the Northwest Territories, 1926–1948', *Histoire Sociale/Social History* 49, no. 99 (2016): 431–52.
[112] Prince of Wales Northern Heritage Centre, 'Timeline: 1928 A.Y. Jackson and Frederick Banting', www.nwttimeline.ca/1925/1928JacksonBanting.htm; J. M. Bell, Diary and Field Notebook Great Slave Lake Trip, RG 45 GSC Vol. 182, NS 1182, LAC.

about August 20'.[113] Patterson's description of important and less important news underscores the callousness of many sojourners towards northern peoples. In Fort Liard, when the treaty party arrived in late July, people were already sick with the flu, and six would die from the illness before the end of August.[114] For these researchers, tourists, and explorers – even those with medical expertise – the epidemic was little more than a footnote to their summertime adventures.[115]

Tulita and Blondin's Histories of the Flu

For people along Dehcho, the four weeks in July were stunning in the speed with which influenza crossed the region and overwhelmed families and communities. North of Fort Simpson, the role of the *Distributor* in carrying the disease became more distinct, as more people on the boat fell ill and then disembarked. But it is also from the Dene of Tulita and Sahtú (Great Bear Lake) that there comes one of the most powerful origin stories about the influenza epidemic. This story situates the genesis of the epidemic not in a virus that travelled on a boat down a river but in a great medicine power battle. George Blondin told this story in detail in both *When the World Was New* (1990) as 'A Conflict in Great Medicine Power' and in *Trail of the Spirit* (2006) as 'The Story of Bechachy'. This is not the only story of the epidemic rooted in northern Indigenous ways-of-knowing, but it is the most widely shared. I draw on the advice Annie Ned shared with Julie Cruikshank, to 'listen for different stories', to offer my observations about what I understand from these stories about the origins and significance of the 1928 epidemic.[116]

The stories begin before 1928 with the son of a powerful medicine man named Bechachy. The son participated in the debt system that underpinned the fur trade, supplying trappers in the fall and collecting payment in the spring. One spring, he went to collect a debt from 'an Elder and very strong medicine-power person named Bahwar'.[117] Bahwar negotiated with the younger man, asking to pay his debt later. Bechachy's son showed him no grace, 'You are

[113] R. M. Patterson, *Nahanni Journals: R.M. Patterson's 1927–1929 Journals*, ed. Richard C. Davis (Edmonton: University of Alberta Press, 2008), 114.

[114] Extracts from Report of Inspector W. J. Moorhead, 1 Sept. 1928, file 6099, LAC.

[115] Also Alf Erling Porsild and his brother Bob, with the anthropologist Cornelius Osgood, there to study the Sahtu Dene, working for Porsild to earn money while he pursued his research. Wendy Dathan, *The Reindeer Botanist: Alf Erling Porsild, 1901–1977* (Calgary: University of Calgary Press, 2012), 187–8.

[116] Julie Cruikshank, *Do Glaciers Listen? Local Knowledge, Colonial Encounters, and Social Imagination* (Vancouver: UBC Press, 2005), 76.

[117] The men have different names in the two versions of the story; in the earlier version Blondin calls the first man Salie, the powerful Elder Onzie, and Salie's father, Polee. In the second version, the first man does not have a name, the powerful Elder is Bahwar, and Salie's father is Bechachy. All quotations from Blondin, *Trail of the Spirit*, 133–40, unless otherwise indicated.

poor, but it is not my fault. You have to pay your bill like anyone else', writes Blondin. The two men grew angry at each other, and Bahwar threatened Bechachy's son. By the autumn, Bechachy's son was dead. Winter passed, and the spring of 1928 arrived. Dene went to Tulita to sell their fur, and a big feast was prepared. Before people could eat, there were speeches. Bechachy asked to speak, saying he had heard Bahwar killed his son with medicine power. Bahwar acknowledged the truth of this, and Bechachy became very angry. People in the crowd became scared and tried to calm things down, but Bechachy said he would kill Bahwar, to which Bahwar replied, 'If you kill me, I will take all your medicine people with me'. The crowd dispersed. Three days later, Bahwar died in the morning and Bechachy in the evening – a sudden loss of important people which happened along Dehcho that summer. 'From then on', Blondin continues, 'people died every day for a whole month. Over half of the people who went to Tulit'a to sell their furs that year never got back home.'[118] This story explains why it was that elders and adults died in disproportionate numbers, and how it came to pass that the Dene lost their medicine power in the modern world.

Blondin also offers other explanations. The battle between the powerful medicine men is the proximate cause, but that conflict was underpinned by a deeper tension arising from the historical experience of colonialism. These deeper roots are conveyed in the first instance by the longer temporal setting of the stories – it is not just 1928 that matters, but what came before. Bechachy's son is an agent of the HBC; he was 'one of the few English speaking Dene' at the time, he was also 'spoiled, proud, and a show off'. A transitional figure who lived between the world of the Dene and the world of the colonizer, Bechachy's son is not a good person. He had a lot of material wealth, 'and he had no respect for Elders'. Bahwar is in debt to him and to the HBC. Material poverty was a construction of colonialism, as was linking poverty to immorality or bad character. By contrast, Blondin writes, 'some Indians were poor . . . others were dishonest'.[119] Blondin draws attention to Bechachy's son refusing to help Bahwar as contrary to the 'sacred laws that were taught to the people by Yamoria', so that they could live safely in a world with powerful medicine. The callousness of Bechachy's son, his failure to show respect and care, reverberated in the devastation brought by the epidemic. Blondin also writes about the failure of the colonial state – not its failure to abide by Dene laws, but its failure to keep its own promises. Treaty 11 guaranteed help in times of sickness and famine, but in 1928, 'no help came'.[120]

Bechachy came from Fort Good Hope and lived his life on the lands around Tsiigehtchic. Bahwar was at Délı̨nę when he first met with Bechachy's son, and

[118] Blondin, *When the World Was New*, 175. [119] Blondin, *Trail of the Spirit*, 134.
[120] Blondin, *Trail of the Spirit*, 138; *When the World Was New*, 176.

the feast where Bahwar and Bechachy quarrelled was at Tulita, west of Délı̨nę on the main stem of Dehcho. Blondin's stories are from the Dene of those lands. To the north, the epidemic continued at Fort McPherson and Tsiigehtchic, in Aklavik, and along the coast.

Fort McPherson and Tsiigehtchic

Fort McPherson and Tsiigehtchic had very different experiences with the influenza, even though the communities are close together and were visited by the *Distributor* in quick succession. Thirty-five people died at Fort McPherson, about 12 percent of the population, whereas there were nine deaths at Tsiigehtchic, about 5 percent of the population.

Hyacinthe Andre remembered 1928 as the 'time that I left my father and mother's house' and began to work for himself.[121] He married Eliza Sam on 2 July 1928, and together they would go on to raise twelve children.[122] The day after their wedding, the *Distributor* arrived in Tsiigehtchic with many sick people on board. Within two weeks, the flu had spread through the community. When Andre caught the flu, 'Everyone said I may not recover, I was going to die too. There was a time when I thought, I was just sleeping, I had just slept. Then I woke up, and on my left ear I was deaf!'[123] It was after this that Andre began to feel better, although his recovery took some time. He was anxious to leave Tsiigehtchic and return to Tree River. Andre recalled that there were two policemen in town, Constables A. S. Wilson and C. J. L. Johnstone, who did not fall ill.[124] Andre helped others and remembered Wilson and Johnstone also gave care and assistance to the sick. Wilson had medical training and provided detailed description of symptoms. He noted that the first symptom was a headache, 'followed by vomiting and bleeding at the nose, then a racking cough'. Wilson wrote that it was curious how after a nosebleed, 'they began to get better, but they suffer most from weakness, which apparently lasts for some time'.[125] Andre described his own experience of this weakness, 'I really had no strength'. Wilson 'helped me up and I tried to walk. "Try not to fall I am helping you, if you fall and hurt yourself you will be in bed for another week"', Wilson said to Andre.[126] Andre remembered that 'most of the Elders died', including Eliza's father Sam, who passed suddenly.[127]

[121] Hyacinthe Andre, interview 19 Jun. 1999, GSCI, Gwich'in Elders' Biographies Research Project.
[122] Heine et al., *Gwichya Gwich'in Googwandak*, 247.
[123] Andre interview, Gwich'in Elders' Biographies.
[124] Andre interview, Gwich'in Elders' Biographies.
[125] A. S. Wilson to Officer Commanding, 31 Jul. 1928, file 6099, LAC.
[126] Andre interview, Gwich'in Elders' Biographies.
[127] Andre interview, Gwich'in Elders' Biographies.

From Tsiigehtchic, the *Distributor* detoured up the Peel River to deliver goods and drop off passengers at Fort McPherson, before heading back to the main stem of Nagwichoonjik. Sarah and James Simon returned home on the *Distributor*, arriving on 4 July. Everyone in the family fell sick with influenza, either on board the ship or after they arrived home. The sickness spread rapidly through the village, and people did what they could to help care for the sick, but compared to other communities there were fewer people well enough to provide care. Sarah Simon recalled, 'They no police, nothing . . . People just whoever could do it they help one another.'[128] On 22 July, a schooner arrived in Aklavik with a letter from J. I. Owen, a divinity student working as missionary at Fort McPherson that summer, requesting help. RCMP Corporal Belcher left the next day for Fort McPherson.[129] A trapper, Frank Carmichael, went with him. Johnny Kyikavichik spoke about the help given by Carmichael and Belcher, who 'did a lot for our people'. Upon their arrival at Fort McPherson, they turned the church into a hospital, 'it was filled with patients and there were a lot more sick people who had to stay at home'.[130] Having a hospital made caring for the ill much easier. For some of those who stayed at home, Belcher purchased blankets. Many were too ill to keep fires going, and it rained almost every day for a week during the epidemic.[131]

There was little food in Fort McPherson, and Johnny Kyikavichik recalled, 'this made everything seem worse'.[132] Belcher reported that when he arrived, he found people very sick and hungry. Then Abraham Stewart and two boys then went down to Black Mountain.[133] Although caribou were scarce, Stewart 'managed to get one and with this, they came back to McPherson'. Stewart gave the meat to Paul Nieman, who ran a little restaurant in the village, 'and he made soup with the caribou. The soup was given out to everyone in the settlement.'[134] Nieman spoke about this too: 'I made soup, cooked some meat, made stew, baked bread, and served lots of canned fruit.'[135] Kyikavichik remembered the caribou though, and how soup was made 'until the whole caribou went, and it really helped in getting the patients back on their feet'.[136] This was in keeping with Gwich'in understandings of good health as linked to eating caribou especially, but also other country

128 Simon interview, Gwich'in Elders' Biographies.
129 V. A. M. Kemp to Officer Commanding, Edmonton, 30 Jul. 1928, file 6099, LAC.
130 Johnny Kaye [Kyikavichik], 'The Flu – 1928', in 'Gwich'in COPE stories', 284.
131 A. T. Belcher to Officer Commanding, Edmonton, 6 Aug. 1928, file 6099, LAC.
132 Kaye [Kyikavichik], 'The Flu – 1928', 284.
133 Black Mountain or Chigwaazraii is in the Richardson Mountains, located west of Big Eddy on the Husky Channel. See GSCI, *Gwich'in Place Names Atlas*, https://atlas.gwichin.ca/index.html.
134 Kaye [Kyikavichik], 'The Flu – 1928', 284.
135 Paul Nieman, 'Pioneering in the Canadian North in the Land of the Midnight Sun', Paul Nieman Fonds, MSS 109 (80/79), YA.
136 Kaye [Kyikavichik], 'The Flu – 1928', 284.

foods.[137] Belcher witnessed the importance of the food, noting that 'I thoroughly believe that the food cooked did more to check the epidemic than the medicines we used'.[138] By the beginning of August, young boys and girls were well enough to fish and look after the older adults.

Aklavik, the Delta, and the Coast

Aklavik was a meeting place for Gwich'in, Inuvialuit, Métis, sojourners, and settlers. A trading post established by the HBC, Aklavik thrived in the early twentieth century with the rise of muskrat hunting in the wetlands of the delta. The dance that Julienne Andre remembered was recalled by others as well. Laura Raymond (b. 1922) and Edgar Kotokak (b. 1918) spoke about Inuvialuit Elders Ayaqak and Sanikpiaq who died that year. Raymond remembered carpenters building a platform in preparation for the dance, with the large canvas tarp to shade the dancers from the sun. Ayaqak had come to Aklavik from Baillie Island (about 350 kilometres to the east). He drum danced for two days; on the third day, he was dancing and then minutes later he died. Raymond remembered many Elders, including her grandparents, 'All died really quick. ... Start to get sick and never last a day.'[139] People had come to Aklavik for the dance, to feast, and to trade. They arrived before the *Distributor*, and David Roland (b. 1922) remembered how he 'could see the big smoke coming down, you know the *Distributor* is coming'. People were excited for the goods the ship brought. 'When it comes, when it unloads, everybody used to go for fresh stuff. It's only about over month old some of it', joked Roland.[140] The boat arrived on 5 July, just past midnight, and by 10 July – the same day Sarah Simon noted the epidemic broke out in Fort McPherson, the same day Harriet Denethlon died suddenly in Fort Simpson – the epidemic had appeared in Aklavik as well.[141]

As elsewhere, the whole community seemed to fall ill at once. Julienne Andre remembered how 'ones that were well worked with the sick'. There were two Inuvialuit men, Ovavak and Piouk, who 'went to every house helping people. They really liked the people.' By this, Andre was emphasizing how even though the men were Inuvialuit they cared for the Gwich'in. Andre and

137 Gwich'in Elders, *Nành' Kak Geenjit Gwich'in Ginjik/Gwich'in Words About the Land* (Inuvik, NT: Gwich'in Renewable Resource Board, 1997), 24–5.

138 Belcher to Officer Commanding, 6 Aug. 1928.

139 Laura Raymond, Sarah Mangelana, Norman Felix, Edgar Kotokak, interview with Florence Nasogaluak and Cathy Cockney, 11 Jul. 1996, Kitigaaryuit, tape 5A, transcript, in *Kitigaaryuit Oral Traditions Project 1996*, 72–3.

140 David Roland, interview by Agnes Gruben White and Murielle Nagy, Inuvik, 21 Feb. 1996, tape Aulavik 5A, in Murielle Nagy, ed., *Aulavik Oral History Project* (Inuvik: Inuvialuit Social Development Program, 1999), 9.

141 Codex Historicus, Aklavik, 10 Jul. 1928, OMI, PAA.

her mother were both sick. 'Ovavak's wife dried some meat and my mother put it in the water and cooked it and brought the broth to us. By acting that way, the Ovavaks saved us. We ate just a little meat, that's how we got our strength back.'[142] Sarah Meyook had come to Aklavik with her family that spring from the east. She was just a small child at the time, only two or three years old, and she was the only one out of her family who did not fall ill. 'My sister must have told me to give my brother a spoon to feed him', Meyook said. 'That's how he is alive now. He would have died if he'd starved if I didn't give him a drink. I don't remember how I looked after him.' She saved her brother, but Meyook herself was still very small.

> I would go on to my mom and dad. When I got on them I would find my mom's breast. I didn't know they were dead. I try to wake up my dad. They never moved. All that time they were both dead. I didn't know. My older sister and my brother were both very sick, so they never bother to check my mom and dad. They said only me was walking around.[143]

Her mother's friend, Sarah Ross, looked in on them. Finding Meyook's parents dead, Ross called on the minister who came and took the children.

Diamond Klengenberg remembered the heat. Although it still fell below zero sometimes at night, during the days it could get into the low twenties Celsius. The heat, 'made it worst. The river was hot and thick', recalled Klengenberg.[144] Archdeacon Fleming complained about the mosquitoes, which made 'life miserable outside so we all try to keep indoors as much as possible'.[145] Fleming fell ill, as did Geddes. Nurse McCabe was still sick on arrival in Aklavik. Although there were two hospitals, the Roman Catholic hospital filled quickly with the thirty children and staff from the Catholic residential school.[146] Klengenberg recalled, 'when the people got sick, there weren't many good doctors. There were doctors but they never really helped, when people got sick and started dying.'[147] There was some medicine in store, which the police quickly depleted. Corporal A. Fielding estimated that only six people in Aklavik did not fall sick during the epidemic. Klengenberg 'got sick for just one night'. When he awoke, he was better and brought water to others. He also helped the ministers to dig graves and bury people.[148] North of the treeline, and with people dying every day, they soon ran out of wood to make coffins. Sarah Meyook's parents were wrapped up 'with cloth around them but they never had coffin on them'.[149] Fleming helped to dig

[142] Julienne Andre in *Gwichya Gwich'in Googwandak*, 272.
[143] Sarah Meyook in *Yukon North Slope*, 57.
[144] Diamond Klengenberg in *Yukon North Slope*, 56. [145] Fleming Diary, 13 Jul. 1928.
[146] A. Fielding to Officer Commanding, Edmonton, 27 Jul. 1928, file 6099, LAC.
[147] Diamond Klengenberg in *Yukon North Slope*, 56.
[148] Diamond Klengenberg in *Yukon North Slope*, 56.
[149] David Roland and Sarah Meyook, interview with Renie Arey and Murielle Nagy, 19 Jul. 1991, Qargialuk (Ptarmigan Bay), tape 28A, transcript, in *Yukon North Slope Cultural Resources Survey*, book 2, 4.

graves, 'a very dirty muddy job'. They buried four people in one grave because there were no coffins left. 'It is a terrible business', Fleming observed.[150]

On 24 July, Anglican bishop Isaac Stringer and the Yukon Gold Commissioner each contacted the police and Finnie asking for a quarantine to protect the Yukon Territory.[151] Belcher, sent to McPherson to help, was instructed to prevent people from leaving McPherson, and in particular 'from crossing into the Yukon . . . until the epidemic is over'.[152] Finnie wired Bourget in Fort Resolution, and the hospitals in Aklavik and Fort Simpson, asking whether settlements in the Mackenzie district needed to be quarantined. In each instance, the response was that 'quarantine would be too late'.[153]

Having initially underestimated the severity of the sickness ('an epidemic of colds, from which recovery would be a simple matter'), RCMP Inspector Kemp wired Commissioner Cortlandt Starnes on 24 July to inform him that he was imposing a quarantine along the Arctic Coast.[154] There were at least thirty-five boats that regularly plied the waters along the coast, from Alaska to the Coronation Gulf, half of which were trading steamers and the other half family vessels (Figure 7.5).[155] As Laura Raymond remembered, 'That time, people always travel by boat. They hunted caribou in July by boat.'[156] The police were concerned about the need to deliver supplies to the east during the short window for navigation. Kemp reported to his superior that 'it is out of the question to hold up the boats till the epidemic is over'.[157] Instead, Kemp detailed restrictions on who could board or disembark from any boat, restrictions on where they could go on shore, and rules about wearing clothing that had not been previously worn in the infected areas. These measures had to account for the fact that there was no sulphur on hand, nor 'disinfectant sufficient to fumigate vessels'. On 27 July, Kemp met with Fleming at Herschel Island, 'about the Eastern Trip and prevention measures. As few services as possible! And none where there is sickness [and] to not go into houses (Natives).'[158]

[150] Fleming Diary, 21 Jul. 1928; on Great Slave Lake, Bourget describes burying people 'in shrouds like in the war', *Douze ans*, 200.

[151] R. Field to Commissioner, Ottawa, 24 Jul. 1928 and G. I. MacLean to O. S. Finnie, 26 Jul. 1928, file 6099, LAC.

[152] Kemp to Officer Commanding, 30 Jul. 1928.

[153] C. Bourget to O. S. Finnie, 2 Aug. 1928 and Father Moison to O. S. Finnie, 4 Aug. 1928, file 6099, LAC.

[154] Kemp to Officer Commanding, 30 Jul. 1928; Cortlandt Starnes to O. S. Finnie, 28 Jul. 1928, file 6099, LAC.

[155] Cortlandt Starnes to O. S. Finnie, 17 Jan. 1927, G-1979-043, file 7-24, NWTA.

[156] Laura Raymond, Sarah Mangelana, Norman Felix, interview with Florence Nasogaluak and Cathy Cockney, 12 Jul. 1996, Kitigaaryuit, tape 8B, transcript, in *Kitigaaryuit Oral Traditions Project* 1996, 128; see Ruben interview, *Paulatuuq Oral History Project*, 240–1.

[157] Kemp to Officer Commanding, 30 Jul. 1928. [158] Fleming Diary, 27 Jul. 1928.

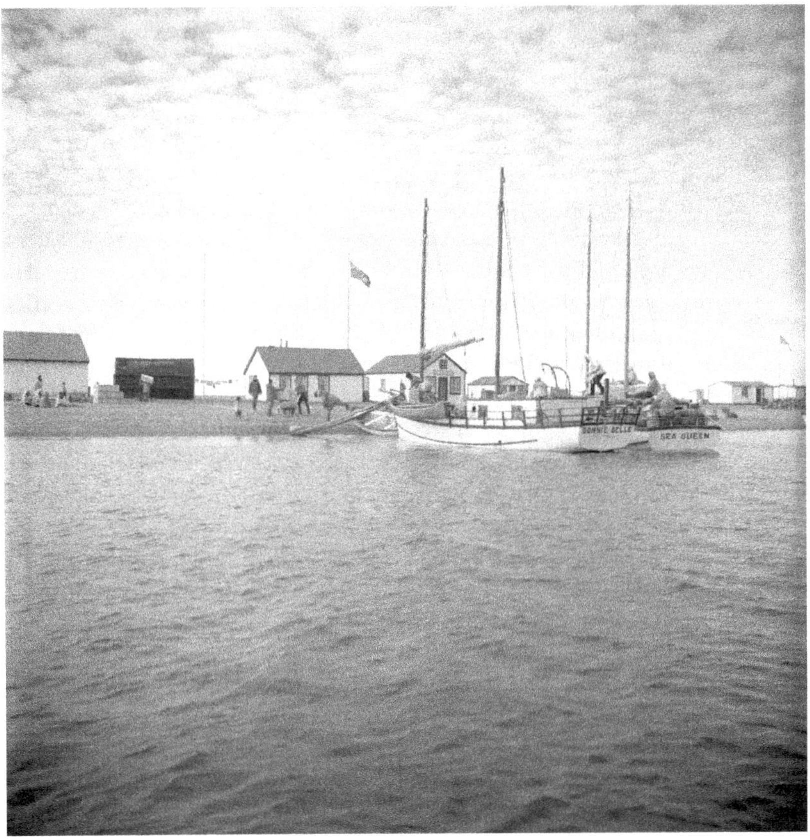

Figure 7.5 Inuit schooners at Tuktoyaktuk, 1936. Photograph by Richard Hourde while on an assignment for *The Beaver* magazine, HBCA 1987/271/NAC6, Hudson's Bay Company Archives, Archives of Manitoba.

With these and other restrictions, the police played a significant role in the epidemic at Aklavik and along the coast. Persis Gruben, who visited Qikiqtaryuk (Herschel Island) with her parents during the epidemic, remembered how 'we were not allowed to go around them [those who were sick] so that we would not catch it'. This also meant that she did not know where people who died that summer were buried, 'we didn't see, so we won't catch the flu'.[159] Corporal Fielding at Aklavik noted that he was 'taking every possible measure to prevent the natives from congregating in each other's tents and

[159] Persis Gruben in *Yukon North Slope*, 57.

houses'. Kemp reported that the Anglican hospital 'has been watched day and night by either a member of the Force or another white man', in order to keep patients from leaving. Kemp further noted that 'we have used one or two natives to do the orderly work'.[160] The racialized distribution of labour, the restrictions against gathering deployed specifically against 'the natives', and the prohibition against leaving hospital, all amounted to a much more intensive policing of the epidemic in the delta. No other communities in the Mackenzie district saw this level of police enforcement. Billy Ruben, who lived at Paulatuk, remembered the police in the 1920s enforcing new hunting regulations that reshaped Inuvialuit relationships with the land. He said, 'Pretty strict police that time. Springtime we couldn't hunt anything couldn't hunt caribou. They were real strict. We used to hide whatever you get when hunting.'[161] The role of the police in controlling the epidemic in the delta came about as part of the racialized approach to the epidemic, discussed further in Chapter 8, which perceived 'Eskimos' as more vulnerable to disease than 'Indians', and both as more vulnerable than 'whites'. Colonial authorities were also more concerned about asserting Canadian sovereignty along the coast.

Flu spread to Shingle Point and Herschel Island to the west, and to Kitigaaryuit, Tuktoyaktuk, and as far as Paulatuk in the east. People were travelling before the quarantine and infection-control measures were put into place, and 'they were sick everywhere', Raymond remembered.[162] Ruben named those who died at Paulatuk, including Elders and Billy Thrasher's son Tapqaaryuk (George Thrasher); he 'was already big when he got sick, nice boy and he died'. Ruben's mother helped care for people who were sick.[163] During the epidemic, so many adults fell ill that nursing care also fell to older children. Kathleen Hansen was thirteen years old in 1928 and with her parents at Qikiqtaryuk (Herschel Island). 'Only me was left when everyone got sick of flu.' Hansen continued: 'My mom and dad also my brothers. Everyone was in bed with flu. Because I was only one not sick, I look after the dogs, cook for them. My dad said he was so lucky to have me for not having the flu. I also get wood for them.'[164] She remembered a doctor visiting with Fred Wolki and Suzie, who brought soup 'in this kind of pail, and they hand out Soda Biscuits with soup'. The doctor also brought some medicine. The epidemic spread no

160 Kemp to Officer Commanding, 30 Jul. 1928.

161 Billy Ruben Isuqtaaq, interview with Lena Ruben and Cathy Cockney, 27 Jan. 2000, *Paulatuuq Oral History Project*, 140.

162 Laura Raymond, Sarah Mangelana, Norman Felix, Edgar Kotokak, interview with Florence Nasogaluak and Cathy Cockney, 12 Jul. 1996, Kitigaaryuit, tape 8A, transcript, in *Kitigaaryuit Oral Traditions Project 1996*, 126.

163 Isuqtaaq interview, *Paulatuuq Oral History Project*, 144.

164 Kathleen Hansen, interview with Renie Arey and Murielle Nagy, 7 Jul. 1990, Aklavik, tape 1B and 2A, transcript, in *Qikiqtaqruk Cultural Study*, 8, 1.

further along the coast that summer, although its repercussions would be felt for months and years going forward.

The East End of Great Slave Lake

At the east end of Great Slave Lake, the influenza continued its spread in the weeks after the treaty gatherings. Dene gathered at Fort Resolution included Wiiliìdeh Yellowknives Dene and Dënesųłiné who came from the east and who traded with the HBC, NT, and independents like Peter Baker at Rocher River, along the Taltson River, on the east arm of the lake at Łutselk'e and Reliance, and on the north arm of the lake, at Yellowknife River.[165] It was at Fort Resolution that Bourget delayed treaty payment waiting for more people to arrive; meanwhile, the flu was spreading among those already gathered. Dene from the Yellowknife River left Fort Resolution early after receiving their treaty payment but before collecting supplies, because of the sickness.[166] They carried the flu with them, and some fell sick before reaching their village. Others who lived around Łutselk'e and Taltson River and who had come to Fort Resolution also got sick. Families spent July with the few who were well caring for others on the islands and shores of the east end of Great Slave Lake.

On 18 July, the geologist Bell reached the entrance to Yellowknife Bay, where he met two Wiiliìdeh Yellowknives Dene men who told him a 'harrowing story of the decimation of the population of Yellowknife Village by the pneumonic flu, which is now raging, and asked for paper to write a letter to the priest at Fort Resolution'.[167] Bell also met up with the police later that day; but the police were preoccupied searching for Philip Godsell, whose boat had gone missing. In the days to come, the police distributed flour, bacon, tea, and medicines to the Dene camps where people were sick. On his return to Behchokǫ̀, Corporal J. L. Halliday reported that nineteen people had died by late July, including headmen and chiefs, and a further eight were not expected to survive.[168] At Reliance, on the eastern tip of the lake, sick families arrived at the police detachment on 31 July looking for help. They got medicines (quinine for fevers, calomel and soda – a purgative and decongestant, and magnesium sulphate – a laxative), fish netting, blankets, tea, and flour. Most of the survivors (more than forty people) continued on to Pikes Portage, to the east towards Artillery Lake, to hunt caribou.[169] Helge Ingstad was trapping near Łutselk'e and fell sick with the flu, as did the Dene families living on nearby islands. Ingstad only sometimes interacted with the Dene; he did not speak their

[165] Usher, *Fur Trade Posts*.
[166] J. L. Halliday to Officer Commanding, 28 Jul. 1928, file 6099, LAC.
[167] Bell, Diary and Field Notebook, 18 Jul. 1928.
[168] Halliday to Officer Commanding, 28 Jul. 1928.
[169] R. A. Williams to Officer Commanding, Fort Smith, 16 Aug. 1928, file 6099, LAC.

language. Nevertheless, in his memoirs, Ingstad told of conversations with Chief Marlo and watching children play.[170] Ingstad helped bury an old man before his elderly wife and surviving family members moved on to the east. Among the hardest hit were families living at Charles Goulet's camp. When a police patrol and then Bourget visited the camp in early August, it was empty. As many as twenty-six people had died, buried at a cemetery not far from the lake.[171] Seven survivors, two women, four men, and a ten-year-old child, left for the safety of the lands beyond the treeline.

Along Dehcho, around the large lakes, into the delta, and across the lands of the Mackenzie district, the 1928 influenza created a shared, regional epidemic at a scale – spatial and in lives lost – that had not been seen since the 1865 scarlet fever. While each village, trade post, and camp had its own experience of the influenza that year, the speed with which the virus travelled, borne by the SS *Distributor* north and radiating outwards from seasonal gatherings, created a shockwave across the land and deepened the epidemic's impact. Where this chapter has charted the experiences of influenza in 1928 and in the decades prior, the chapter to come turns to account for why the influenza travelled as it did at that time; to try to understand the dynamics – ecological, demographic, and social – that shaped its course; and to begin to assess the profound consequences of that devastating summer.

170 'Red Neighbours', in Helge Ingstad, *The Land of Feast and Famine* (Montreal: McGill-Queen's University Press, 1992), 145–55.

171 Bourget, *Douze ans*, 203–4; Bourget, Medical Report, 19 Sept. 1928.

8 Colonial Ecologies

From the nineteenth century onwards, colonial logics, processes, and power remade interrelationships between humans and the rest of nature in the Yukon and Mackenzie district, producing colonial ecologies knit through natural and social worlds. Linda Nash wrote of the 'inescapable ecologies' that keep disease situated in place, even if 'modernist amnesia' obscures these relations in favour of locating disease in sovereign bodies.[1] When it comes to directly transmitted, acute infectious diseases such as influenza, the ecological relationships at work in epidemics or pandemics are elusive. There is, of course, the distant instigating moment when a swine or avian influenza virus mutates and becomes transmissible among humans. From that mutation forth, however, human relationships with the virus and with each other are what shape the course of disease. This is in contrast to many other diseases that involve vectors (malaria, yellow fever, Lyme disease), that require human-built environments (Legionnaire's disease), or that are a product of environmental disruption and change (allergies, toxins).[2] Even without swamps, rats, or pesticides involved, influenza is as situated in ecological relationships as any other disease, and there is a materiality to experiences of influenza that shapes every outbreak, epidemic, and pandemic. This materiality lies in human relationships to each other and to pathogens through space and time. These relationships can confer specific immunity – or not – and can allow a pathogen to travel more easily between people and communities or can disrupt its transmission. The virulence, or severity, of disease produced by a virus is also part of that material relationship. Virulence arises from the nature of the pathogen, from the presence or

[1] Nash, *Inescapable Ecologies*, 6, 199.

[2] See among others McNeill, *Mosquito Empires*; Paul S. Sutter, 'Nature's Agents or Agents of Empire? Entomological Workers and Environmental Change during the Construction of the Panama Canal', *Isis* 98, no. 4 (2007): 724–54; George Dehner, 'Legionnaires' Disease: Building a Better World for You', *Environmental History* 23, no. 3 (2018): 522–44; Michelle Murphy, *Sick Building Syndrome and the Problem of Uncertainty: Environmental Politics, Technoscience, and Women Workers* (Durham, NC: Duke University Press, 2006); Nancy Langston, *Toxic Bodies: Hormone Disruptors and the Legacy of DES* (New Haven: Yale University Press, 2010); Gregg Mitman, *Breathing Space: How Allergies Shape Our Lives and Landscapes* (New Haven: Yale University Press, 2007).

absence of other pathogens, and the health of the bodies encountered. Colonialism shaped these material relationships, while also offering up and formulating new ideas about race to explain the severity of disease that accompanied settlers and sojourners. These are the colonial ecologies at work and which are the subject of this chapter, which traces the contours and effects of the 1928 influenza epidemic. Owsei Temkin writes that through the ancient global history of conceptualizing health, 'disease receives meaning when placed in man's moral universe, when its occurrence within a scheme of creation and right and wrong actions is accounted for'.[3] Blondin's histories of the 1928 epidemic offer a clear moral accounting that point directly to the effects of colonialism in northern lands and how it remade relationships among the Dene, with dire consequences. I build on this work by thinking further about the ways that influenza, a disease caused by a highly mutable virus, and its cataclysmic effects along Dehcho and the Arctic Coast in 1928 show how northern colonialism reshaped relationships, while feeding into understandings of 'race' and 'racial' difference.

Vulnerabilities

Ideas about race were imported to the Yukon and Mackenzie district as part of settler culture, while northern Indigenous bodies were simultaneously used to advance the construction of race science. When the *Distributor* stopped in Fort Simpson, on its second round trip of the season, on board was 'Prof. Gates of London'. This was R. Ruggles Gates, a eugenicist described by historian Elazar Barkan as 'among the most radical racists in British science', whose research that summer would inform the 1939 Supreme Court of Canada case over whether 'Eskimos' were 'Indians'.[4] Interested in blood groups, Gates and his student assistant Kenneth Mellanby worked out of 'missionary hospital[s]' and the residential school at Hay River and visited people in their tents as they travelled down the Mackenzie River to the delta.[5] Gates noted in his published research how 'the difficulties were also increased by the fact that all the Indians were either ill or just recovering from a severe epidemic of influenza'. For Gates, the flu epidemic was simply part of the challenges of his research: the

3 Owsei Temkin, *The Double Face of Janus and Other Essays in the History of Medicine* (Baltimore: Johns Hopkins University Press, 1977), 421.

4 Elazar Barkan, *The Retreat of Scientific Racism: Changing Concepts of Race in Britain and the United States between the World Wars* (Cambridge: Cambridge University Press, 1992), 170; L. Baker, 'Gates, Reginald Ruggles', http://eugenicsarchive.ca/discover/tree/512f9fab34c5399e2c000004; Backhouse, *Colour-Coded*, 45–6.

5 There was no discussion of consent. For the broader context of northern health research and ethics, see Tess Lanzarotta, 'Ethics in Retrospect: Biomedical Research, Colonial Violence, and Iñupiat Sovereignty in the Alaskan Arctic', *Social Studies of Science* 5, no. 5 (2020): 778–801 (p. 783).

'conditions under which the blood tests were carried out', as he wrote.[6] Gates obtained his samples by puncturing the left ear lobe with a surgeon's needle. He also physically examined those he tested – with attention to 'racial' characteristics – and elicited information about where they had been born and their families. He tested seventy-one 'Indians' and sixteen 'Eskimos'; Gates had hoped to collect more blood samples but ran out of supplies. Test subjects included Gwich'in, Inuvialuit, and Dene children at the Hay River residential school, as well as Dehcho Dene families living in Hay River, Tłı̨chǫ at Tulita, K'áhshó Got'ı̨nę at Fort Good Hope, Gwich'in at Tsiigehtchic, and Inuvialuit at Aklavik. On what was described in his obituary as an 'extensive expedition', Gates and Mellanby spent a fortnight in the Mackenzie, coming and going with the *Distributor* on a single round trip.[7]

The influenza epidemic shaped Gates's travels, even as Gates's research and the lens of race – specifically the categories of 'whites', 'Indians', 'Eskimos', and 'half-breeds' – were integral to the discourses used by settlers, sojourners, and colonial administrators to understand the severity of the 1928 epidemic.[8] On hearing of the epidemic in the Mackenzie, O. S. Finnie asked 'whether this epidemic is general or is [it] confined to Indians?'[9] When Ingstad fell ill, he wrote 'I learned from experience that the disease which had afflicted the Indians could attack the white man as well'.[10] Police reports made specific distinctions, as from Resolution on 21 July, when Sergeant Clifford described deaths he noted, 'six are half-breeds and the remaining 15 were indians'.[11] Race was also tied directly to outcomes, as when Dr Arthur Truesdell wrote that in Aklavik, 'the Eskimos are peculiarly susceptible to Influenza and gave up very easily'.[12] There are countless examples of these kinds of characterizations that circulated during the epidemic and in memoirs and correspondence thereafter.

The degree of racialization employed in 1928 was greater than that seen in earlier epidemics. Racial categories had been employed from the outset of colonial interactions around health, for instance, in the ways that Petitot constructed two different epidemics from the scarlet fever of the mid-1860s – one for Inuvialuit and one for Gwich'in as explored in Chapter 2. Categories were reified in the early twentieth century through new census definitions of race introduced in 1901, and through treaties that set 'half-breed' people apart

6 R. Ruggles Gates, 'Blood Groups of Canadian Indians and Eskimos', *American Journal of Physical Anthropology* 12, no. 3 (1929): 475–85 (p. 479).
7 J. A. Fraser Roberts, 'Reginald Ruggles Gates. 1882–1962', *Biographical Memoirs of Fellows of the Royal Society* 10 (1964), 90.
8 Capitalization here is consistent with the use commonly deployed at the time.
9 O. S. Finnie to Deputy Superintendent General, DIA, 16 Jul. 1928, file 6099, LAC.
10 Ingstad, *Land of Feast and Famine*, 152–3.
11 J. Clifford to Officer Commanding, 21 Jul. 1928, file 6099, LAC.
12 W. A. M. Truesdell to O. S. Finnie, 28 Sept. 1928, file 6099, LAC.

from their 'Indian' or treaty counterparts, with different rights and a different relationship to the state. These distinctions were reinforced along the coast where Inuit chose not to sign treaties and had still-different relationships with the federal state before and after 1939.[13] Lest we dismiss 'Indian' or 'Eskimo' as bureaucratic categories, there are many examples from the 1920s of racist ideas shaping beliefs about biological difference and social hierarchy. Frederick Banting was in the Mackenzie in 1928 and remains a highly respected figure in Canada's medical history. In 1927, he offered his expert advice to government officials regarding recent sickness among the Inuit, including the observation that, 'the Eskimo does not suffer from tonsillitis. I was told by a number of observers that the tonsils are invisible.'[14] Representations of not just different but inferior Indigenous peoples appeared in memoirs published by sojourners about their formative Arctic adventures and authored for southern audiences. Those which circulated into the post-war years have been examined critically by historian Joan Sangster.[15] In *I Was No Lady* (1959), Jean Godsell used racist pidgin to convey how the 'redskin' spoke, employing language that mimicked degrading depictions of African Americans. In one passage, Godsell writes of the popularity of 'skin bleach' at Fort Smith, portraying a Métis woman coming into her kitchen saying '"Dat damn stuff no good . . . I'm use all dem jars an' my skin . . . 'stead o' being white like yours" she jumped in fury, "is still lak damn black Injun's!"'[16] Racist beliefs, imagery, and cultural tropes were imported by settlers and sojourners to the Yukon and Mackenzie district in many ways, nowhere more so than in the residential schools where, in December 1927, boys performed a minstrel show as part of the seasonal celebrations.[17]

In 1928, 'race' mattered significantly in the influenza epidemic. Only two 'white' deaths were reported, one of whom was Arden A. Carroll, a fifty-two-year-old trader at Shingle Point.[18] The racial origins table from the 1921 census combined with the mortality estimated in the 1928 epidemic suggests that if this mortality were evenly distributed across the entire population, then we could expect anywhere from 79 to 149 'whites' to have died, where only two did.[19]

[13] Backhouse, *Colour-Coded*, 27.

[14] F. G. Banting to O. S. Finnie, 14 Sept. 1927, RG 85 vol. 1128, file 250-1-1, vols. 2–13, LAC.

[15] Joan Sangster, *The Iconic North: Cultural Constructions of Aboriginal Life in Postwar Canada* (Vancouver: UBC Press, 2016). Sangster discussed Godsell's writing specifically, pp. 40–2, 63–4.

[16] Godsell, *I Was No Lady*, 191, 202.

[17] St Paul's Daily Journal, 19 Dec. 1927; St Peter's Daily Journal, 5 Dec. 1927; see also blackface photos from Dawson, NA-4412–34 and PB-121–1, GM.

[18] Bishop Stringer to Rev. G. E. Merritt, 10 Oct. 1928, COR 263, file 3, Anglican Church, Series 1, YA; V. A. M. Kemp to Officer Commanding, Edmonton, 30 Jul. 1928, file 6099, LAC. Carroll appears in the 1921 census for Bernard Harbour.

[19] Table 27 in *Sixth Census of Canada, 1921*, vol. 1, 'Population' (Ottawa: F. A. Acland, printer, 1924), 540–1.

The Indigenous population essentially bore the entire weight of the deaths brought by the influenza in 1928, even as settlers and sojourners made up more of the population in Mackenzie district communities than ever before. 'Lack of resistance' was a common racist refrain in colonial reports about why so many northern Indigenous people died, but 'race' does not explain different experiences with the 1928 influenza.

From Fort McPherson, Johnny Kyikavichik recalled the epidemic: 'we lost a number of well-loved friends and neighbours. Some lost their small babies, grandparents, mothers, and fathers.'[20] Age and gender information is available for sixty-four of the 1928 influenza deaths, all but one of whom were Métis, Dene, Gwich'in, or Inuvialuit. Fifty-seven of the sixty-four deaths occurred between 10 July and 29 July 1928 – the height of the epidemic across the region. From these records, an equal number of men and women died. The more significant variation was in age groups, where the very young (under five) and the older (sixty and up) were at much greater risk of dying from influenza than other age groups. Elders in particular were vulnerable in 1928, as many observers noted at the time and as figured significantly in memories of survivors. For the group for whom age information exists, twenty-nine men and women over sixty died, compared to twenty-five between the ages of six and sixty, and eighteen deaths of children five years old and younger (see also Figure 8.1). There was nevertheless a significant number of adults under forty

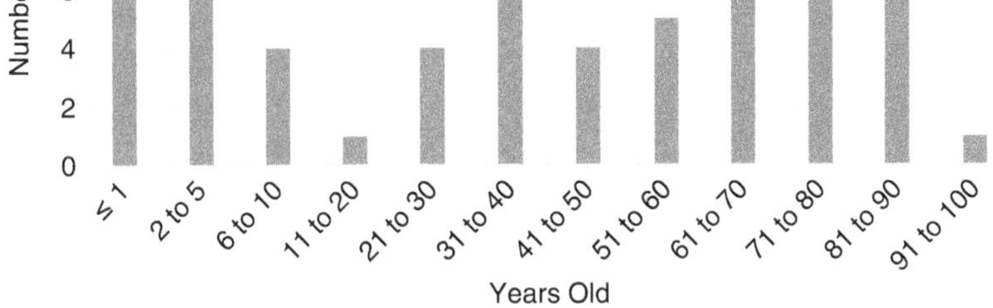

Figure 8.1 Age at death, influenza, 1928. Source: COD Database.

[20] Kaye [Kyikavichik], 'The Flu – 1928', 284.

who died. Looking at the relationship between age and gender, among the very young, boys and girls were equally vulnerable. Among adults aged twenty to sixty-five, women in their thirties were significantly more vulnerable than men. And among elders, men in their seventies saw the greatest number of deaths.

The significant effect of age on risk of death during this epidemic offers our first insight as to why fewer whites died in 1928, namely because far fewer whites grew old along Dehcho. Although there were those who spent their old age in the Mackenzie district and those who died and were buried in the North, many of the whites who appear in the census were traders, trappers, prospectors, missionaries, and government officials who returned south after a period of time. The pull to return south at times of ill health was apparent from the first newspaper story about the 1928 epidemic, which described the *Distributor* as full of people fleeing sickness. Not everyone who left on the *Distributor* were fleeing from the flu, however. Some, like Ward, were leaving because this was the first trip of the *Distributor* southwards, and it was the most efficient, direct, and comfortable of the steamboats travelling the river. The very idea of fleeing south in the face of sickness was a product of sojourning and settler culture. For the majority of northerners, whether Tłı̨chǫ, Gwich'in, Tagish, K'áhshó Got'ı̨nę, Inuvialuit, or Métis, it made no sense to leave their homelands when confronted with ill health. Nor would it make sense in the decades to come when evacuations for medical treatment became commonplace. For those for whom the North was a job, a station, a post, or an opportunity, however, leaving in the face of illness was a long-standing, deeply ingrained response.[21]

Census records give further evidence of this pattern. In the Fort Simpson census record for 1921, out of a total population of 507 there were twelve people of European or British origin over the age of fifty. Only two of these were over sixty: a prospector and Flynn Harris the Indian Agent.[22] Harris stayed in the North into the 1930s but moved to Cold Lake, Alberta in his old age and died there in 1943. Given close family connections and long-term residence in the North, Harris was among those most likely to stay, and still he left. There is a similar pattern in the 1921 census record from Tulita, which had only seven people who were of European or British racial origin over the age of fifty, and none over the age of sixty.[23] It is also significant, in this context, that of the two whites who died in 1928, the one whose age and gender we know was a man over fifty. The fact that the population in the Mackenzie district aged sixty and older would have been almost entirely Indigenous and that it was this

[21] See also L. Piper, 'Chronic Disease in the Yukon River Basin', in *Locating Health: Historical and Anthropological Investigations of Place and Health*, ed. E. Dyck and C. Fletcher (London: Pickering and Chatto, 2011), 129.

[22] 1921 Census Schedule for Simpson, N.W.T., 25.

[23] Whites and Indigenous people were enumerated separately in the 1921 Census. D. L. McKeand enumerated the whites at Fort Norman, District 231, Subdistrict 4, 27–9.

age group most at risk of death during the epidemic, helps to account for why Indigenous peoples disproportionately bore the burden of mortality in 1928.

Gender also had a part to play. There was a higher death rate among women in their thirties apparent in the detailed mortality evidence from 1928. Colonial record-keeping was relatively indifferent to women in this period, which makes understanding why these women were more vulnerable to the flu challenging.[24] However, pregnancy may have been a factor in some of these deaths. Mortality rates among pregnant women during the 1918 and 1957 pandemics were 'abnormally high'. In the 2009 influenza pandemic, the risk was highest in the later stages of pregnancy.[25] Among the deaths at Fort McPherson during the epidemic, there were two stillbirths recorded. The mother of one was recorded as dying in childbirth, and the second mother was recorded as dying from influenza.[26] Both women were in their thirties, and both may have had influenza, even though only one of the deaths was attributed to this cause. There was also a woman from Taltson River who died from the flu, with her infant stillborn 'at the mother's death', according to a police report.[27] Sarah Meyook's mother, who died in Aklavik, had very young children at her death and was likely part of this same adult cohort that saw higher mortality in 1928. Southern women living in the Mackenzie district at this time often sojourned as nurses or school teachers, spending months or a few years in the North before they returned home. Southern women who lived longer in the Mackenzie included many nuns. Although there were important exceptions – wives of police officers or Anglican missionaries, for instance – the occupational categories that brought young women north often also meant that these women were less likely to be pregnant or raising small children than women born on these lands.

There were, as we saw in Fort McPherson, problems with securing food – especially fresh meat – during the epidemic. This arose foremost from the 'weakness' described by those who fell ill. Jimmy Sabourin spoke of how people were so sick 'hardly anyone could stand'. His parents were 'too sick to even move. They couldn't even sip water.' His grandmother 'tried to crawl out', to help light a fire, 'but she was too weak'.[28] Hyacinthe Andre was so weak he could hardly walk to the entrance of his house, let alone leave to hunt or fish.[29] Virginie Beaulieu recalled how the 'sick people couldn't cook for themselves'.[30] When Ingstad fell ill, he was unprepared and 'living from hand

[24] See Appendix.

[25] William M. Callaghan, Susan Y. Chu, and Denise J. Jamieson, 'Deaths From Seasonal Influenza Among Pregnant Women in the United States, 1998–2005', *Obstetrics & Gynecology* 115, no. 5 (2010): 919–23, http://doi.org/10.1097/AOG.0b013e3181d99d85.

[26] COD Database IDs 2269, 2270, 2281, 2292.

[27] Extracts from Report of Inspr N. Royal Gagnon, Fort Smith, 11 Aug. 1928, file 6099, LAC.

[28] Sabourin in *Nahecho Keh*, 59–60. [29] Andre interview, Gwich'in Elders' Biographies.

[30] Virginie Beaulieu in *That's the Way We Lived*, 75.

to mouth'. He had to catch fish to eat but felt so sick that he wanted to just let it rot in the nets, 'for I was unable to swallow a mouthful of food in any event'.[31] Fleming observed how 'this Flu leaves people so weak', even after they started to recover.[32] This weakness, though, was a product of the flu infection – not a pre-existing condition. More white trappers in the Mackenzie district, people like Ingstad, created greater competition for resources and declines in fur bearers as a result. There had been reports of caribou not coming to their usual places in 1927.[33] But in general there was no more evidence of hardship and hunger preceding the 1928 flu than in any other year; no exceptional weather conditions, no population crashes, and few failed hunts that meant people were malnourished before the flu arrived. In 1928, Sabourin remembered how his family 'were great trappers and had good luck'. Joe Bayah (b. 1910), remembered his father going into Tulita to trade that spring with '45 beaver skins. And they had 450 muskrats. And a lot of other furs.'[34] The flu did not come in a year of pre-existing widespread hardship; some people struggled (as in Blondin's story of Bahwar), but others were prospering. Across the Mackenzie, it was the flu that left great adversity in its wake.

Age also appears to have been a more significant factor in shaping influenza mortality in 1928 than tuberculosis co-infection. Deaths reported from Fort Simpson, Reliance, Herschel Island, and Fort Resolution identified tuberculosis as a complicating cause in some deaths. There are twelve deaths in the database attributed to tuberculosis that occurred during the epidemic, although only one death in the burial registers is attributed to both tuberculosis and influenza. In all of the cases where age information was available, these tuberculosis deaths were in children or younger adults – not elders, although as we will see in Chapter 9, this was consistent with tuberculosis mortality in the North in these years. In speaking about her mother's death, Rose Fabien described how, 'my mom spit blood and she was sick for a long time and then she died'.[35] This suggests that Fabien's mother was sick with tuberculosis before she caught the flu. Some of those whose deaths were attributed to tuberculosis and influenza during the epidemic were described as emaciated at the time of death.[36] At Herschel Island, three of the seven who died were people who 'were ill with tuberculosis before the epidemic reached here'.[37] Long-term or advanced tuberculosis infection appears to have contributed to deaths, as did other co-infections. 'Other complaints besides the flu', including

[31] Ingstad, *Land of Feast and Famine*, 153. [32] Fleming Diary, 14 Jul. 1928.
[33] J. Clifford to Officer Commanding, 19 Mar. 1927, RG 10, vol. 6742, file 420-6 1, part 2, LAC.
[34] *MVPI Fort Franklin, NWT* (26 June 1975), vol. 9 (testimony of Joe Bayah), 783.
[35] Rose Fabien in *That's the Way We Lived*, 76.
[36] R. A. Williams to Officer Commanding, Fort Smith, 16 Aug. 1928, V. A. M. Kemp to Officer Commanding, Edmonton, 30 Aug. 1928, file 6099, LAC. COD Database ID 6277.
[37] Canada, Parliament, Sessional Papers, 'Report of the Royal Canadian Mounted Police, 1928' (Ottawa, 1929), 58.

one child in Aklavik with 'a severe dysentery', caused higher mortality in 1928, especially among younger people.[38] Pneumonia is the most significant co-infection that kills during influenza epidemics, as was apparent in 1928.[39] Children in residential schools would have been at risk, given widespread tuberculosis infection in these institutions in the 1920s. In 1928, there were 173 children reported in attendance at the four residential schools in the NWT. Almost all of these children fell ill during the epidemic, and while there were 'many complications', only one schoolchild died from the flu that summer.[40] We will return to the relationship between tuberculosis and influenza again in Chapter 9. That children in the schools were less vulnerable to influenza in 1928 points primarily to the lower risk of death in this epidemic for their age cohort, people between five and twenty years old.

Immunities

Influenza is a highly contagious, acute, viral disease that attacks the respiratory tract. The virus might incubate in a body for one to three days, and recovery usually occurs within a week. Deaths from influenza can result from organ failure or sepsis, but most commonly arise from pneumonia, which can be a consequence of influenza infection on its own or co-infection by the influenza virus and bacterial pneumonia. The three types of influenza that cause disease in people are designated A, B, and C, a sequence which reflects both the order of their discovery and decreasing severity. Influenza A is the type that has been associated with pandemics and major epidemics and can cause significant morbidity and mortality.[41] Influenza type A is further distinguished by numerous subtypes based on the pattern and shape of proteins (**h**emagglutinins and **n**euraminidases) on the surface of the virus. These are what designate **H**1**N**1 or **H**3**N**2 influenzas, the prevailing subtypes that circulate in human populations. Human bodies have defences against influenza viruses in the form of innate (general) immunity and immune memory (specific), where the body is able to more quickly fight off a virus that it has previously encountered. But perhaps the most important defining feature of influenza is that it is not a stable virus, and because it is constantly changing it can evade immune defences.[42] Antigenic drift is the process whereby small mutations in influenza virus genes produce different patterns in the defining H and N surface proteins that

[38] A. T. Belcher to Officer Commanding, Edmonton, 6 Aug. 1928; Truesdell to Finnie, 28 Sept. 1928, file 6099, LAC.

[39] Fleming Diary, 24 Jul. 1928; Andrew Noymer, 'Influenza Analyses Should Include Pneumonia', *American Journal of Public Health* 98, no. 11 (2008): 1927–8.

[40] C. Parker report to D. C. Scott, cited in Fumoleau, *As Long as This Land Shall Last*, 358; Bourget reported on his visits to Providence and Resolution 19 Sept. 1928; St Peter's Daily Journal, 4–23 Jul. 1928; Truesdell to Finnie, 28 Sept. 1928.

[41] Dehner, *Influenza*, 23. [42] Dehner, *Influenza*, 25.

mean the body's defences no longer recognize the viral invader. This drift is why we need annual influenza vaccinations: the virus changes from one year to the next, and the vaccine targets the newest version, updating the body's defences at the start of flu season. A greater, abrupt change in the influenza virus is referred to as antigenic shift. The 1957 pandemic arose when the prevailing H1N1 viral strain was replaced by a new H2N2 strain that spread rapidly. In 2009, antigenic shift produced a new H1N1 virus that differed from the prevailing H1N1 types then in circulation and became pandemic.[43] These more significant mutations in influenza viruses arise in the crucible of human relations with birds and swine especially, as it is the intermingling of human influenza viruses with those from other species that encourages genetic re-assortment.[44]

Any population can become immunologically naïve when confronted with a novel pathogen, and with influenza this process happens over and over again.[45] Nevertheless, relations between this virus and human bodies are shaped by past encounters. Even in 1918–19, people over sixty-five appeared to have protective immunity during the pandemic, presumably conferred by exposure to a virus that had circulated before 1889.[46] The importance of such previous exposures to specific immunity or immune memory encourages modes of analysis that point to so-called isolated populations – like those in the North – and argue that their vulnerability to epidemic influenza was rooted in fewer previous encounters with circulating flu viruses.[47] On one level, this reasoning makes sense. As Mathews et al. write, 'in the highly connected modern world, most populations are regularly exposed to non-pandemic viruses, which can even boost immunity without causing influenza symptoms'.[48] But this line of analysis, I argue, mis-imagines so-called isolated populations and their historical relationships with cosmopolitan pathogens. In 1986, Alfred Crosby wrote about an Amazonian Indigenous community, 'contacted for the first time' who 'lost at least 15 percent of their people in a single brush with common influenza. The evidence is that when isolation ceases, decimation begins.'[49] There are problems with this line of reasoning, from the notion of

[43] Gavin J. D. Smith, Justin Bahl, Dhanasekaran Vijaykrishna, et al., 'Dating the Emergence of Pandemic Influenza Viruses', *PNAS* 106, no. 28 (2009): 11709–12, http://doi.org/10.1073/pnas.0904991106; Centers for Disease Control and Prevention, '2009 H1N1 Pandemic (H1N1pdm09 virus)', www.cdc.gov/flu/pandemic-resources/2009-h1n1-pandemic.html.

[44] See also Taubenberger and Morens, '1918 Influenza'; Mathews, Chesson, McCaw, and Vernon, 'Understanding Influenza Transmission'.

[45] Hackett, *Remarkable Sickness*, 88. [46] Taubenberger and Morens, '1918 Influenza'.

[47] Mathews, Chesson, McCaw, and Vernon, 'Understanding Influenza Transmission', 147; G. D. Shanks and J. F. Brundage, 'Pacific Islands Which Escaped the 1918–1919 Influenza Pandemic and Their Subsequent Mortality Experiences', *Epidemiology & Infection* 141 (2013): 353–6.

[48] Mathews, Chesson, McCaw, and Vernon, 'Understanding Influenza Transmission', 143.

[49] Crosby, *Ecological Imperialism*, 197.

'common influenza' to the conclusion that imagines isolation as a threshold that is crossed: from isolation to connection; from 'virgin soils' to acquired immunity. Examining the 1928 influenza epidemic shows the limits of such analysis and offers other ways to historically imagine relationships between pathogens and small populations living on large territories distant from, but connected to, dense population centres.

After 1919, H1N1 became the prevailing seasonal influenza, and some years the flu was more lethal than others. Of course, this was not understood at the time as the influenza virus itself was not discovered until 1933, and early research was muddled by disagreements over the possible role of bacteria or a virus.[50] In their 1940 textbook, *Virus Diseases of Man*, C. E. Van Rooyen and A. J. Rhodes noted significant influenza epidemics repeatedly in the 1920s, albeit with mortality well below the 1918–19 pandemic.[51] Historians and northerners described these epidemics in the 1920s (Table 8.1) as they pulsed through the North, sometimes characterizing them as the 'Spanish flu'.[52] This term was used in these contexts by northerners and historians alike to link the severity of specific outbreaks in the early 1920s to the well-known lethality of the 1918–19 pandemic. These were not the regular flu, they say, they were the 'Spanish flu'. This usage was at once inaccurate and apposite. It was inaccurate because there were marked differences between the virus that circulated the globe in three waves in 1918–19 and those that came after. Mortality in 1918–19 was much greater, and the proportion of young adult deaths much higher. More importantly, the virus drifted after 1918. So if we are imagining influenza's global travels in and after 1918, calling influenza in 1920 or 1922 the 'Spanish flu' gives the impression that a disease that was circulating in the urbanized south in 1918–19 just took that little bit longer to arrive in the North. Instead, the influenza outbreaks in 1920, or 1921, or 1922 are better understood as seasonal influenzas that reached northern communities from southern outbreaks in years when the protective measures deployed in 1918–19 were absent. The characterization is apposite because after 1918, seasonal influenza viruses were H1N1, and in that sense different from the viruses that had circulated before.

The relationship between the influenza in 1928 and previous influenzas is an important one (Figure 8.2). Before 1918, influenzas circulated frequently in the

[50] See for example, 'File: Miscellaneous influenza in Canada', 1920, RG 29 vol. 186, file 310-10-1, LAC; Dehner, *Influenza*, 48–50, 59; Michael Bresalier, 'Uses of a Pandemic: Forging the Identities of Influenza and Virus Research in Interwar Britain', *Social History of Medicine* 25, no. 2 (2011): 400–24.

[51] C. E. Van Rooyen and A. J. Rhodes, *Virus Diseases of Man* (London: Oxford University Press, 1940), 577; Selwyn D. Collins, 'Influenza-Pneumonia Mortality in a Group of about 95 Cities in the United States, 1920–1929', *Public Health Reports* 45, no. 8 (21 Feb. 1930), 364–5.

[52] McCarthy, *Great River*, 206; 'The diary of Victor Mercredi', Acc.# 71.369, PAA; Mercredi interview, MHAF; McCormack, *Fort Chipewyan*, 268; Johnnie Johns interview; Fumoleau, *As Long as This Land Shall Last*, 355.

Table 8.1 *Influenzas 1920–7*

Area of Outbreak	Year	When appeared	Specific locations	Deaths	Ages at death
Yukon	1920	Mar.–Jul.	Carcross	4	One infant, three elders
			Chooutla School	1	Thirteen-year-old Tutchone boy
			Whitehorse	1	Adult
			Dawson	3	Adults including two women in their thirties
Lake Athabasca	1922	Mar.–Apr.	Fort Chipewyan	20	
			Fond du Lac	88	
Yukon and Alaska	1925	Jun.–Aug.	Mayo	3	Elders, two in seventies, one in nineties
			Fort Selkirk	5	One seven-year-old, four adults
			Dawson	6	One adult male from Moosehide; others born outside Yukon, forties and older
			Moosehide	1	Teetł'it Gwich'in man in fifties
			Fort Yukon	12	
			Whitehorse	1	Male in his sixties from Little Salmon
			Champagne/ Haines Junction	1	Male in his forties
Arctic Coast	1926	Spring and summer	Bathurst Inlet	2	Adults
			Bernard Harbour	20	All ages
			Coppermine River	13	All ages
			Inland Tree River	3	One adult, others unknown
			Krusenstern	3	One adult, others unknown
			Lady Franklin Point	2	
			Prince Albert Sound	3	One elder, two adults
			Rymer Point	2	
			Tree River	7	Adults, youth, and unknown
			Victoria Island	5	Adults, youth, and unknown
	1927	Aug.–Sept.	Bernard Harbour	6	One elder, two adults, one child, two infants
			Rymer Point	4	Two elders, one child, one infant

Sources: COD Database; Skookum Jim Oral History Project Fonds, YA; Linklater Fonds, YA; Canada, Parliament, Sessional Papers, 'Report of the Royal Canadian Mounted Police, 1928'. Ottawa, 1929; McCarthy, *Great River*; McCormack, *Fort Chipewyan*.

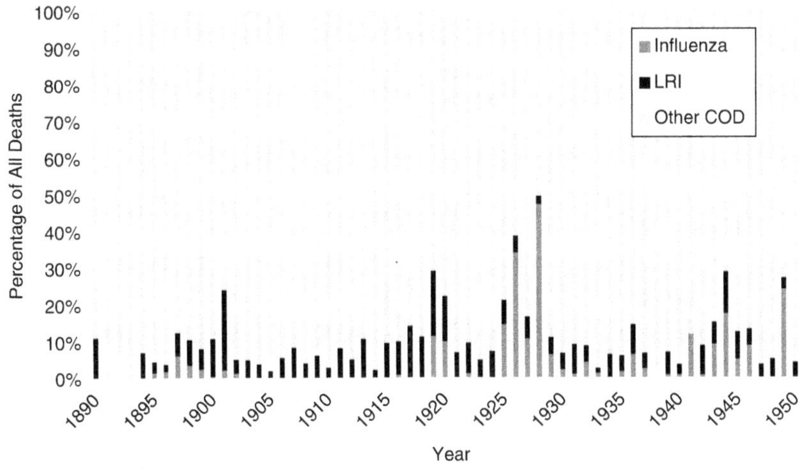

Figure 8.2 Mortality from influenza and lower respiratory infections (LRIs) relative to all other causes of death, 1890–1950. Source: COD Database.

Mackenzie district. Between 1890 and 1910, they did so with a pattern that approximated influenza outbreaks in other more populous and connected places. Although the 1918–19 influenza pandemic only reached the edges of the Yukon and Mackenzie district, specifically with mortality in northern Alberta and the southern Yukon, H1N1 did not otherwise travel the length of the Mackenzie River that year. There were several significant outbreaks between 1920 and 1928: at Fort Chipewyan, at Fort Selkirk in the Yukon, and in the Coppermine River region of the Arctic Coast. These outbreaks were at times linked to the 'Spanish flu' and were outbreaks of seasonal influenza. The geography of these 1920s outbreaks informs our understanding of the geography of the 1928 epidemic. In 1928, influenza did not travel eastward beyond Paulatuk on the Arctic Coast. While this can be attributed to quarantine and isolation measures imposed by Inspector Kemp, the devastating influenza of 1926 surely also played a role. Sixty people died in 1926, an estimated 7 percent of the population recorded in the 1921 census. As Bishop Stringer wrote about the 1928 epidemic, 'It was very hard on the natives, especially just as apparently *the same kind of epidemic* carried off so many around your district last year at Coronation Gulf'.[53] People who had survived the previous influenza epidemic may have been more cautious in 1928, particularly if they knew there was another flu circulating. And those who survived the flu in 1926

[53] Stringer to Merritt, 10 Oct. 1928. Emphasis added.

may have had greater immunity to the flu in 1928, lessening the chance of serious disease or death. This latter effect would apply if we knew that the influenza reached people near Kugluktuk in 1928, and that we cannot say for certain. The archival evidence goes no further east than Paulatuk. However, to the south, Fort Chipewyan saw influenza in 1922 and 1928. In Table 7.1, we see that mortality at Fort Chipewyan in 1928 was significantly lower (around 1 percent of the total population) than the mortality anywhere else in the Mackenzie district, with the exception of Fort Smith. This was still a significant influenza epidemic for Fort Chipewyan but with lower mortality.

In 1928, there were significant influenza outbreaks elsewhere in the North: at Wakeham Bay/Kangiqsujuaq in Nunavik, where eight adults died, and another in Labrador.[54] Neither was connected to travellers from the west but rather came directly from the south. Research on influenza epidemics done in the 1940s repeatedly pointed out that 1928 was a particularly bad year for influenza. The severity of 1928 was more apparent at mid-century, before the influenza pandemics of the late 1950s and 1960s offered new perspective on how bad influenza could get. In the 1940s, the Minnesota State Board of Health identified 1928 and 1929 as 'the most serious outbreaks' since 1918–19. The physician and immunologist Rufus Cole gave a speech in 1946 on 'the Etiology and Prevention of Influenza'. In it, he noted that an epidemic in the winter of 1943–4, while of short duration, 'was the most extensive and serious that had occurred since 1928, which was the worst since 1918'. Cole continued with statistics to support his claim, 'The excess mortality in 90 large cities in 1943–44 was 50, in 1928–29 was 65 and in 1918–19 was 598'.[55] Van Rooyen and Rhodes emphasized the severity of epidemics in the decade after 1918, with particular note 'of 1922, 1923, 1926, and spring 1928', where there were 150,000 deaths in excess of the expected seasonal rates.[56]

Influenza actually broke out twice in 1928, first in the spring and then again in the winter of 1928–9.[57] Several people who survived the 1928 epidemic commented on how normal it was for the first boat of spring to bring colds to posts along the river. But in most years, these were just that – colds. It was rare for influenza to be circulating globally in the spring, and so it was also unusual

[54] See Ralph Parsons to O. S. Finnie, 10 Aug. 1928, RG 85 vol. 1128, file 250-1-1, vols. 2–13, LAC; S. G. Coward to O. S. Finnie, 10 Dec. 1928, and 'Account of Supplies Furnished . . . Aug. 1928' in file 6099, LAC; W. G. Smillie, 'An Epidemic of Influenza in an Isolated Community – Northwest River, Labrador', *American Journal of Epidemiology* 11, no. 2 (1 March 1930): 392–8.

[55] 'Report of the Minnesota State Board of Health and Vital Statistics, 1922–1943', 30–1 and Rufus Ivory Cole Papers, BC 671, 12, both in *American Influenza Epidemic of 1918–1919: A Digital Encyclopedia*, www.influenzaarchive.org. See also Collins, 'Influenza-Pneumonia', 364–5.

[56] Van Rooyen and Rhodes, *Virus Diseases of Man*, 577.

[57] John Hawksley, 'Report on the Carcross Indian Residential School', 9 Jul. 1929, RG 10 Vol. 6479 File 940-1, parts 1, C-8794, LAC.

for it to come into the Mackenzie district with the first boat. A decade earlier, in March 1919, with the prospect of the influenza pandemic in the North looming and quarantine planning on his mind, Inspector Anderson warned about the dire consequences should pandemic flu arrive in the Mackenzie district in the spring: 'The Flu is most likely to strike there when the boats commence running, and the warm weather arrives', wrote Anderson. He continued by observing 'The boats can not be stopped as the supplies has to get into the country, as if they did not the country would starve.'[58] In 1928, this timing came to pass, and the decision to let the boats continue on had devastating effects.

It would appear from Fort Chipewyan that a previous encounter by the community with H1N1 influenza softened the impact of the 1928 influenza. Survival and recovery from the 1918–19 influenza pandemic may also help to account for some of the disparities in who died in 1928. People living in the Mackenzie district in 1918 were not exposed to the flu virus that year. Those who came to the Mackenzie later may well have encountered and survived the 1918 flu. The majority of people who immigrated to the Mackenzie were not Indigenous. This included the prospectors and government officials who came in the wake of the oil strike at Norman Wells and the signing of Treaty 11. But Indigenous people also travelled in and out of the region, like Mackenzie Joe, who died of the flu in Fort Selkirk in 1925. No systematic records exist of previous influenza exposures. The only person who made explicit reference to their own experience of the 1918 pandemic was Clermont Bourget. He closed his September 1928 report to O. S. Finnie with the observation, 'I had six months of experience with the flu in France, and this epidemy [*sic*] was severe evn [*sic*] among the whites who were real sick and the recovery has been long and tedious'.[59] In 1928, Bourget was very sick, unable to care for himself for at least four days. He emphasized, as is supported by other evidence, that the flu in 1928 was not just a regular influenza but very severe, even among those people who had experienced the 1918–19 pandemic. Some protection may have been offered to a very small portion of the population by previous exposures to the influenza, and this would have been a greater factor among recent immigrants to the Mackenzie, who were predominantly white.

All that said, proximity in time between 1918 and 1928 and the frequency with which flus circulated in the North belie the significance of the protection offered by immunity acquired in that decade. Had the 1918–19 influenza reached the Mackenzie district, many people, possibly far more than in 1928, would have died then. That would have been a different epidemic with different character and effects, and in that instance neither whites nor Indigenous

[58] K. F. Anderson to 'N' Division, Peace River, 8 Mar. 1919, file G6, LAC.
[59] C. Bourget, Medical Report, 19 Sept. 1928, file 6099, LAC.

northerners would have had immune protection – that was the nature of the 1918 pandemic. Immunity as shaped by previous exposure to influenza had a role to play in 1928, but it is just one piece of a complex puzzle when it comes to understanding the course and consequences of the epidemic.

Choices

George Blondin wrote how in the spring of 1928, people were happy and well-off when they gathered on Sahtú for a drum dance and games, 'but the Elders warned that a great disaster was coming'.[60] Inspector Anderson did not have their foresight, but in 1919 he did anticipate the impacts of flu arriving in the spring, when the boats would carry it downriver. His warning points directly to one decision that produced the 1928 epidemic, namely that the *Distributor* was not halted in its first trip downstream because of the need to get supplies 'into the country, as if they did not the country would starve'.[61] This proposition in itself was the product of colonial anxieties around subsistence in the North and the creation of food economies predicated on importing southern foodstuffs that permitted the reproduction of Euro-Canadian diets, fundamentally disconnected from the land. Dene, Gwich'in, Inuvialuit, and others had subsisted off the land since time immemorial. Into the twentieth century, they made nets for fishing and snares for trapping. The fur trade brought dependence on guns; imported twine was more durable and easier to use than willow-bast netting; people adapted their annual rounds to the rhythm of the fur trade; and flour and tea especially had been integrated into northern diets. But in a year when trapping and hunting had been good, in a place where sharing and care for others in times of hardship was a core value, and where people had lived off the land for thousands of years, the idea that delaying the *Distributor* would produce starvation is an idea generated from a singular, colonial perspective. It was an idea borne of a stomach that, like Fleming's, consumed bread, tea, dried figs and pears, rice pudding, peaches, apricot pie, egg omelette, and apples while in Aklavik and on Herschel Island (although Fleming was excited to have 'venison' one day for tea). The health of the trade was what was at stake. Anderson was not the only one who connected the need to allow vessels to travel on to the need to restock the posts. Kemp had made this same point in permitting vessels along the Arctic Coast, albeit with isolation measures ('in view of the number of people dependent on the traders for supplies, and the short period of navigation, it is out of the question to hold up the boats till the epidemic is over', Kemp wrote). This same discourse was also apparent in the police reports of Dene who had starved on the east end of Great Slave Lake. No supplies, no annual outfit produced hardship, there is no doubt about that.

[60] Blondin, *When the World Was New*, 169. [61] Anderson to 'N' Division, 8 Mar. 1919.

But the *Distributor* made at least three trips a season, and when it stopped running, the motor boats (the *Liard River* for example) continued to barge needed goods into communities along the river until freeze-up.[62] The *Distributor* was the flagship of the HBC's transportation operations and the main tourist boat, as well as a supply vessel. The impetus that drove the *Distributor* forward in July of 1928 was decidedly a colonial one.

Other critical decisions made more than once hinged on the perception that the sickness that year was not serious, just another spring cold. Bourget accounted for his decision to leave Resolution, writing 'I hated leaving so many sick at the fort, but it was imperative that we get to Rae. Besides, we had these flus . . . every summer on the same date without any disastrous consequences; the nurse would stay at the fort and visit the sick.'[63] People – Inuvialuit, Dene, Gwich'in, and Métis – who came to summer gatherings, even though they heard reports about a sickness, might have made a similar assumption, that it was a mild illness as in years past. Up to a point, these decisions reinforce the significance of the spring timing of the flu virus that year in producing the epidemic. But only up to a point.

There were those, like the Dene who left the treaty gathering early without waiting for supplies and rations, who made other choices once they saw the sickness for themselves. What the Dene saw that the physicians Bourget and Truesdell failed to see amounts to a difference rooted in beliefs about the racial character of disease and, with it, a different valuation of the importance of Indigenous lives. Where Bourget was the government physician assigned to the southern Slave, Truesdell was responsible for the people at Fort Simpson north; he also filled in the gap between Ward's departure from Aklavik and the arrival of his replacement, J. A. Urquhart. Bourget and Truesdell were, then, the medical authorities in the region at the time. Truesdell was the doctor who sent the *Distributor* on from Fort Simpson, even though there were 'several cases of Influenza aboard among whites and Indians'. Truesdell continued: 'these seemed of such a mild variety that I deemed it sufficient to keep them separate from the rest and to warn the other passengers and crew to give them a wide berth'.[64] This may seem in line with the other early assessments of the disease, but Truesdell wrote this at the end of September, after the epidemic had run its course, and offered no revision or comment on his original decision.[65] Instead, Truesdell reinscribed the role of racial difference, describing the disease as 'a mild form, for whites, of Influenza'. Bourget disagreed, as would have other whites who fell very sick, including the missionary

[62] See St Peter's Daily Journal, 14 Aug. 1926.
[63] Truesdell to Finnie, 28 Sept. 1928; Bourget, *Douze ans*, 198.
[64] Truesdell to Finnie, 28 Sept.1928.
[65] Vernon A. M. Kemp, *Without Fear, Favour or Affection: Thirty-Five Years with the Royal Canadian Mounted Police* (Toronto: Longmans, Green and Company, 1958), 122.

Franklin Clarke and his wife at Fort Simpson, both of whom were hospitalized. Or Arden Carroll, who died. Or William Geddes, who first fell ill on 11 July and had the flu 'very bad', according to Fleming. Geddes's recovery was slow and uneven. Even after the first sickness passed, Geddes remained weak and relapsed at Herschel Island on 24 July and was tended by the wife of Inspector Kemp with mustard plasters and soup. Geddes recovered somewhat but continued to have health problems in the months to come, including 'a sudden attack of appendicitis and . . . neuralgia'. 'The doctor ordered him to come out', reported Bishop Stringer in October of that year.[66] Geddes had no choice but to leave the Mackenzie district because of the longer-term deterioration of his health as a result of the flu.

For Truesdell, it was, quite simply, a matter of race. When people died at Tulita after he had 'treated 187 cases of Influenza' at the post, he noted, 'it is hardly to be wondered at as the Indians have so little natural immunity to any new disease of this kind'.[67] It was not just their lack of 'natural immunity' though. Truesdell went on: 'Also they insisted, when their temperature was high, in sitting or lying outside their tents on the cold wet ground.' As in the nineteenth century, it was the perceived ignorance of proper treatment that made Indigenous people ultimately responsible for their own ill health. Further on in his report, Truesdell described Fort McPherson where the 'Indians [are] of a better type than those in the upper river posts, although the same fatalism exists among them about death as in the other posts – the utter lack of combativeness against disease, so preeminent among most white races'.[68] Truesdell's understanding of race-based vulnerability to disease thus consisted of a 'lack of natural immunity', wedded to ignorance of medicine, further combined with 'fatalism' and a 'lack of combativeness against disease'. Fatalism refers to a belief in the inevitability of a certain outcome, a submission to disease in this instance, and ultimately to death. It is a characterization that is profoundly at odds with the actual responses of people during the epidemic, the children who looked after their parents and grandparents who lay sick; those who hunted and fished to feed others; those who worked to bury the dead; those who prepared medicines for their families; and those who asked for help, such as the Wiiliideh Yellowknives Dene men who asked Bell for paper to write to the priest at Resolution. Truesdell saw weakness and vulnerability as intrinsic to Indigenous peoples, and their deaths in this epidemic as, essentially, inevitable. The tone of his September report shows a shocking level of callousness, no more so than where he concludes:

> Our trip down the river was a decided success, although our labors were heavy at times and during rainstorms we went through many contortions to avoid the many little

[66] Stringer to Merritt, 10 Oct. 1928. [67] Truesdell to Finnie, 28 Sept. 1928.
[68] Truesdell to Finnie, 28 Sept. 1928.

> streams that dropped in, around and up on our bedding. We all acquired a beautiful sunburn and took our tricks at the wheel like real deep sea men.[69]

That was Truesdell's assessment of the summer when 500 people died.

What about the medical care Truesdell provided? In his report, Truesdell tallied those he 'treated' at each post north of Fort Simpson. He travelled initially on the *Distributor* but got off at Tulita and continued downriver on the *Ptarmigan* with Charles C. Parker with the DIA and John Moran with the NWT and Yukon Branch of the Department of the Interior. Truesdell stopped anywhere from twenty-four hours to six days at each post, inspecting sanitary conditions including refuse piles and dogs and offering what could not have amounted to more than cursory medical care given the short time he spent and the numbers of people he treated. 'At Arctic Red River I treated 112 Indians ill with Influenza in the 28 hours we spent there', went a typical description of his visit to a post. Truesdell and the others spent more time in Aklavik, where 'in all I had 206 patients in Aklavik and made 894 visits'. He was there during the height of the epidemic and visited patients more frequently. Truesdell did not elaborate on what medical treatments he offered, aside from a mention of mustard plasters. But at Fort Good Hope, when he stopped there, the RCMP constable observed how 'treatment was given them with quinine and cathartics but the disease was not checked to any appreciable extent'.[70] From Tsiigehtchic, Wilson wrote, 'All help possible was rendered to the sick, but very little could be done except in giving them something to relieve their throats'.[71] The help that worked was nursing care and providing food, water, and warmth.[72]

John Moran's assessment of Truesdell's skills was highly complimentary. Moran arrived at Tulita to meet Truesdell on 7 July, 'and found that there was an epidemic of light 'flu in the settlement'. But he noted: 'It is really a Godsend that Truesdell had some spare time here otherwise there might have been many deaths . . . The Indians have no resistance whatever.'[73] Moran clearly echoed Truesdell's own racist perceptions of a 'lack of resistance'. His comments were also premature, as people began dying soon after Truesdell left. At the next stop to the north, Fort Good Hope, Father Antoine Binamé described to Gabriel Breynat how 'the very night the devoted doctor left us, some began to die'.[74] Charles Parker, on board with Truesdell and Moran, expressed a very different

69 Truesdell to Finnie, 28 Sept. 1928.
70 J. D. Cummings to Officer Commanding, Simpson, 30 Jul. 1928, file 6099, LAC.
71 Wilson to Officer Commanding, 31 Jul. 1928.
72 For example, Johnny Kaye [Kyikavichik], 'The Flu – 1928', in 'Gwich'in COPE stories', 284–5, or F. Cook to Officer Commanding, Fort Smith, 12 Sept.1928, file 6099, LAC.
73 Extract from Mr. J. F. Moran's letter, 7 Jul. 1928, file 6099, LAC.
74 Gabriel Breynat, *Bishop of the Winds: Fifty Years in the Arctic Regions*, trans. A. G. Smith (New York: P. J. Kenedy, 1955), 180.

perspective on the journey down the river. 'One cannot but recall, however, the gruesomeness of the journey from Ft. Norman on. As we progressed down stream the disease became more serious owing possibly to delayed attention.'[75] Archdeacon Fleming, who passed almost a week with Truesdell at Aklavik, was explicit in his criticism. They, with Moran as well, had supper together in the community on 17 July. 'The Dr. is very nice. Moran I know from Ottawa', wrote Fleming afterwards. But by 22 July, having spent his days digging graves for the dead, and with the recent news of twenty-eight deaths at McPherson, Fleming's opinion of the doctor plummeted: 'Dr. Truesdale [Truesdell] is not on his job. He and the Corporal RCMP, Mr. Parker the officer for the Dept of Indian Affairs do a lot of drinking and that does not help matters.'[76] This casts a different light on what Truesdell reported to Finnie: 'It was really refreshing to meet Mr. Moran again, and we spent many an enjoyable hour together. Mr. Parker too was the best of company and helped pass the time very pleasantly.'[77]

Dr J. A. Urquhart arrived only after the main epidemic wave had passed. When Ward left the Mackenzie district, Finnie scrambled to find a replacement. The response to an initial call for applicants 'was not encouraging'. But after reports appeared in newspapers 'to the effect that medical men had no desire to serve in the North West Territories', more applicants came in and from these by 26 July Finnie was able to select a 'very well recommended' candidate, Dr W. M. Wilkinson.[78] Wilkinson was a graduate of McGill and Johns Hopkins, a returned soldier who was practising at a mining camp in Northern Ontario. Unfortunately, he died of a heart attack in an Edmonton hotel room on his way north. As Truesdell noted, 'was sorry to hear of Dr. Wilkinson's death but better in Edmonton than on the way to Aklavik'.[79] Urquhart was sent in as the replacement, arriving by the summer's end. Steeped in the same racialized ideology of the time, Urquhart nevertheless was remembered positively by Kathleen Hansen as coming with Fred Wolki to Qikiqtaryuk (Herschel Island) during the epidemic, bringing medicine and food.[80] It was also Urquhart who advocated keeping the second hospital at Aklavik in the wake of the epidemic.

What people needed most during the epidemic was care. During the epidemic, a moment of 'severe crisis', to quote Truesdell, many people came together and helped out by sharing food, visiting the sick, carrying wood and

75 For contrast in tone, see Parker to Scott, in Fumoleau, *As Long as This Land Shall Last*, 357.

76 Fleming Diary, 16 and 21 Jul. 1928.

77 Truesdell to Finnie, 28 Sept. 1928.

78 O. S. Finnie to Lt. Col. A. W. Duffus, 25 Jul. 1928, O. S. Finnie to W. W. Cory, 3 Aug. 1928, file 6099, LAC.

79 Truesdell to Finnie, 28 Sept. 1928; Vanast, 'Arctic Bodies', 155.

80 J. A. Urquhart, 'The Most Northerly Practice in Canada', *Canadian Medical Association Journal* 33, no. 2 (1935): 193–6; 'Doctor Auker', in Hansen interview, *Qikiqtaqruk Cultural Study*, 1.

water, catching fish, hunting to share meat, and digging graves.[81] As in the past, moral communities were not formed exclusively around categories of race. However, others did less because of their perception of the relative value of different lives and in this manner fell short of delivering the quality of care they would expect for themselves. There were too few doctors, nurses, hospital beds, and medications on hand in 1928, a consequence of the inadequate infrastructures of care erected in the Mackenzie district. Settlers and sojourners had greater access to hospitals and nursing care, whether because more of them lived at the posts than out on the land or because they were more likely to go to hospital when they fell sick. When the temporary hospital was put into the church at Fort McPherson, Johnny Kyikavichik – sick with the flu – 'did not want to go'.[82] He stayed at home, and his family looked after him. Going to a hospital could represent a loss of autonomy for Indigenous peoples in the North in this period, and specifically during this epidemic. In his memoirs, RCMP Inspector Kemp described how hospital patients were given combination woollen underwear from which 'escape was impossible' – in other words that they could not throw off like blankets.[83] It was also Kemp who posted a guard so that, should people get out of their beds, they could not leave the hospital. And caring for the sick elicited disgust from Kemp and others: 'Mrs. Murray and Nance bathed the bodies of the women and their report of the disagreeable task was as distasteful as was our own experience in performing a similar office for the men.'[84] For people like Kyikavichik, it is not surprising that a hospital was not viewed as a place of care. For whites, though, hospitals were just that. Franklin Clarke and his wife were grateful for the care they received at the Fort Simpson hospital. Jean Godsell fell ill in Fort Smith with the flu in 1928. As she recalled in her memoir, while at the Grey Nuns hospital in Fort Smith, she overheard two women 'arguing hotly downstairs as to which of them was going to nurse me'. While it was 'touch and go' for a while, Godsell concluded, 'I lacked for nothing in the way of care'.[85]

There was nothing exceptional in the eventual arrival of the H1N1 influenza in the Mackenzie district. That it was kept out in 1918–19 was remarkable, but in the years that followed, the virus reached into the Yukon and along the Arctic Coast with significant effect. When it arrived in the summer of 1928, the devastating epidemic that ensued was a product of material circumstances, namely the severity of the seasonal flu circulating that year and the fact that its appearance in spring allowed the virus to reach the Mackenzie in time for the open-water season. This circumstance was then joined to the

[81] V. A. M. Kemp to Officer Commanding, Edmonton, 5 Sept. 1928, file 6099, LAC.
[82] Kaye [Kyikavichik], 'The Flu – 1928', 284. [83] Kemp, *Without Fear*, 122.
[84] Kemp, *Without Fear*, 122. [85] Godsell, *I Was No Lady*, 189.

swift movement of the *Distributor* and treaty gatherings to spread the virus farther, faster, and among far more people than would otherwise have been the case. The epidemic was produced by steamboats, the commercial demands of the fur trade, and the social importance of summer gatherings that had been wedded to the newer rituals of annually acknowledging treaties. It was these colonial relationships that created an epidemic effectively spanning the entire region all at once. The timing was critical to the scale of the epidemic, as people did not realize the severity of the flu until it was too late, and then there was less opportunity for people in one part of the district to offer care to others. Bourget wrote that they were unable to offer as much care as they could have because they 'were traveling between posts when the great demand would have been for us at the posts. The distances to cover are so great that when we were most needed at the post we were on the lake.' But these material conditions should not be allowed to obscure the choices made in 1928 that most certainly caused more people to die than might otherwise have been the case and contributed to the remarkably disproportionate mortality between 'whites' and the majority Indigenous population. These choices were both initial choices – to send the *Distributor* on, or to continue with treaty gatherings in the face of sickness – and persistent, repeated choices about how to properly care for people and who to care for.

Close reading of Truesdell's, Bourget's, and Kemp's reports and memoirs is essential because of the responsibility these three men had for medical care in the Northwest Territories. Their decisions reverberated across the Mackenzie district as a whole, from Bourget south of Great Slave Lake, to Truesdell along the length of the Mackenzie River, to Kemp along the Arctic Coast. But these documents are as much works of persuasion and justification as they are accounts of 'what happened', and they need to be interpreted as such. Combined with other materials, we see their omissions; read closely and in context, we see their ideological underpinnings; and ultimately, we interpret these records against the consequences of their decisions, 500 lives lost – close to one in every ten people, in one short month.

Consequences

Such devastating loss had deep, long-term effects for people along Dehcho and the coast. Certainly, while the epidemic wave peaked and passed by August, many people were still sick in the weeks and months that followed. In burial registers, deaths were attributed to influenza as late as November 1928. William Geddes departed in the fall, having never fully recovered from his illness. Sarah Simon in Fort McPherson nursed people into the next year. George Sanderson Sr, who had accompanied Bourget on his treaty payments across Great Slave Lake, fell ill during the epidemic, 'stayed in bed all winter', and died in the spring.[86] Children at the school in Hay River recovered from the flu, but in November, Singleton wrote in the mission diary 'some serious chest conditions. We fear much weakness following the flu.'[87] In the burial register from Hay River, more deaths from tuberculosis were recorded in 1929 than any other year since 1920, more even than in 1925 when there was a tuberculosis 'epidemic' at the school. While tuberculosis infection may have been less of a factor in causing deaths during the epidemic than might have been expected, intensified tuberculosis sickness leading to death was a clear consequence of the flu after 1928.[88] Bourget suggested that these health effects, 'pneumonia and lung diseases', were felt for years to come.[89]

The deaths of adults and the disruption to normal activities during the summer months affected people's health and well-being through autumn and winter. From Herschel Island, Thomas Umaok wrote to Bishop Stringer in the autumn of 1928 that there were fewer people – 'only three hunters' who had gone for caribou (and got fourteen) – and there were few people in for Christmas.[90] This was because of both deaths and the decision by survivors to leave Herschel Island and move elsewhere. During the epidemic, dogs starved in some places as no one was well enough to feed and care for them. The police shot over 100 dogs, including fifty at Fort McPherson and sixty at the Goulet Camp on Great Slave Lake.[91] Without these dogs, the work of winter would have been that much harder. There were reports that traders at the east end of Great Slave Lake refused to give credit that autumn, leaving people without supplies needed to prepare for winter.[92] At the posts, summer was when gardens were planted and nets and boats repaired. At Hay River, Singleton noted that 'everything received a set back due to the epidemic'. He relied on the schoolchildren to weed the potato gardens, but many were still weak and could not work. He could not find anyone to fish for the mission until later in August, and then windy weather led to poor catches. By late October, Singleton reported that they were already eating the 'hung fish' meant for winter, and he feared a food shortage. By December, he wrote: 'All are short of fish this year. We at the school will have to spend more money on deer meat.' Yet amid the struggle that year, people and communities also began to recover.

86 'Sarah Simon', Life Histories of Elders; George Sanderson in *That's the Way We Lived*, 16–17.
87 St Peter's Daily Journal, 24 Nov. 1928.
88 This is consistent with what Robert Fortuine found in Alaska, *'Must We All Die?*, 26.
89 Bourget, *Douze ans*, 204–5.
90 Thomas Umaok to Bishop Stringer, 27 Nov. 1928, COR 251 file 15, Anglican Church, YA.
91 At McPherson, Belcher shot the dogs, but it was left to another RCMP officer, Const. Wilson, to burn them on a later trip. Belcher to Officer Commanding, 6 Aug. 1928; 'Patrol to Macpherson', 18 Aug. 1928, file 1928, G-1979-043, NWTA; J. L. Halliday to Officer Commanding, 6 Aug. 1928, file 6099, LAC. The year 1928 also saw the introduction and enforcement of a new law that dogs needed to be tied up, see Truesdell to Finnie, 28 Sept.1928 and St Peter's Daily Journal, 9 Nov. 1928.
92 Bourget, Medical Report, 19 Sept. 1928.

John Martin, Gwich'in from Fort McPherson, wrote to Bishop Geddes in January 1929 and told him that while some people were still unwell, others were healthy, and no one had died in the winter. The Christmas celebration had been a success and had raised $55 to buy a gravestone for Edward Sittichinli.[93]

In the wake of the epidemic, people – both Indigenous people and government officials, namely Bourget and DIA inspector Charles Parker – called for better healthcare in the North. The people at Behchokǫ̀ had already asked for a nurse to be stationed at that post even as the epidemic was underway. René Fumoleau noted that 'every band asked for a resident doctor'.[94] When Finnie came to Aklavik to seek Inuvialuit signatories to Treaty 11, he met there with Mangilaluk from Tuktoyaktuk, Nuligak, and others (Figure 8.3). As Nuligak described it, the Inuvialuit declined to sign the treaty, 'Keep your five dollars. Instead of distributing it to everyone, put that money to some purpose.

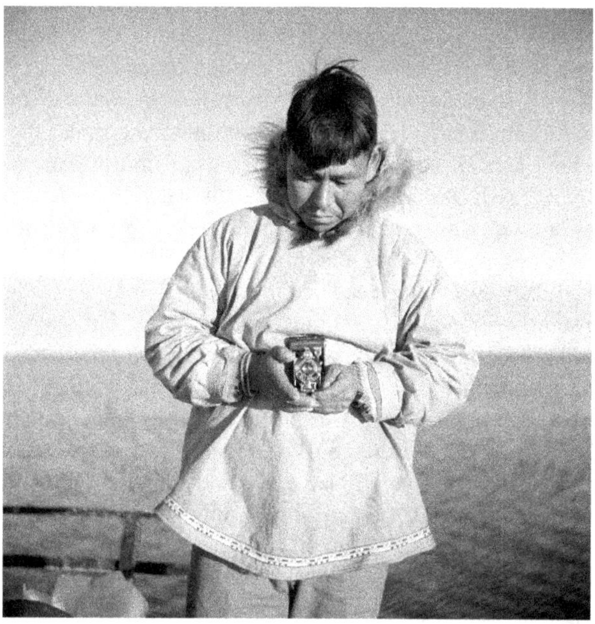

Figure 8.3 Bob Cockney or Nuligak, 1936. Photograph by Richard Hourde while on an assignment for *The Beaver* magazine 1987/271/NAA61. Name provided by Cathy Cockney. Hudson's Bay Company Archives, Archives of Manitoba.

[93] John Martin to Bishop Geddes 23 Jan. 1929, COR 251 file 22, Anglican Church, YA.
[94] Fumoleau, *As Long as This Land Shall Last*, 358.

Everything costs so much here, and five dollars will not help us. It would be better to feed those who are in misery, the widows, the blind, and the sick.'[95] Although not explicitly connected in Inuvialuit histories to the 1928 epidemic, it is significant that in the wake of that epidemic, the Inuvialuit called for the government to spend their money caring for those in need. In his 1928 report to D. C. Scott, Parker asserted that 'expenditures, in recent years, on medical attention and care for aged and destitute have undoubtedly increased'. But from Parker's inspection, this money was all well spent and fully accounted for. He went on: 'If an increased expenditure is regrettable we can only regret that it is necessary and assure ourselves that what is being done now should have been done in the past and must be done in the future.'[96] At the end of his report to Finnie, Bourget called for a larger stock of medicines everywhere, so that there were reserves in case of an epidemic. Bourget further suggested that 'wireless sub stations of one man or two should be installed at the larger posts or the very isolated posts like Rae'.[97] This suggestion aimed to ensure the capacity to immediately impose a quarantine when infectious diseases appeared in future. Some additional resources were directed to health care in the Northwest Territories in the wake of the epidemic. The government agreed to fund the second, Anglican hospital at Aklavik. Additional physicians were posted to the Central Arctic and the area around Hudson Bay in 1929. As the economic contraction and ecological crisis of the 1930s deepened, the federal government cut spending on Indigenous health care across Canada.[98] These funding cuts arrived as the scale of tuberculosis illness and death in the Northwest Territories and Yukon accelerated towards the end of the decade. But that is the story of the next chapter.

There was for many years a brochure available at the Prince of Wales Northern Heritage Centre in Yellowknife that described the Wìiliideh Yellowknives Dene as 'extinct', 'the last having died in the influenza epidemic of 1928'.[99] At a public hearing held in Dettah in 1996, Fred Sangris spoke about the purported extinction of his people, emphasizing that 'we have survived through epidemic and we are still a surviving nation today'.[100]

95 Arnold et al., eds., *Taimani*, 102; Nuligak, *I, Nuligak*, 163.

96 As cited in Fumoleau, *As Long as This Land Shall Last*, 359.

97 Wireless stations proliferated across the North in the 1920s, and one was built at Stoney Island in 1929. For more see Dianne Green, *In Direct Touch with the Wide World: Telecommunications in the North 1865–1992* (Whitehorse: NorthwestTel, 1992), chapter 3 and Fumoleau, *As Long as This Land Shall Last*, appendix I.

98 Fumoleau, *As Long as This Land Shall Last*, 358.

99 Yellowknives Dene First Nation, 'Our People Who We Are', https://ykdene.com/about/our-people/, last accessed 28 Sept. 2022.

100 'Federal Environmental Assessment Panel Review of BHP Diamonds Inc. Northwest Territories Diamonds Project', Public Hearing, Dettah, NWT, 3 Feb. 1996, English transcript, p. 8.

This was not the first assumed 'extinction' of an Indigenous people in a major epidemic that we have seen – there was also the 'extinction' of the Birch Creek Gwich'in in the 1865 scarlet fever epidemic. Anthropologists had a role to play in both of these 'extinctions', as did the larger edifice of settler colonialism in the North. The Wìlıìdeh Yellowknives Dene write in their own history that, after the epidemic, 'survivors ... stayed in camps below the treeline or in the barrens year-round until they felt it was safe to return'. They returned to find that many families around Wìlıìcheè (Yellowknife Bay) had died and 'newcomers in their traditional lands'.[101] Lands that would go on to become the epicentre of the Yellowknife gold-mining industry. Gros Cap, near to where Charles Goulet's camp was located and which was so hard-hit in the epidemic, was a rich fishing site – an ideal location to access the wealth of freshwater fish in Great Slave Lake. Indigenous camps and villages were often sought after by newcomers and settlers; brush would be cleared in these places and cabins built, with trails. These were good sites with choice access to resources and clean water. While denigrating Indigenous camps and property as less valuable, settlers and sojourners coveted these same locations. When Great Slave Lake opened to commercial fishing in the 1940s, McInnes Fisheries established a fish camp and a 'floating fish factory' at Gros Cap to harvest the rich resources of the lake.[102]

In the immediate aftermath of the epidemic, the police assumed the role of arbiters of property left by those who had died.[103] Some property was burned, as in other epidemics. Where people had died in communities with kin at hand, claims had to be made to the police. At the Goulet camp, where many had died and the survivors had left, police took matters into their own hands. A patrol led by Corporal Halliday went to the camp in the first week of August. There they found and shot sixty dogs 'on their last legs for want of food'.[104] Halliday described in his report that there were five houses at that place, of which one was locked and the other four had their contents heavily damaged by the dogs. The locked house was left alone, 'it being considered that it belonged to the remainder of the band' who the police knew had fled the sickness. Nevertheless, the police took other belongings back to their storehouse at Behchokǫ̀. These included '50 traps, 4 Sewing Machines, 2 Gramophones, 5 sets Dog Harness, 6 strings Dog Bells, 5 Dog Collars, 5 Shotguns, 3 Rifles, 2

[101] Weledeh Yellowknives Dene, 'Weledeh Yellowknives Dene: A History' (Dettah: Yellowknives Dene First Nation Council, 1997), 49. Also told in a newer exhibit at the Prince of Wales Northern Heritage Centre, YDFN and PWNHC, *This Land Is Our Home.*

[102] Liza Piper, *The Industrial Transformation of Subarctic Canada* (Vancouver: UBC Press, 2009), 181.

[103] See also Clifford to Officer Commanding, 21 Jul. 1928.

[104] They did not bury the dogs either, and Bourget later reported having to shoot two more that had been living off the carcasses.

white Deerskins and one small canoe'.[105] Another seven canoes they left at the camp. Police looked for two motorboats, but these 'could not be located'. Halliday wanted to turn the goods over to Bourget to 'despose [*sic*] of in whatever way has been the customary manner'. Halliday acknowledged that relatives of those who had died might come looking for their property. This was precisely what then happened. When Bourget went himself to see the Goulet camp, he described six or seven houses at that place and decided to touch nothing of what remained, 'knowing that 3 or 4 persons were still alive and gone east'.[106] As he visited with other survivors on Great Slave Lake, those who had lost their headman 'Johny Benaya [Johnny Beniah], the head Chief Dry Geese and brother', Bourget heard complaints about the police. Halliday had refused help offered by one man 'to show what to take and what to leave'.[107] There was, as a result, a lot of confusion about what had been taken and where it was to be found. Traps had been given to one man by another before his death, guns and a sewing machine also belonged to people still living. Bourget emphasized that 'the whole thing was a mistake to remove any of these articles before ascertaining if the people were dead or not, or these articles were not given'. With winter coming, difficulties in securing their property made it that much harder for the survivors 'who had already lost so much in relatives etc. to go without their traps and guns until the error is corrected'.[108] What Bourget characterized as a 'mistake' and an 'error' was never acknowledged as such by the police. To the contrary, Halliday described how 'none of the goods are really of much value'.[109] But in removing property, not only did the police keep it from the survivors to whom it belonged, they also undermined Dene claims to the camp. If everything left behind was, as Bourget described, 'abandoned, wrecked, ruined', that made it that much easier for settlers and sojourners to occupy the land.[110]

Struggles against colonial power underway in the 1920s, including new game and fish regulations, were shaped by the effects of the 1928 epidemic, which saw many Elders and leaders perish.[111] Blondin described the loss of those with medicine power. Abe Okpik, born in January of 1929, was named for his uncle 'Auktalik . . . one of the last medicine men', who died in the flu epidemic.[112] In Fort McPherson, in addition to the death of Edward Sittichinli, Sarah Simon

[105] Halliday to Officer Commanding, 6 Aug. 1928; Bourget, Medical Report, 19 Sept. 1928.

[106] Bourget, Medical Report, 19 Sept. 1928.

[107] Bourget, Medical Report, 19 Sept. 1928; Sangris describes Johnny Beniah's old campsite and the gravesites there since the epidemic, see 'Federal Environmental Assessment', Public Hearing, Dettah, NWT, 3 Feb. 1996, English transcript, pp. 11–12.

[108] Bourget, Medical Report, 19 Sept. 1928.

[109] Halliday to Officer Commanding, 6 Aug. 1928.

[110] Bourget, Medical Report, 19 Sept. 1928.

[111] Abel, *Drum Songs*, 196; Fumoleau, *As Long as This Land Shall Last*, 365–9; Norn interview, MHAF; Sandlos, *Hunters at the Margin*, 159.

[112] Okpik, *Survival*, 75–6, 27–9.

spoke about how in 'one month we lost 35 people and all the Church workers Gwich'in, Church we call them Church leaders. They all gone.'[113] Treaty chiefs and headmen, such Chief Sìzeh (Joseph) Drygeese, died. Drygeese had led opposition to new game laws in the 1910s and 1920s.[114] As Kemp wrote from Herschel Island, describing the deaths of some of those who were 'well-known characters', including Peter Cheechuck and old man Pokiak, 'it will be next to impossible to get a guide next winter here'.[115] These Elders and leaders, in addition to being those at the forefront of navigating relationships with colonial authorities, were also parents and grandparents. It was within their own families that their loss had the greatest effects and was most deeply felt.

Men and women aged sixteen to sixty made up 31 percent of the influenza deaths (where age information was available). If these proportions held in the wider population, as many as 150 adults, aged sixteen to sixty, may have died in the epidemic: men and women responsible for hunting, snaring, fishing, and harvesting plants for food and medicine for their families. Many survivors spoke of losing one or both parents in the epidemic (Figure 8.4). There were those, like Sarah Meyook, who were very young when their parents died.[116] The pain experienced by children was expressed by Julie Lacorne, born in 1921 at Horn River. She spoke of how her mother died in the epidemic, and then 'my little sister died that same summer out of grief over the loss of my mother'.[117] Virginie Calumet, who had spent time at the mission school before 1928, returned there after her mother's death in the epidemic.[118] Some children went to residential school for the first time in the wake of the flu. Jimmy Jacobson, who was four years old in 1928, lost his adopted parents at Qikiqtaryuk (Herschel Island) in the epidemic. He spoke of how after 'every body died, Bishop Geddes, an Anglican Bishop took me and Eddy, Pat, Maggie, Adam, Nellie, Lena and Ruby they took us to Hay River'.[119] Jacobson recalled his time at the Hay River school: 'I cut wood all those five years! Cut wood and pack wood for kitchen 'cause that time there's no fuel of any kind no saw mill . . . . After five years they sent me home. Right now I still don't know how to read and write.'[120]

113 Simon interview, Gwich'in Elders' Biographies.

114 Fumoleau, *As Long as This Land Shall Last*, 153–9.

115 Kemp to Officer Commanding, 30 Jul. 1928; Amanda Nettelbeck, 'On the Side of Law and Order: Indigenous Aides to the Mounted Police on the Settler Frontiers of Australia and Canada', *Journal of Colonialism and Colonial History* 15, no. 2 (2014), http://doi.org/10.1353/cch.2014.0031.

116 See also Rose Fabien, *That's the Way We Lived,* 76.

117 Julie Lacorne in *Nahecho Keh*, 102.

118 Virginie Calumet in *That's the Way We Lived*, 21, 71.

119 Jimmy Jacobson interview with Agnes Gruben White and Murielle Nagy, 27 Jun. 1991, Qikiqtaryuk, tape 10B, transcript, in *Yukon North Slope Cultural Resources Survey,* book 1, 5; See also Kemp to Officer Commanding, 30 Aug. 1928.

120 Jacobson interview, 5–6.

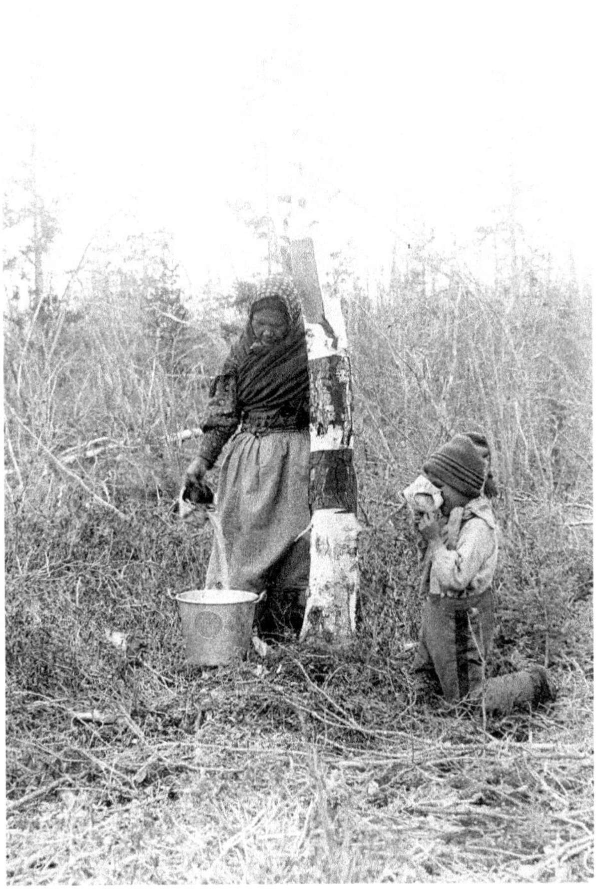

Figure 8.4 Charlotte Sarcelle Jones tapping a birch sap for syrup. Her son Fred is drinking from a birchbark cup. Near Fort Resolution, *c.*1910–17. Charlotte Sarcelle Jones died of influenza in 1928. NWT Archives/Henry Jones/N-1981-001-0065.

The epidemic, like the 1865 scarlet fever before, prompted greater government and missionary attention to schools. The Shingle Point residential school opened in 1929 (there had previously been a day school). Kathleen Hansen remembered that 'most children had no home so they brought them here then'.[121] Children came to the Shingle Point school from the east as well, but

[121] Kathleen Hansen and David Roland, interview with Renie Arey and Murielle Nagy, 19 Jul. 1991, Coal Mine Lake and Tapqaq, tape 27A, transcript, in *Yukon North Slope Cultural Resources Survey,*

the school closed within the decade when a new residential school opened in Aklavik instead.[122] Having been unable to recruit children for the residential school at Resolution during the epidemic, Bourget resumed his efforts soon after, even as he offered care and supplies to parents who were still recovering from the flu. Among Tłı̨chǫ whom he visited 'camped among the islands' at the east end of Great Slave Lake, he noted that 'they gave us the only four children of school age there were in the old whole band'. These were the families who had not been able to secure credit and supplies from traders that year. But some parents were even more reluctant to send their children away to residential school in the wake of the epidemic. Already in 1926, Teetł'it Gwich'in and Inuvialuit parents had lobbied the Anglican Church and DIA for schools in their home communities because of the great distance that their children had to travel to Hay River, and in particular, 'their inability to see their children in times of sickness'.[123] Such concerns intensified after 1928. Truesdell wrote that a day school needed to be opened in Tulita, because parents were unwilling to send their children all the way to the residential school at Fort Providence.[124] When children at Hay River were laid up with a cold in October 1928, Singleton noted that 'the local parents become very anxious and generally want to take their ailing children home for a spell'. The fear that people felt that year would have been overwhelming.

Police and other colonial officials also continued to refuse to acknowledge adoptive relationships within Indigenous communities. When Bourget went east on the lake and visited the Goulet camp and others, he had been instructed by the police that there were fourteen children orphaned in the epidemic whom he was to pick up and bring to the school. What Bourget found was that

> there were no orphans whatever except two children from Francois Dry Geese and wife who died, and had given before their death their children to a relative at Rae. The fourteen children counting babies had their father and mother every one of them, the error of the Police was not to have an interpreter with them and they did not understand the Indians.[125]

Many children were adopted across the Mackenzie district when their parents died or the surviving parent could not care for the children alone. Sarah Simon adopted one of the Inuvialuit children sent from Tuktoyaktuk to the Hay River school, one of five adopted children and eight children altogether whom she and her husband raised.[126] Nuligak and his wife adopted two children orphaned in the epidemic.[127]

book 1, 12–13; See also Fred and Lucy Inglangasuk, interview with Renie Arey, Murielle Nagy, and Bill Schneider, 10 Jul. 1990, Aklavik, tape 5B, transcript, in *Qikiqtaqruk Cultural Study*, 3–4.

122 Okpik, *Survival*, 96.

123 Extract of Commissary's Report Aug. 1926 and petition, RG 10 vol. 6476, file 919-1, part 1, c-8792, LAC.

124 Truesdell to Finnie, 28 Sept. 1928.

125 Bourget, Medical Report, 19 Sept. 1928.

126 Simon interview, Gwich'in Elders' Biographies; 'Sarah Simon', Life Histories of Elders.

127 Nuligak, *I, Nuligak*, 167.

In other families, the older children took over responsibility for caring for the smaller ones. Testifying at the Berger Inquiry in Hay River, Dean Sabourin spoke about losing both parents in 1928: 'I was the oldest and I didn't have no money and I didn't have nothing, and I had five others beside me to look after, he said.' Sabourin did not own a boat, or have a dog team. But he worked hard, hunting and trapping 'to bring the others up beside him'.[128] Deaths of parents and Elders represented a loss of knowledge and skills too. Mary Firth Sr was born in 1916, and her mother Lillian Wilson died in the flu epidemic. Mary was left to raise her brother and sister, while her father continued to trap. She taught herself to tan moosehides, sew, and do bead and quill work. She recalled how, 'I used to try hard to work and set a trap with my other friends. We know if we catch a fur it will be good for us to buy something from the store at Christmas time. That's how people use to work, and people never use to think how hard I work or get tired.'[129]

Life became harder for many, as there were fewer adults and Elders to help raise children. Beatrice Daniels (Métis) lost her father, while Jeanette Mandeville, who was interviewing Daniels, spoke of how her father had lost his mother in 1920 and then his father in 1928.[130] Philip Buggins lost both his grandfathers. George Sanderson lost uncles and aunts, and his father died within a year.[131] So many perished in the epidemic, Sanderson recalled, 'I used to think all the people were going to die'.[132] Pierre Benoit was seven years old at the time. He emphasized how at Fort McPherson, Tsiigehtchic, and at Aklavik, it was 'lots of Elders, mostly Elders . . . So that's why I don't remember none of them much at all'.[133] For some, the loss of their grandparents was felt powerfully even late in life. Jimmy Sabourin at Providence spoke of losing his grandmother. His father, while still very sick, had laid out his own mother. For Jimmy, 'I was so sad and there were tears in my eyes. Who could I call granny now?'[134] In an interview in the 1990s, nearing the end of her own long rich life, Sarah Simon spoke about the loss of her grandmother decades earlier in the 1928 epidemic, saying, 'I miss my grandmother very, very much'.[135]

Conclusions

To understand the relationships – between people, the land, pathogens, and power – that shaped the 1928 influenza requires situating that epidemic not just in place, but more importantly in time. The longer history of influenza along

[128] *MVPI Hay River, NWT* (May 30, 1975), vol. 6 (testimony of Dean Sabourin), 579.
[129] Mary Firth Sr, interview 1989, GSCI, GLC files. [130] Daniels interview, MHAF.
[131] Philip Buggins and George Sanderson in *That's the Way We Lived*, 16–17, 75, 77.
[132] George Sanderson, interview with Doris Beck, June 1984, English transcript, N-1993–016: 2–5, Fort Resolution Community Education Council, NWTA.
[133] Pierre Benoit, interview 7 Jul. 2000, GSCI, Gwich'in Elders' Biographies Research Project, tape 5.
[134] Jimmy Sabourin in *Nahecho Keh*, 61. [135] Simon interview, Gwich'in Elders' Biographies.

Dehcho, Chu kon' dëk, their tributaries, and beyond provides a temporal perspective to understand the dynamics shaping the 1928 epidemic and its effects. Influenzas travelled frequently to northern lands from the late nineteenth century onwards. These historical encounters gave northern peoples experience: immune experience with the pathogen and practical experience in dealing with it, whether by staying away from trade posts or knowing the most effective medicines needed to help care for the sick. Changes over time in the virulence of influenza, particularly with the 1918–19 pandemic, combined with the ways that outbreaks in the North were not always in sync with those elsewhere, helped to shape the unique character of the flu in 1928. People underestimated the seriousness of the flu that year, allowing it to rapidly spread downriver and out on the land, creating an epidemic remarkable for its synchronous impact across an enormous territory. That synchronicity deepened the severity of the epidemic – at times keeping care and medicines from those in need, and shaping the long-term impacts of losing so many Elders and adults in such a short time. But, in colonial context, we cannot brush past that failure of judgement – that disregard for the seriousness of what was happening – for it was that failure, that disregard, which deepened the severity of the flu and its awful effects. Individual personalities and ignorance shaped those failures. So too did collective racist ideas about Indigenous 'lack of resistance' and 'fatalism' that were in the making during these years, mixing old colonial stories about vulnerability to disease with new scientific and bureaucratic indifference.

9 A Smouldering Fire

At the turn of the twentieth century, Alex was in his thirties and had been working for the HBC since he was a teenager. He married a young woman, Mary, from a northern fur-trade family like his own: Alex's mother was Métis, and his father was born in Sri Lanka, son of a British army officer. Mary's mother was Gwich'in, and her father, born in Orkney, worked for the HBC for thirty years; he ached to leave the North towards the end of his life. When Mary was a child, her mother had taken her and her siblings, the 'youngest not 20 days old and Nootlevin with her son Peter . . . to cross the mountains'. It was mid-November, and Robert McDonald wrote in his diary that there was 'a strong north wind and snow falling' at their departure from Fort Yukon.[1] Alex and Mary had three children when Mary fell sick. In 1904, she was travelling with Alex to Edmonton for her health when she died from 'childbirth and consumption'. Mary was buried in the municipal cemetery, far from the lands where she had lived, but in a city Alex would visit in the years to come. The daughter born just before Mary's death lived a few months before she too passed away. Alex and Mary had lost a baby to 'consumption' in 1903. And so, within three years of his marriage, Alex found himself widowed with a little boy to raise on his own.[2]

In 1908, when his son was six years old, Alex remarried. Ruth was a young Dene woman whose family became Anglicans in the late nineteenth century. Ruth's mother died during an 1898 influenza outbreak. Her father lived into his eighties, dying of influenza in 1928. Ruth and Alex had five children together before Ruth died in 1919, days after delivering a stillborn child. Alex and Ruth had already lost a baby boy to tuberculosis in 1910. A month after Ruth's death, Alex lost their four-year-old daughter in a whooping cough outbreak. It was far more common in the early twentieth century for women to lose their lives in

1 McDonald Diary, 13 Nov. 1873.

2 'Alex', 'Mary', and 'Ruth' are pseudonyms used to preserve the anonymity of real people whose relations are otherwise accurately described. The causes of death are taken from the COD Database IDs 6414, 6411; family relationships have been reconstructed using the 1891, 1901, 1911, and 1921 censuses; HBC biographical sheets; and 'Declaration', in RG 15, series D-II-8-d, vol. 1372, reel C-15011, file ******, ******, LAC.

childbirth and for families to lose children under the age of five, in the North as elsewhere. Steep declines in maternal, infant, and childhood mortality have been among the most valuable medical advances of the past hundred years.

Alex enrolled two of his daughters in the Hay River Anglican residential school. The younger one died from tuberculosis after a month's illness in the summer of 1925. That year, tuberculosis tore through the school, killing a quarter of the children in a profound episode of loss. Like many parents, Alex withdrew his surviving daughter from the school and did not let her return. His younger son, aged eight, passed away from tuberculosis only a month after he buried his daughter. A note in the burial register observed that there was a 'large crowd' at the son's funeral 'both Indian and white'.[3] The family had deep community connections, people who were acknowledging the tragedies that Alex and his children had faced. The two surviving children – a boy and girl, one from each marriage – would live long lives, as would Alex himself. In his ninety years, he carried the loss of two wives and six of eight children, with at least five of these deaths attributed to tuberculosis. We can see from this family's experience the toll of tuberculosis in the North. If this book up to now has shown the role of epidemics and infectious diseases in creating moments of extreme grief, tuberculosis was a smouldering fire – lit in the fur trade, and which burst forth with a vengeance in the 1920s and 1930s, before dying down again, but never extinguished entirely.

Tuberculosis was 'the quintessential family disease'.[4] Into the twenty-first century, the household has been the most important place where *Mycobacterium tuberculosis* spread – through the air, borne by droplets – from infected to susceptible bodies. Before Robert Koch's identification of the bacterium in 1882, tuberculosis was understood as a hereditary disease.[5] The existence of a germ shifted attention to sanitation and environment in the bacterium's spread, but over a century of biomedical research shows the role of genetic susceptibility to tuberculosis infection and progression to active disease.[6] Thus, familial relations within the home and genetic relations within a family influenced exposure and susceptibility to tuberculosis. In the early twentieth century, residential schools must be understood as 'household' environments, even though they were a stark departure from the homes where children were loved and cared for. The schools were, however, shared residential spaces – where

[3] COD Database IDs 5044, 6287.

[4] Jeffrey R. Starke, 'Tuberculosis: An Old Disease but a New Threat to the Mother, Fetus, and Neonate', *Infections in Perinatology* 24, no. 1 (1997): 107–28 (p. 107).

[5] Michael Worboys, 'Was There a Bacteriological Revolution in Late Nineteenth-Century Medicine?' *Studies in History and Philosophy of Biological and Biomedical Sciences* 38 (2007): 20–42 (p. 23).

[6] Marlo Möller, Craig J. Kinnear, Marianna Orlova, et al., 'Genetic Resistance to *Mycobacterium tuberculosis* Infection and Disease', *Frontiers in Immunology* 9 (2018), http://doi.org/10.3389/fimmu.2018.02219.

children ate, worked, and slept together – creating countless opportunities for the spread of disease. While this book cannot trace each family's experience in the way that is possible for Alex, Mary, Ruth, their parents, and their children, by situating the experience of tuberculosis within families we see the role of this disease in tearing through the dense webs of kinship that made up northern communities. It was not just tuberculosis the disease that did this, but the way tuberculosis interacted with other infectious diseases, and more importantly, the way it was interwoven with key features of the colonial project.[7] This chapter shows the role of colonial relations, institutions, and responses in the amplification of tuberculosis in the Yukon and Mackenzie district in the 1920s and 1930s.

Health of the Land, Health of the People

Trapping thrived across the Yukon and Mackenzie district in the 1920s and 1930s. The drought and depression that shaped southern Canada and the western provinces in the 1930s did not extend north. Instead, wetter conditions contributed to the thriving trade, making Aklavik the 'Muskrat Fur Capital of the World' (Figure 9.1).[8] Edward Nazon, recalling 'life on the land in the 1930s', did well in 1929, with two white foxes, a cross fox, a red fox, and four marten: 'I had quite a bit of money and really enjoyed myself'.[9] Of course, and as Nazon himself emphasized, some years trapping went well, and other years it did not. Southern economic pressures affected northern economies. In 1930, traders in the delta stopped giving out credit to trappers, and at Fort McPherson the usual dances and feasts were subdued. Smaller catches and low fur prices meant 'they have no surplus with which to celebrate'.[10] But there was no prolonged hardship. Arthur Ray showed how prices for fur across Canada as a whole fluctuated significantly in these years.[11] As Peter Josie said, 'Even

[7] Lux, *Separate Beds*; Qikiqtani Inuit Association, *Qikiqtani Truth Commission: Community Histories 1950–1975* (Iqaluit: Inhabit Media, 2014); chs. 1 and 2 in Frank J. Tester and Peter Kulchyski, *Tammarniit (Mistakes): Inuit Relocation in the Eastern Arctic* (Vancouver: UBC Press, 1994); Stevenson, *Life beside Itself*, ch. 2; Laurie Meijer Drees, *Healing Histories: Stories from Canada's Indian Hospitals* (Edmonton: University of Alberta Press, 2013); Tess Lanzarotta, 'The Disappearing Clinic', *Modern American History* 2 (2019): 257–64; Fortuine, *Must We All Die?*

[8] Alunik, Kolausok, and Morrison, *Across Time and Tundra*, 117–18; Canada, *Historical Climate Data*, Monthly Data for Aklavik A, Fort Good Hope 2, Fort McPherson, Fort Simpson, Hay River, 1929–1937.

[9] Edward Nazon in *Gwichya Gwich'in Googwandak*, 290.

[10] RCMP Patrol to Aklavik, 16 Apr. 1930, and Patrol to Fort MacPherson, 24 Apr. 1930, file 1930, G-1979-043, NWTA.

[11] Ray, *Industrial Age*, 200–9; Erin Sherry and Vuntut Gwitchin First Nation, *Jii Nành Tth'aih Hèe Gıinkhii/The Land Still Speaks: Gwitchin Words About Life in Dempster Country* (Old Crow, YT: Vuntut Gwitchin First Nation, 1999), 138–41, 152, 156–7; Dick Nukon in *People of the Lakes*, 204

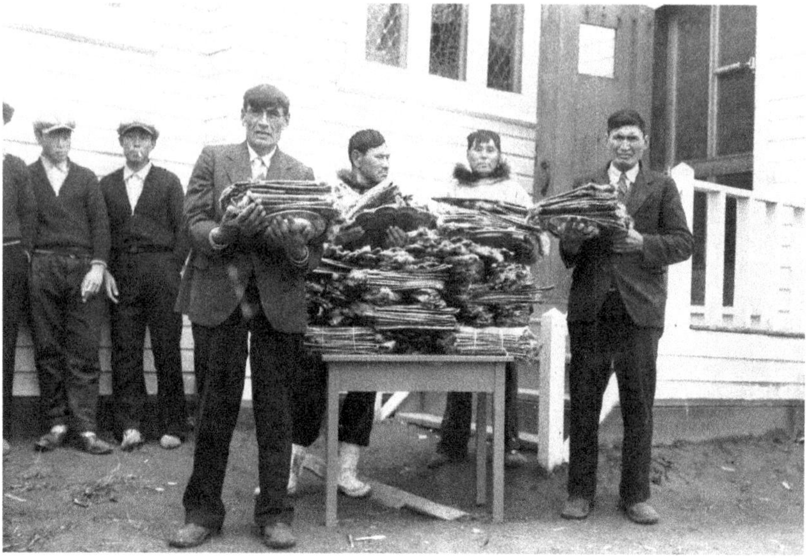

Figure 9.1 Muskrat skins were put on the collection plate, Sunday 1933. NWT Archives/Archibald Fleming/N-1979–050: 0092.

when the fur price is down, they go out. That's our life. . . . You feel good out on the land, having a good time.'[12]

There were new expenses too. By the 1930s, outboard motors were common on Lake Athabasca, Great Slave Lake, and Great Bear Lake, with small 'kickers' hooked on the back of boats. Motors needed gasoline. Snowmobiles would not be adopted until the 1950s. In the meantime, dogs could be powered by fish, and store-bought fish nets were a common purchase at this time. Buying kickers, canvas boats, and nets was possible with greater disposable income in these years. Most Indigenous northerners hunted, fished, and gathered berries for food; they did not depend solely on the prices secured from the sale of pelts for subsistence. Flour, tea, lard, and some dried fruit were the main store-bought commodities, and even then people made their own grease as well.[13] Alfred Charlie remembered that the HBC at Fort McPherson continued to buy meat and fish from the Gwich'in up to 1940 and would sell it back making '10 per cent on it in the summertime'. It was only after that time that the HBC brought in meat, including canned meat, from the outside.[14] The 1930s also

[12] Peter Josie in *Jii Nành Tth'aih Hèe Gwinkhii*, 158.

[13] Archie Roberts, interview by Anne-Marie Miller, Dawson City, YT, 1994, Tape/Transcript #93–09A-C, Tr'ondëk Hwëch'in Heritage Department.

[14] Alfred Charlie in *People of the Lakes*, 199; Frederick F. Tisdall and Associates, *Your Food and Health in the North* (Winnipeg: Hudson's Bay Company, 1940).

saw growth and expansion in the northern mining industry. While farms failed in the prairie west, the price of gold soared and the pitchblende mined on Great Bear Lake kept its value. These opportunities brought prospectors, mine workers, and white trappers northwards in the 1930s, creating new tensions and pressures within communities and out on the land.

Elders in the late twentieth century consistently shared memories of joy and satisfaction from their lives and work, as well as the richness and beauty of the land. Some described in detail the seasonal round that governed their travels and work in those years. In the delta, Abe Okpik and his family would spend the summer on the coast, whaling and making dry fish and blubber for winter. In autumn, when not travelling, they would go back to camp and fish to get ready for winter. They would not see other families until after freeze-up. Okpik's father went inland to trap at the beginning of November, which lasted until 'the 21st or 25th of December, and they got loads of furs ... They would take their catch to Aklavik around Christmas.' Okpik said they only travelled to town four times a year, 'in September, December, Easter and June', by dogsled in winter and by boat in summer.[15] In the spring and summer along the coast, Mary Evik Ruben remembered that while the men were hunting geese, she and other women would look for eider duck eggs. When they moved inland along the rivers and lakes, they would trap siksik squirrels to make parkas.[16] Ellen Bruce, the baby born during the 1911 smallpox epidemic, spoke about going into the mountains after New Year's to hunt and dry meat. When Easter came, the families would go down to Van Tat (Crow Flats) with dog teams. In the summer, people made rafts to go to Rampart House; travel at other times of the year was with dogs or on foot. In later years, they used canvas boats. In the autumn, people fished, and women tanned and smoked the autumn caribou hides to sew parkas for their children. Bruce spoke of how families did not all stay together, 'families stayed here and there ... on this side of the mountain and all over ... At that time ... the willows weren't very big, nor the trees. Everybody could see each other clearly and what they were doing.'[17]

Born in the 1910s where Tucho meets Dehcho, Adeline Constant and Marie Gargan each gave birth to fifteen children, all but one of whom were also born out on the land. For Gargan, her 'biggest happiness was living in the bush'.[18] Children learned from their grandparents: skills at how to live and stories about their people and values. Mary Louise King from Fort Resolution spoke about her grandmother showing her how to set rabbit snares: 'She taught me things like that, just like teaching me in school.'[19] Travelling together meant that the babies and smallest children had to be packed. When Ishmael Alunik was four

[15] Okpik, *Survival*, 31–5. [16] Ruben interview, *Paulatuuq Oral History Project*, 214–15.
[17] Ellen Bruce in *People of the Lakes*, 180, 164–6, 215.
[18] Marie T. Gargan in *Nahecho Keh*, 91.
[19] Mary Louise King in *That's the Way We Lived*, 32.

years old, he walked with his family over the mountains from Crow Flats. His grandmother 'packed me over rough areas but because she was old she would let me walk. I held her hand but after a few days I walked on my own. It was tough walking and my grandmother always encouraged me even though it was really tough going.'[20] As in earlier generations, life on the land was life travelling. Constant remembered going to the mountains in the spring when 'water ran around us like so many creeks'. Some days they waited until evening, when the water froze again, before continuing on. 'We walked, even my mother who was with child, walked to the mountains.'[21] During winter, travelling with dogs sometimes meant one team went ahead to make a trail in the snow. Elsewhere there were big trails that the dogs would anticipate and then race along.[22] Mary Louise King's grandfather dug a potato garden in Fort Resolution, but they did not plant every year, 'because we travelled all the time'.[23] And people came together at the trade posts for Easter, Christmas and New Year's, and at treaty time or other summer gatherings.[24]

The geography of the early twentieth century was different from that which came before and that which came after. South of Great Slave Lake was a network of thriving communities: Fort Resolution, Rocher River, Rat River, Fort Fitzgerald, Salt River, and Fort Smith. Fred Dawson, born in 1916, described Fort Fitzgerald and Salt River as towns with lots of houses, Fitzgerald was the larger.[25] People would go to Fort Smith to get their treaty payments and then leave. People who lived at Rat River and Fort Resolution would gather at Rocher River for dances at Christmas and New Year's before going home.[26] Caribou 'used to come right into Rocher River, then travel down to Fort Smith', recalled Francois King.[27] Beatrice Daniels ran a bake shop and restaurant in Rocher River with her husband and described the town as 'still going strong' when she left in 1942. The community at Rocher River arose around the trading post during the trapping boom years of the 1920s, but by the late twentieth century it had ceased to be.[28]

Further north, there was a similar network of villages built as part of the thriving trapping economy. In addition to the larger centres at Fort Yukon, Fort McPherson, and Herschel Island, there were smaller settlements – Rampart House, Old Crow, Bluefish River, Lapierre House, Whitestone Village,

[20] Alunik, Kolausok, and Morrison, *Across Time and Tundra*, 145.

[21] Adeline Constant in *Nahecho Keh*, 75. [22] Van Bibber, *Born Under a Spruce Tree*, 72.

[23] Mary Louise King in *That's the Way We Lived,* 45.

[24] Mary Kassi, Andrew Tizya, and Ellen Bruce in *People of the Lakes*, 187, 202, 256; Margaret Sabourin Sr and Madelaine Canadien in *Nahecho Keh*, 9–11, 71; Caroline Fabien in *That's the Way We Lived*, 29; Joseph Masuzumi, interview with Tom Kakfwi, n.d., N-1997–012, MHAF.

[25] Fred Dawson, interview, 3 Jun. 1993, Fort Resolution, English transcript p. 5, Salt River Settlement Oral History Project, N-1997–009, NWTA.

[26] Fred Dawson in *That's the Way We Lived*, 9.

[27] Francois King in *That's the Way We Lived*, 31. [28] Daniels interview, MHAF.

Johnson Creek, and others – some of which were occupied seasonally, others year-round. Some of these communities were a handful of cabins, but they acted like villages – as sites of commerce, exchange, and socialization.[29] Hannah and Joe Netro ran a trading post at Whitestone Village, where J. J. Van Bibber remembered buying shells, trading marten, and sleeping in the store.[30] Edward Nazon described Tsiigehtchic, a larger centre with two trade posts, an RCMP post, and 'about two or three families. Today we would call a place like that a ghost town.'[31] To the east of Tsiigehtchic, at Khaii Luk Tshik a trader named William Clark set up a trading post. With his Gwichya Gwich'in wife Vileh' or Agatha Bluecoat, Clark raised a family and grew impressive gardens. As Gabe Andre recalled, 'Yeah, [Bill Clark] made big garden with shovel. No machine them days. Big garden too. Grow potatoes, cabbage, turnips, beets. Everything. Work hard you know that old man.'[32] The Clarks had fresh vegetables and chickens as well. That these were new gathering centres or sites of trade does not mean that Inuvialuit, Gwich'in, Dene, or Dënesųłıné did not know or move around these lands since time immemorial. Aklavik flourished in the 1930s, but John Joe Kyikavichik figured that the trail from Fort McPherson to Aklavik through Rat Pass had been used for '1,000 years or more'.[33]

When Gwich'in came together at Crow Flats in the springtime, 'some families would get thousands of muskrats, 1,500 muskrats, 900 muskrats, 1,900 muskrats', remembered Charlie Thomas, who went on to observe that 'muskrat skins are heavy, too'.[34] Travel on the land, trapping, hunting, fishing, and gathering berries and plants was hard work. As Ellen Bruce said, 'all our lives we never had a rest'.[35] Elders remarked on the physical strength of their parents, family, and friends.[36] Long after Robert McDonald had returned to Winnipeg, his wife Julia stayed in her homeland. Charlie Thomas remembered she 'worked as hard as a man for her livelihood, trapping'.[37] Julia Kutug died in 1938 after a long life.

Many who were adults in the 1930s celebrated the independence and freedom of life on the land, trapping and hunting. Some people had cabins. Ishmael Alunik's family travelled each year from Crow Flats to their camp on the other

[29] Vuntut Gwitchin First Nation and Smith, *People of the Lakes*, 173.
[30] Hannah Netro, Dick Nukon in *People of the Lakes*, 209, 205; Van Bibber, *Born Under a Spruce Tree*, 74.
[31] Edward Nazon in *Gwichya Gwich'in Googwandak*, 292; Sherry and Vuntut Gwitchin First Nation, *Jii Nành Tth'aih Hèe Gıinkhii*, 136.
[32] Cited in Kristi Benson, *Nomination Form for Territorial Historic Sites: Khaii Luk Tshik (Travaillant Creek)* (Fort McPherson: GSCI, 2009), 12.
[33] John Joe Kyikavichik in *People of the Lakes*, 198.
[34] Charlie Thomas in *People of the Lakes*, 168. [35] Ellen Bruce in *People of the Lakes*, 166.
[36] Van Bibber, *Born Under a Spruce Tree*, 105; Marie T. Gargan in *Nahecho Keh*, 91.
[37] Charlie Thomas in *People of the Lakes*, 168. See also COR 252 file 29, Anglican Church, YA.

side of the mountains. It took two weeks for the multigenerational family and fifteen pack dogs to reach their cabin, made from driftwood on the Yukon coast. Hannah Netro remembered the cabins where white trappers Rube Mason and Frank Foster lived. 'We Gwich'in didn't have cabins', Netro said. 'We just camped anywhere we wanted, at a good place. And then we took the tents down and went again the next day.'[38] Adeline Constant, born in 1913 near Burnt Island, remembered the moosehide tents she lived in. 'They never let mosquitoes or the rain in and I loved the smell of tanned hide. The tents were made by hand but a woman never had to make one alone.'[39] Edward Nazon remembered how 'in those days, people who had no house to live used to pitch a tent and live their own life'.[40] Many others emphasized the freedom to go wherever they chose on the land, in the words of Willie Minoza (born in 1924), to 'be our own masters than be governed by the will of others'.[41] Trapping and hunting were hard work, and sometimes it was luck more than anything that decided the outcome, but it gave people 'a feeling of self worth', said Jean Marie Sabourin; 'nobody was the boss of us when we trap', recalled Alfred Charlie.[42]

There were new opportunities for wage labour, in the summer months especially. Men found work loading and unloading freight, cutting brush, and harvesting cordwood for sternwheelers. They worked as pilots on boats or as special constables or guides for police on patrol as well as for the prospectors and explorers who came north in greater numbers than ever.[43] Some found work in mining operations. Charlie Johnson of Fort Selkirk worked on dredge No. 4 in the 1930s.[44] J. J. Van Bibber's brother Abe was on his way to work at the radium mine on Great Bear Lake when he drowned in a storm.[45] For the most part, however, Indigenous men were excluded from the new mine operations that opened in the 1930s on the grounds that they were not suited to industrial labour. They could find work at the surface of the mines and in construction; Dene men would bring meat and fish to sell to workers at Cameron Bay. Gwich'in carpenters, who helped build the new school building at Aklavik in the 1930s, were praised for their highly skilled work.[46] Some women, like Hannah Netro or Beatrice Daniels, ran businesses with their husbands. Most women who found wage work in these years were employed

38 Hannah Netro in *People of the Lakes*, 208. 39 Adeline Constant in *Nahecho Keh*, 75.
40 Edward Nazon in *Gwichya Gwich'in Googwandak*, 290.
41 Willie Minoza in *Nahecho Keh*, 31.
42 Jean Marie Sabourin in *Nahecho Keh*, 78; Alfred Charlie in *Jii Nành Tth'aih Hèe Gwinkhii*, 159; see also Edward Nazon in *Gwichya Gwich'in Googwandak*, 293–4.
43 Dick Nukon in *People of the Lakes*, 207; 'Working for Wages' in *That's the Way We Lived*, 61–6.
44 Charlie Johnson, interview with H. Doborowolsky, 21 Jul. 1985, tape 1, side 2, transcript, in *Fort Selkirk Elders Oral History Project* (1987), 117.
45 Van Bibber, *Born Under a Spruce Tree*, 13.
46 T. B. R. Westgate to Secretary, DIA, 25 Jul. 1936, RG 10, vol. 6476, file 919–1 part 1, c-8792, LAC.

as domestics. Dora Tourangeau, a Métis woman born in Fort Fitzgerald, travelled to Aklavik and Herschel Island while working as a housekeeper for a doctor in the mid-1930s.[47]

White trappers were a significant new group of settlers and sojourners in these years. They included people who made the North their home, and others who came for shorter periods – to take advantage of high fur prices for instance – and then left. White trappers were not a uniform group. Some married into Indigenous families and shared in their values and ethics. Charlie Thomas spoke about Victor Peterson at Black Fox Creek: 'Peterson was a good man. ... In those days, when the people came to Van Tat, there wasn't much food. Sometimes the dogs were hungry before the muskrats came out on the ice. He gave out fish for dog food. He really helped the people, Peterson.'[48] Len Heron, a Métis man from Fort Smith, remembered lots of white trappers in the delta by Fort Chipewyan: 'White trappers got along very well with the native people, they done pretty much what the native were doing, they would share like anything that they had.'[49] Others did not fit in so well. Nazon recalled 'a Mr. McBride, a man undersize who as everybody knows, was not a very clean man but who could make a violin sing when he took hold of it'.[50] Others still infringed on treaty rights, violated social norms, displaced Indigenous peoples from their own lands, and threatened the health of the land and of the people.

In 1923, there were over 200 white trappers in the Mackenzie district with more than half concentrated around Fort Smith and Resolution.[51] Albert Fabien at Fort Resolution said that, before they were replaced by white traders, 'it was mostly natives or Metis people who looked after the stores'.[52] George Minoza, from Fort Providence, 'knew some of the white people who used to trap among the Dene. We did not own many traps, but they did. We could not travel as easily as they could and they chased us off our land. It was not good when they did that.'[53] Alexander King and James Balsillie spoke with René Fumoleau, telling him, 'White trappers spoiled the country. Had too many traps, 600, 500, like that. Us natives, well, my brother had 35 and that the most any had, most had 18, 19, 20, like that.'[54] Around Whitestone and Eagle River, Dick Nukon described how white trappers – Rube Mason, his brother Billy Mason, and Frank Foster – used poison: 'The poison is left on the river after it is used. Also,

47 Dora Tourangeau, interview with Sister Agnes Sutherland, 31 Mar. 1992, Fort Smith, N-1997–012, MHAF.
48 Charlie Thomas in *People of the Lakes*, 168.
49 Len Heron, interview with Joe Mercredi, 5 Feb. 1992, Fort Smith, N-1997–012, MHAF.
50 Edward Nazon in *Gwichya Gwich'in Googwandak*, 296.
51 As cited in Fumoleau, *As Long as This Land Shall Last*, 319.
52 Albert Fabien in *That's the Way We Lived*, 36. 53 George Minoza in *Nahecho Keh*, 109.
54 Fumoleau, *As Long as This Land Shall Last*, 321.

other animals came by traps and carcasses and died.'[55] Nukon emphasized that 'they pretty well spoiled the land', and animals stayed away for decades.[56] Although they relied more on canned food than Indigenous trappers, white trappers also depended on game animals and fish to sustain themselves.[57] Competition for food resources led to local depletion, as in 1932 when the Carcross band petitioned the government to restrict white fishing and hunting in Little Atlin Lake after Tagish Lake was 'about fished out'.[58] There were many reports of the decline and depletion of fur bearers and game animals, especially on the lands closest to the main communities. As Fumoleau observed in the southern Slave region, 'White trappers argued that a few hundred of them could never exhaust the fur resources of an area of one and a quarter-million square miles'.[59] But these trappers were not spread over the whole country; they used the same trails and took advantage of the same rich sites for sustenance. While the land is geographically large, it sustained people who travelled long distances. This was extensive, not intensive, land use, and white trappers competed directly with Indigenous trappers even as they failed to practise the conservation strategies that had ensured the long-term health of the land.

Instead, conservation of animal populations – like public health – became a site for the articulation and elaboration of colonial control.[60] The early twentieth-century political debate over the enforcement of new conservation regulations and its effects on Indigenous peoples revealed a profound gulf in values that is important to understanding the history of disease and the effects of the tuberculosis epidemic. Enforced restrictions on hunting and trapping were perceived as necessary and fair by colonial authorities because they included exceptions that allowed for harvesting in case of 'dire need'.[61] Indigenous political leaders maintained that by treaty their hunting and trapping rights were protected from restriction, but colonial authorities deemed restrictions necessary in the interests of conservation – a perceived common good and

55 Dick Nukon in *People of the Lakes*, 212, and also *Jii Nành Tth'aih Hèe Gıinkhii*, 137.

56 Dick Nukon, Alfred Charlie in *People of the Lakes*, 212, 227, 262; this poison was different from that used by federal wildlife officers in the later twentieth century, see also *MVPI Fort Franklin, NWT* (24 Jun. 1975), vol. 7 (testimony of Joe Naedzo), 604, 607, *Rae/Edzo, NWT* (11 Aug. 1976), vol. 72 (testimony of Jim Erasmus), 8121–2; Karen Jones, '*Never Cry Wolf*: Science, Sentiment, and the Literary Rehabilitation of *Canis lupis*', *Canadian Historical Review* 84, no. 1 (2003): 65–93.

57 Hannah Netro in *People of the Lakes*, 228.

58 John Hawksley to A. F. Mackenzie, 26 May 1932 and J. Hawksley to D. C. Scott, 21 Aug. 1931, Gov 1619 1490 J file 2, YRG 1, series 1, vol. 9, YA.

59 Fumoleau, *As Long as This Land Shall Last*, 319.

60 Peter Keith Kulchyski and Frank J. Tester, *Kiumajut (Talking Back): Game Management and Inuit Rights, 1900–70* (Vancouver: UBC Press, 2007); Tina Loo, *States of Nature: Conserving Canada's Wildlife in the Twentieth Century* (Vancouver: UBC Press, 2006); Sandlos, *Hunters at the Margin*; Nadasdy, *Hunters and Bureaucrats*.

61 Quoted in Fumoleau, *As Long as This Land Shall Last*, 398.

one where colonial authorities, informed by Western science, asserted that they knew best.

It is in the category of 'need' that the imagined poverty of northern Indigenous populations took shape. There were larger colonial ideas about the relative value of Indigenous property, on display in the decision to destroy cabins and caches at Rampart House in 1911 (see Chapter 6), or in handling Dene belongings in the aftermath of the 1928 flu (see Chapter 8).[62] Then there was the leverage created by Indigenous leaders claiming need or privation when arguing for individual or collective exemption from the enforcement of hunting regulations, regulations they considered illegitimate in the first instance. These claims of need – of hunger – reach back to the discourses of starvation that circulated in the fur trade. In the early twentieth century, the government had replaced the HBC as the main colonial power in the North, and so the discourses of hunger and need were extended to them.

Indigenous northerners were perceived by colonial authorities to have few means to get food. Small-scale gardens saw considerable success in the North, but the model of settler market-based agriculture was not something that would thrive. Wage labour was limited, and Indigenous peoples often were denied the opportunity to participate in this kind of work, even when they wished to. Emphasizing the need for Indigenous northerners to hunt and trap to survive gave their advocates (including white advocates such as Bishop Gabriel Breynat and J. K. Cornwall) leverage in conversation with government officials. But Indigenous northerners did not eat caribou, moose, dry fish, smoked fish, fresh fish, porcupine, beaver, duck, eggs, blubber, squirrels, rabbits, or berries because they were poor, but because this was their wealth.[63] The richness and beauty of the land, the ways it sustained them and their children and grandchildren, gave them strength and health. In return, Dene, Gwich'in, Tr'ondëk Hwëch'in, Tutchone, Tagish, Tłı̨chǫ, Dënesųłıné, Inuvialuit, and Métis showed respect and love for the land and animals, appreciation for this wealth, and reciprocity among themselves to ensure the collective good.

I write of the 'imagined poverty' of northern Indigenous peoples in this period, because although there were many references in archival documents to destitution and need that accompanied petitions from bands, or RCMP reports, or discussions about relief, there is much less of this in the oral history. In addition to the joy people felt out on the land and when trapping detailed above, when this generation of Elders spoke of being hungry and how hard that was, they told these stories as lessons about how to survive or about their good or ill

[62] John Hawksley to A. F. Mackenzie, 5 Jun. 1930, Gov 1619 1490 J file 2, YRG 1, series 1, vol. 9, YA.

[63] See for example Rosalie Causa, b. 1903, in *Nahecho Keh*, 56.

fortune, not as stories about how the land failed to sustain them.[64] As Monique Sabourin, born in 1926, remembered,

> I was raised in the bush and loved that way of life. I never lived anywhere else or with any other family. . . . I have been very lucky for I have never gone hungry. My parents were good providers. I can't remember a time when we were completely out of food.[65]

Noel Yelle, born in 1910, spoke about how 'The people used to eat good on geese at that time. . . . There weren't any stores in those days so the only way that people made their living was to travel all over the place looking for food.'[66] This generation of Elders highlighted changes in diet and understandings of good food arising from the new trapping economy and changing colonial relations. People had strength because they did not eat 'whiteman's' or canned food.[67] Mary Evik Ruben, born in 1925 across from Tuktoyaktuk, described making *utitchaq*, fermented flippers. She said, 'Everything good to eat. We used to make any kinds of things, now when we try to make some that kind, these young people, "You gonna poison!" There's no poison! . . . All our life we eat anything! Never turn to poison.'[68] Here Ruben expresses how what she knew as good food became remade as unhealthy ('poison') in her own lifetime.

The most significant departure in the stories from the early twentieth century was the new relationship between sickness and hunger. Two Elders from near Great Slave Lake clearly expressed how sickness made for hardship. Monique Providence was born in 1931 in Kakisa. 'My father was a good hunter so we rarely went hungry, though it was a hard time when we did. When my father was sick that was a hard time.'[69] Jimmy Bonnetrouge, born in 1907 at Fort Providence, recalled,

> Life in the bush made me very happy. The land is so beautiful and you can see so far. . . . My life was really happy but between the ages of 25 and 45 I had some bad luck. TB was quite prevalent at that time and I had to go to the hospital for five years.
>
> I remember being hungry, and when I say hungry, I mean in the winter time when there are no rabbits and you can't set nets and you can't get credit at the store. You only used to be able to get credit when you were going trapping.[70]

Julienne Andre, born in an earlier generation, made the connection between poverty and health when she spoke about her early life. 'We never thought we were poor – but today we're poor (always sick, lots of people go to the hospital

[64] Andrew Tizya in *People of the Lakes*, 202; Jean Causa and Harry Minoza in *Nahecho Keh*, 55, 89.

[65] Monique Sabourin in *Nahecho Keh*, 117.

[66] Noel Yelle in *That's the Way We Lived*, 33.

[67] Harold Balsillie in *That's the Way We Lived*, 9; Lazarus Charlie, John Joe Kyikavichik in *People of the Lakes*, 199, 203; Monique Providence in *Nahecho Keh*, 96.

[68] Ruben interview, *Paulatuuq Oral History Project*, 248.

[69] Monique Providence in *Nahecho Keh*, 98.

[70] Jimmy Bonnetrouge in *Nahecho Keh*, 67.

and are operated on – that's the way they are poor)'.[71] Andre's insight that as a Gwichya Gwich'in poverty was not about wealth or property, but about health and well-being, is essential to our understanding of northern poverty in historical perspective. The twentieth-century resource economy constructed Indigenous trappers as 'poor' relative to the standards of wealth that governed colonial power and objectives in the North. Need and hunger also became tools deployed to assert political rights in the context of the Crown's abdication of its treaty promises. That is not to say that people did not go hungry and did not experience hardship in this period, but recognizing these other constructions of poverty brings into clearer relief the central and significant role of sickness and tuberculosis in particular in creating hardship in these decades. Tuberculosis stole away parents, siblings, and children, created physical weakness in a place that demanded such strength and hard work, and pushed people off the land and into hospitals to get care. In the early twentieth century, tuberculosis in the North was not a consequence of poverty, it *was* poverty.

Tuberculosis and Syndemics

Tuberculosis arrived in the lands that became the Yukon and the Mackenzie district borne by fur traders. Along the Alaska coast, Russian traders and ships introduced tuberculosis by the late eighteenth century.[72] There were early reports from explorers and HBC traders of sickness and death from 'consumption'.[73] When Émile Petitot and Robert McDonald arrived in the North in the 1860s, each wrote about people sick with consumption, as well as scrofula and wasting illnesses.[74] Genetic analysis has connected the dominant *Mycobacterium tuberculosis* lineage among present-day Indigenous populations in Alberta, Saskatchewan, and Ontario with a lineage also dominant among French Canadian populations in Quebec. These connections are rooted historically in the fur trade. They support the historical evidence that spans the west and north of a small number of fur traders carrying tuberculosis to their trade partners, which progressed only slowly until 'shifts in host ecology' favoured expansion and more rapid spread.[75]

[71] Julienne Andre in *Gwichya Gwich'in Googwandak*, 270.

[72] Fortuine, *Chills and Fever*, 103.

[73] Krech, 'Influence of Disease', 127; Sir George Simpson and E. E. Rich, *Journal of Occurrences in the Athabasca Department by George Simpson, 1820 and 1821, and Report* (Toronto: Champlain Society, 1938), 308; George Back, *Narrative of the Arctic Land Expedition …* (Edmonton: M.G. Hurtig, 1970, first published 1836), 457.

[74] Petitot, *Autour*, 189; McDonald Diary, earliest examples: 30 May 1868 and 15 Jun. 1873; see also William Hardisty to Strachan Jones, 28 Nov. 1865, B.200/b/35, pp. 62b–62c; HBCA; McMillen, *Discovering Tuberculosis*, 10.

[75] Caitlin S. Pepperell, Julie M. Granka, David C. Alexander, et al., 'Dispersal of *Mycobacterium tuberculosis* via the Canadian Fur Trade', *PNAS* 108, no. 16 (2011): 6526–31.

The bacteria responsible for tuberculosis historically included both *Mycobacterium tuberculosis* (*M. tb*) and the closely related *Mycobacterium bovis* (*M. bovis*). Where *M. tb* spreads from person to person, most commonly via the respiratory system, *M. bovis* infects cattle and spreads to humans when they consume products from diseased animals and in particular when they drink unpasteurized milk. Both kinds of bacteria can infect many different parts of the body: most commonly the lungs (pulmonary tuberculosis, also called phthisis in the past), also the lymph nodes or glands (scrofula), intestines, bones, brain, and spinal cord (tuberculosis meningitis), and the blood (miliary tuberculosis). Infection with *M. tb* or *M. bovis* did not lead directly to tuberculosis (TB) disease; the bacteria could live in the body for years, or even a lifetime, without causing disease. In these cases, the infected person had latent TB and would not show symptoms, nor would they be infectious to others, although a skin or blood test (diagnostic tools developed in the late nineteenth century) would usually be positive for TB infection. Alternatively, infection with *M. tb* or *M. bovis* could lead in short order to active TB disease. Without treatment, active tuberculosis could lead to death very quickly (sometimes called 'galloping consumption'), or through a prolonged, wasting illness.

The course of tuberculosis disease among the communities and people of the Northwest, had a much more attenuated arc – one that stretched over years and decades – as compared to that of an influenza or measles epidemic. Figure 9.2 shows this arc between 1887 (the first records of TB deaths) and 1960. Across the region, TB was without a doubt the most significant cause of death throughout the period, with 969 deaths attributed to this cause, or just over 14 percent of all the deaths recorded.

Subsumed within the larger arc were deaths from tuberculosis disease in families as well as outbreaks where tuberculosis moved swiftly through a local population or institution, causing significant mortality in a short period of time. Residential schools were sites of significant tuberculosis outbreaks. Ten children, including Alex and Ruth's daughter and the infant child of an employee, died from tuberculosis in the 1924–5 outbreak at the Hay River Anglican school.[76] In 1931–2, there was an outbreak at the St Paul's hostel where Métis children lived while attending public school in Dawson.[77] Five children died at the hostel.[78] J. J. Van Bibber had begged his parents not to return him to school and was allowed instead to 'get home schooled' by his sister, Leta. His older sister Helen, however, had returned to Dawson. That year, 'with all the bad nourishment and cold', tuberculosis 'got pretty bad' at the hostel. 'Helen got

[76] Vanast, 'Arctic Bodies', ch. 7.

[77] TRC, *Canada's Residential Schools: The Métis Experience*, vol. 3 (Montreal: McGill-Queen's University Press, 2015), 35–8.

[78] Deaths recorded between October 1931 and June 1932 in the parish burial register.

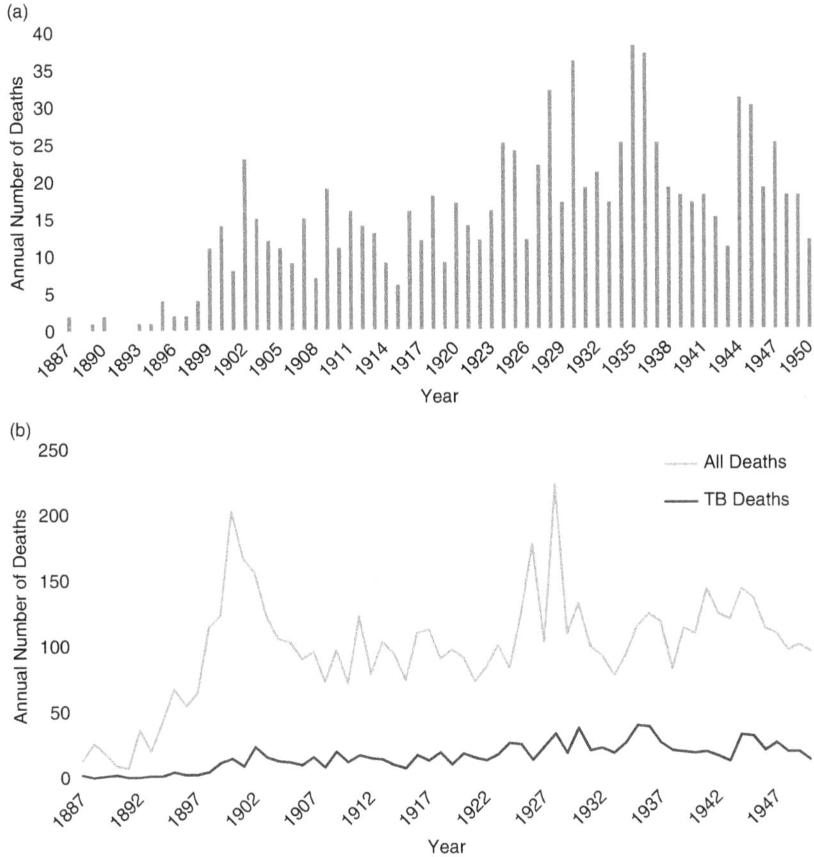

Figure 9.2 (a) Deaths attributed to tuberculosis, 1887–1950; (b) compared to all deaths over same period. Source: COD Database.

sick too, really sick.'[79] Their father went to the school to bring Helen home, and she died a short while later, buried among her family at Mica Creek. Van Bibber describes his father's anger at the deacon, Charles Johnson, who had not even informed the family of Helen's sickness; the news was delivered by an RCMP officer instead. 'None of us ever went back to school', Van Bibber writes. He was twelve years old at the time and soon thereafter started trapping.

There were outbreaks in communities as well. The role of syndemics, involving influenza and measles especially, in activating otherwise-latent TB infections

[79] Van Bibber, *Born Under a Spruce Tree*, 27–9.

and creating higher mortality cannot be understated. In January 1900, Jean Séguin wrote to his sister describing influenza at Fort Good Hope the preceding autumn. Although the influenza had been less serious than other outbreaks in recent years, a 'good number' of Dene then developed tuberculosis and within a short time 'left for the next world'.[80] In December 1925, after an influenza epidemic travelled through the Yukon, several children from Moosehide were admitted to St Mary's hospital with tuberculosis. Deaths from influenza in 1925 and again in 1928 included those already sick with TB. And, as Bourget noted in the aftermath of the 1928 epidemic, there was a marked increase in pulmonary illness and TB deaths. One experience illuminates this pattern and its awful tragedies. A girl from Herschel Island at the Hay River residential school survived the 1928 influenza epidemic but 'did not seem to wholly recover ... and contracted TB'. She was due to travel home to her parents on the *Distributor* in 1929, 'but her fitness to go is very doubtful', wrote W. B. Singleton in the mission journal. Her parents had no knowledge that their daughter was sick, and, while the missionaries intended to send a letter by aeroplane, the girl died and was buried at Hay River.

The synergistic relationship between tuberculosis and measles can be seen clearly in 1935. That year, measles broke out among Inuvialuit, Gwich'in, and Dene along the coast and in Aklavik and Fort McPherson, spreading south to Hay River, Fort Resolution, and Fort Providence in the autumn.[81] The measles itself was severe.[82] Agnes Nasogaluak was born in the spring of that year on the Horton River, between Tuktoyaktuk and Paulatuk. She spoke of how 'when they had measles long ago, my mother passed away'.[83] Sarah Simon from Fort McPherson lost two of her children from measles that year, her fourteen-year-old daughter (who had survived the 1928 flu epidemic) and her five-year-old son.[84] Ishmael Alunik was in residential school at Aklavik. He recalled children getting sick with measles at the school, 'Measles was the first disease I experienced. Some people died from it.'[85] Measles also spread among children and youth in the Roman Catholic hospital at Aklavik. The first measles case was a fourteen-year-old girl admitted on 7 July. By the end of the month, fifteen more children and teenagers had come to the hospital with measles. At the time, there were four TB cases in the hospital already, as well as one child with 'discharging glands'. Notwithstanding rules about isolation, the disease spread within the hospital,

80 Jean Séguin to sister, 4 Jan. 1900, 71.220 / 7347, OMI, PAA.
81 Alfred Gargan in *Nahecho Keh*, 83; Memorandum into Cause of Death of ______ of the Fort Resolution Indian Residential School on 27 Nov. 1935, RG 10, vol. 6475, file 916–23, part 1, c-8791, LAC; St Peter's Daily Journal, 24 Aug. 1935.
82 MacKay interview Parker, 20 Sept. 1978.
83 Agnes Nasogaluak, interview with Agnes Gruben White and Murielle Nagy, 22 Feb. 1996, Inuvik, tape 8B, transcript, in *Aulavik Oral History Project*, 6, 16.
84 Simon interview, Gwich'in Elders' Biographies; St Matthew's Mission Journal, Jun.–Jul. 1935.
85 Alunik, Kolausok, and Morrison, *Across Time and Tundra*, 149.

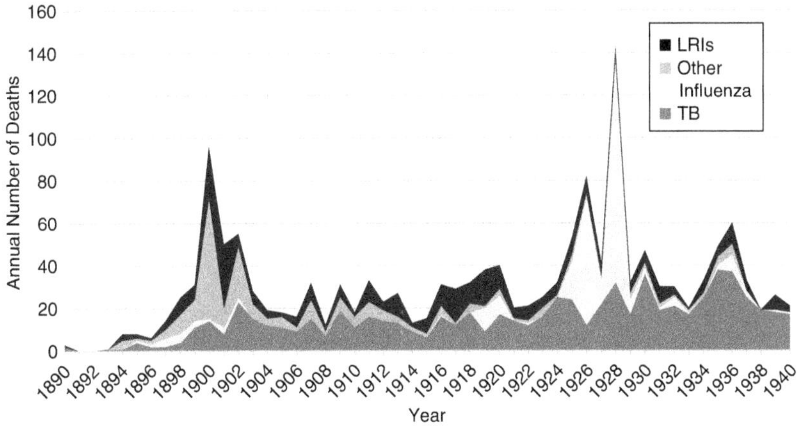

Figure 9.3 Syndemics 1890–1940, showing deaths from tuberculosis, influenza, lower respiratory infections (LRIs), and other infectious diseases (Other). Source: COD Database.

with at least two children contracting measles while being treated for another illness. By September and October, the measles outbreak ebbed, but the number of TB cases doubled. A nine-year-old boy admitted with measles in August passed away in September with TB and measles. Of the eight TB cases in September, five also had measles, and two passed away by the end of October. By the next summer (July 1936), there were ten cases of tuberculosis being treated in the hospital. Measles infection destroys the body's immune memory, making a person more susceptible to tuberculosis as well as activating previously latent TB. Recognizing this mechanism, and the way in which other infectious diseases (influenza especially) also could aggravate existing tuberculosis infections, allows us to interpret most of the peak years in Figure 9.3. These were also years with, or immediately following, significant measles (1902, 1935), or influenza (1925, 1928) epidemics. Although the residential schools reported almost no influenza deaths during the 1928 epidemic, at Hay River the effects were felt over the next two years, when eleven children died from tuberculosis.

Schools

Mary Rose Drybone, born and raised in Fort Good Hope, testified about her early life before the Berger Inquiry:

> In those days there was a deadly sickness called tuberculosis of which a lot of Dene people died and it caught up with my family. It got the best of my father and I am proud

> at this moment to say that my father is a real – or was a real Dene. Because he made his living off the land for us. There was no welfare at that time. He died in 1953 but left a memory for me and my brother to be a true Dene and we are still and we'd like to keep it that way. My mother had left to go to the hospital first for TB and later on my dad and my brother did too, went to the hospital in Aklavik.
>
> They left me all alone with my sister, but my sister and I still returned to the bush with another family. Then I caught TB also and they sent me to Aklavik too.[86]

Mary Rose Drybone clearly described both how tuberculosis affected her family and the ways that it disrupted 'real Dene' life, as people left for hospitals for months or years at a time and their children were sent to residential schools. The experience of tuberculosis in the early twentieth-century North is inseparable from the history of schooling and hospitals, as is the case elsewhere in Canada.[87] Peter Bryce's 1907 report highlighting the death rate from tuberculosis at residential schools did not include northern Alberta, the Yukon, or the Northwest Territories but offers an important framework for recognizing the role of residential schools in amplifying the tuberculosis epidemic.[88] The connections between schools and hospitals were tightly woven in conception, as each worked to advance larger colonial policies of subjugation and assimilation and, in practice, with some children leaving one only to enter the other.

The DIA kept records of the children enrolled in residential and day schools across the Northwest Territories and Yukon (Figure 9.4). Enrolment slowed in the 1930s when parents removed their children from schools or kept them home because of health concerns. Annie Benoit from Fort McPherson left for the Hay River school in 1921 when she was eight years old with her sister Rachel Reindeer and her cousin Mary Koe. Her father brought all three girls home two years later, 'because so many of the children were dying of disease at the school'.[89] There were more fatal outbreaks in schools in the 1930s compared to earlier decades.[90] Reports of children dying from tuberculosis within the schools underestimated the scale of the problem and the role of these institutions in mortality from this disease as children were released from the schools if

86 *MVPI Fort Good Hope, NWT* (7 Aug. 1975), vol. 20 (testimony of Mary Rose Drybone), 1940–1.

87 Crystal Fraser, 'T'aih k'ìighe' tth'aih zhit dìidìch'ùh (By Strength, We Are Still Here): Indigenous Northerners Confronting Hierarchies of Power at Day and Residential Schools in Nanhkak Thak (the Inuvik Region, Northwest Territories), 1959–1982' (PhD diss., University of Alberta, 2018), TRC, Inuit and Northern Experience and Métis Experience; Kenneth Coates, '"Betwixt and between": The Anglican Church and the Children of the Carcross (Chooutla) Residential School, 1911–1954', *BC Studies* 64 (1984): 27–47.

88 P. H. Bryce, *Report on the Indian Schools of Manitoba and the North-West Territories* (Ottawa: Government Printing Bureau, 1907).

89 'Annie (Koe) Benoit', Life Histories of Elders, GSCI, GTC Department of Culture and Heritage, https://gwichin.ca/elders-biographies.

90 TRC, *Inuit and Northern Experience*, 27–31.

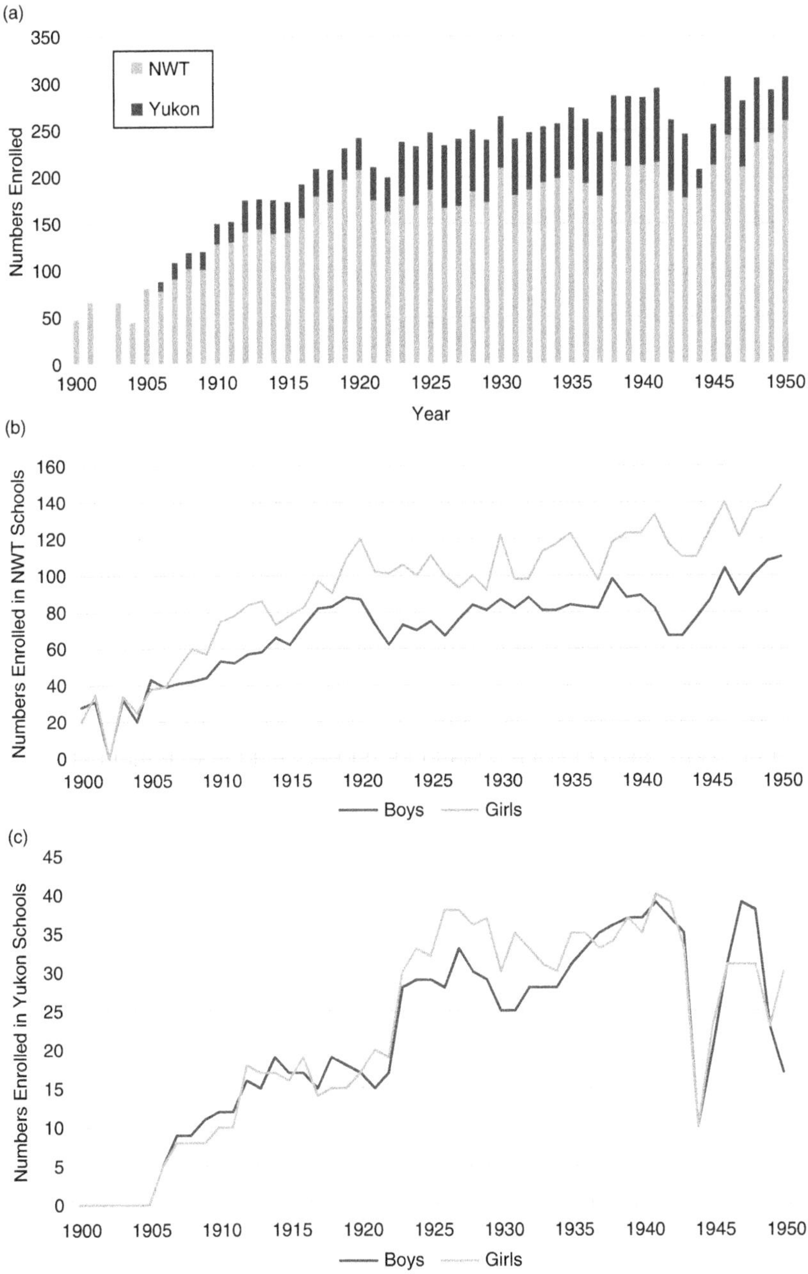

Figure 9.4 Residential school enrolment in the Yukon and NWT, 1900–50. (a) Both territories; (b) NWT by gender; (c) Yukon by gender. Source: Canada, Department of Indian Affairs, *Annual Reports*, 1900–50.

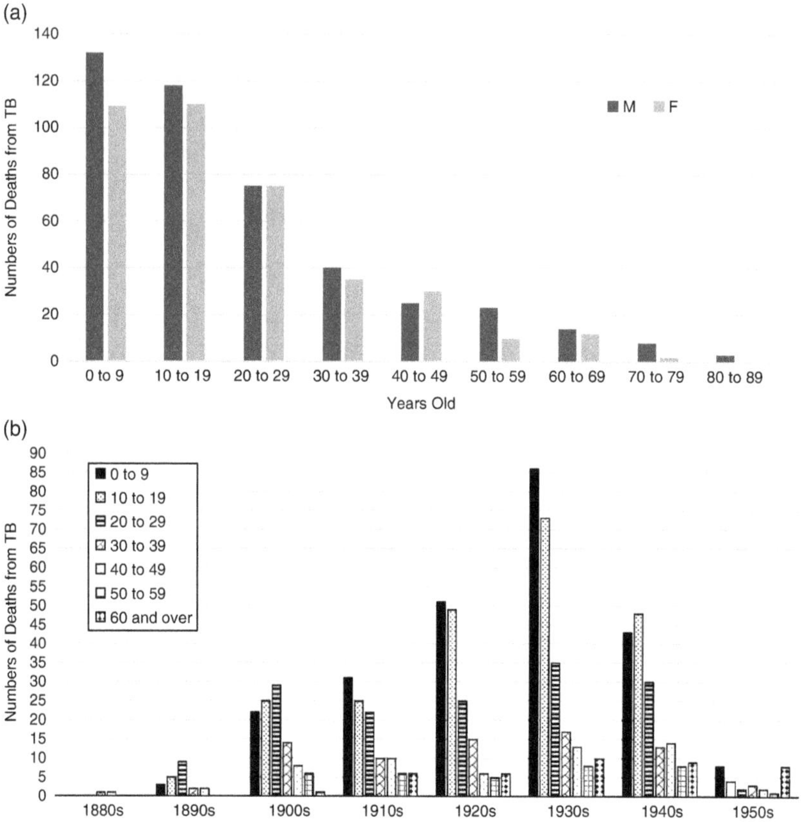

Figure 9.5 Tuberculosis deaths. (a) By gender; (b) age at death from tuberculosis, by decade. Source: COD Database.

they were very sick.[91] After they left, many children died at home where their death might be recorded in the parish burial record.

Tuberculosis had a disproportionate impact on the health of the young (Figure 9.5). People under the age of thirty made up 65 percent of all deaths attributed to tuberculosis. Perhaps even more striking was that people under the age of twenty made up almost 50 percent of all tuberculosis deaths. There is a significant peak among children aged nine to fifteen years, which is connected to the residential school experience. From Hay River, Carcross, and Dawson, there are fifty-nine records of schoolchildren who died from tuberculosis. Most were

[91] Bryce, 18. TRC, *Inuit and Northern Experience*, 30.

between seven and fifteen years old, and twice as many girls than boys died. This last statistic is particularly striking, given that within the total population under twenty, more males than females had deaths attributed to tuberculosis (m=250, f=219). This gendered mortality reflects how more girls attended residential schools than boys in this period (see Figure 9.4). In the Northwest Territories, this was a significant and consistent disparity from 1906 through 1950. In the Yukon, girls outnumbered boys in the system from 1923 until 1935. As a school inspector noted in 1936 while visiting the Providence residential school, 'The boys are generally discharged from school at the age of 13 or 14, which I would say is about the proper time. The girls are kept a little longer, and in cases where they are orphans, of course they have to be kept there until they are able to do for themselves.'[92]

At Hay River, the greater mortality among girls compared to boys is consistent with the level to which girls outnumbered boys at the school and the different age distribution of girls and boys. This speaks to the direct relationship between these institutions and TB mortality. Schools were places where children came together from distant places, contributing to the spread of pathogens. Survivors have said that on arrival at school they were confronted with more people than they had ever seen in one place at one time.[93] As Alice Masak French wondered on her arrival in Aklavik, 'How could there be so many people living in one building?'[94] These memories highlight close living conditions in the schools compared to the villages and on the land. Schools received money for operations through grants paid for each student. Buildings constructed to accommodate a certain number of children deteriorated over time, while administrators constantly recruited more children. A new building was constructed at Fort Resolution in the 1920s. By 1947, it needed to be replaced as the classrooms were 'small and unhealthy'.[95] TB spread more easily among girls because of their higher enrolment. School buildings were designed to segregate children by gender, with equal space allotted. With more girls in schools, each girl had less space. At Hay River in the mid-1920s, girls experienced 'gross overcrowding', and their sleeping quarters received no natural light.[96]

In a 1916 tour of the Mackenzie district residential schools, including the institutions at Fort Resolution and Fort Providence, H. J. Bury reported on the need for medical inspections of children before they were admitted to the schools. From Fort Providence, Bury cited the example of three children from Fort Good Hope, admitted 'without having the necessary health certificate'. Bury observed: 'All of these children developed sickness after being at the school

[92] M. Christianson, to Harold W. McGill, 13 Aug. 1936, RG 10, vol. 6475, file 918–1, part 1, c-8791, LAC.

[93] Thrasher, *Thrasher*, 9–13. [94] Alice Masak French, in *Northern Voices*, 204.

[95] J. W. McKinnon to Mr. Meikle, 9 Aug. 1947, RG 10, vol. 6474, file 916–1, part 1, c-8790, LAC.

[96] Vanast, 'Arctic Bodies', 350.

a short time and in consequence two of them died just prior to my arrival.'[97] Admission rules provided for medical examinations but were not 'rigidly enforced'.[98] By the late 1930s, the Northwest Territories Council was advised that children were being examined after admission, as it was at the point of admission that the schools received their grant money.[99] The timing of medical examinations was only one part of the problem. Doctors performing medical exams lacked effective diagnostic tools. Tuberculin tests were never used, and X-rays were introduced only in the mid-1940s. Doctors relied on physical examinations of children; sometimes they found evidence of active TB, other times they noted a history of family tuberculosis, and other times they used euphemisms – 'weakness', 'not very strong' – to refer to tuberculosis. Children who were perceived to have nowhere else to go were admitted with evidence of active tuberculosis.[100]

There was moreover a hegemonic belief that the schools were safer and healthier for children than their homes and families. This attitude was expressed countless times by administrators, doctors, and advocates for residential schooling in the Yukon and the Mackenzie district.[101] As the doctor at Atlin wrote to Harper Reed in 1932, regarding two children admitted to the Carcross school, 'In my opinion the only chance these Indian kiddies have of keeping good health is to be placed in a school as early as possible'.[102] This attitude was rooted in ideas about Indigenous vulnerability to disease and was widespread across North America, as well as in racist beliefs about Indigenous peoples' poverty and unsanitary 'nature'.[103] Teachers believed that the schools were safer and more sanitary than the children's own homes. At Hay River, the Anglican bishop James Richard Lucas persuaded two families to enrol their teenage children with active tuberculosis, on the grounds that the school provided a therapeutic setting.[104] Doctors argued, even in the face of evidence to the contrary, that the general risk of TB in the North was greater than the risk in the schools. A schoolteacher from Saskatchewan who contracted

[97] Extract from report of H. J. Bury on Boarding Schools of Treaty 8, 6 Oct. 1916, RG 10, vol. 6475, file 918–1, part 1, c-8791, LAC.

[98] Bury, 6 Oct. 1916. [99] TRC, *Inuit and Northern Experience*, 29.

[100] 'Application for Admission', 31 Mar. 1936 and Philip Phelan to Sister Mack, 11 Apr. 1936, RG 10, vol. 6476, file 918–10, part 2, c-8791, LAC.

[101] See comments from Dr Urquhart reported in 'Extract from report of Mr. Mackay Meikle', 30 Jul. 1937, RG 85, vol. 191, file 554/119-1 part 2, LAC. Extract from Annual Report on Fort Resolution NWT Agency, 1947–48, RG 10, vol. 6475, file 916–5, part 3, c-8791, LAC; Bishop Breynat, 'Canada's Blackest Blot', as cited in Fumoleau, *As Long as This Land Shall Last*, 498.

[102] L. G. C. d'Easum to Harper Reed, 11 Apr. 1932, RG 10, vol. 6481, file 940–10, part 4, c-8795, LAC; W. A. M. Truesdell to R.A. Hoey, 15 Jan. 1942, RG 10, vol. 6475, file 918–1, part 1, c-8791, LAC.

[103] Extract from letter from Sister McQuillan, 18 Jul. 1911, RG 10, vol. 6475, file 916–5, part 1, c-8791, LAC; See also McMillen, *Discovering Tuberculosis*, 42; Jones, *Rationalizing Epidemics*, 155.

[104] Vanast, 'Arctic Bodies', 343.

tuberculosis while teaching at the Anglican residential school in Aklavik was 'informed that she incurred no avoidable hazard and was apparently in robust health but the incidence of TB is very high in the McKenzie delta area'.[105] It was not the school, she was told, it was the general environment. Under this logic, residential schools were there to isolate children from an unhealthy environment and to provide them with the food and medicine needed for good health. These beliefs, combined with limited resources, explain the perfunctory medical exams – not only were doctors ill-equipped to diagnose latent or mild tuberculosis infection, but they also assumed that the children had already been exposed to tuberculosis and their time in the schools would make them healthy.[106]

Under this governing logic, the schools became sites of significant medical interventions.[107] Children were vaccinated at the schools, given regular doses of cod-liver oil, and had their teeth inspected and pulled.[108] Tuberculosis therapies included ultraviolet treatments, premised on the value of sunlight for tuberculosis sufferers, introduced at the Fort Resolution school in October 1930. Tonsillectomies were the most common immediate medical intervention in the lives of schoolchildren, justified by the appearance of enlarged tonsils during initial medical exams. Leslie Livingstone, doctor at the Aklavik school from 1938, took the most aggressive approach to tonsillectomies. As he wrote in 1944:

> The first year that I spent here I had a large number of deaths of school children which I attribute to a large extent to infective tonsils which undermined their general health and also was a source of continuous infection among the pupils. Since that time I have removed the tonsils of most of the children on admission or shortly afterwards and the improvement through the years has been quite marked.[109]

Although it was not until the twenty-first century that the medical benefits of routine childhood tonsillectomies were disproved, Livingstone's autonomy in deciding that every child would have their tonsils removed (no other physician pursued this practice) speaks to the power of these physicians as well as the wider paternalistic attitudes towards the well-being of children in the schools.

[105] H. A. Alderwood, 20 Oct. 1945, RG 85, vol. 989, file 15535, LAC.

[106] Coates, 'Betwixt and Between', 38.

[107] Ian Mosby, 'Administering Colonial Science: Nutrition Research and Human Biomedical Experimentation in Aboriginal Communities and Residential Schools, 1942–52', *Histoire sociale/Social History* 46, no. 91 (2013): 145–72.

[108] Catherine Carstairs and Ian Mosby, 'Colonial Extractions: Oral Health Care and Indigenous Peoples in Canada, 1945–79', *Canadian Historical Review* 101, no. 2 (2020): 192–216; W. A. M. Truesdell, 'Monthly Report for Fort Simpson Agency', Oct. 1940, RG 10, vol. 6474, file 916–1, part 1, c-8790, LAC; [List of medicines, n.d.] RG 10, vol. 6475, file 916–5, part 1, c-8791, LAC.

[109] L. D. Livingstone to Harold W. McGill, 22 May 1944, RG 10, vol. 6476, file 919–1, part 1, c-8792, LAC.

Parents, of course, disagreed with the assumption that the schools were healthier than their homes by removing their children in the wake of outbreaks and deaths.

K'áhshó Got'ı̨nę, Tłı̨chǫ, Dënesųłıné, Inuvialuit, Tr'ondëk Hwëch'in, Tutchone and other northern Indigenous peoples – all found strength and health in food they harvested from the land. For their children in residential schools, this food was almost entirely out of reach. Survivors from the Mackenzie district schools recalled a diet dominated by fish and potatoes. One of George Sanderson's clearest memories from his time in school was how children would be given the same piece of fish over and over again at meals until they ate it; even if it was the worst piece of fish (the one with the stick through it) to begin with. This was a memory that Albert Fabien shared.[110] Noel MacKay attended the school at Fort Chipewyan. He described breakfast 'most of the time fish, and one slice of bread and not even butter on it, drank mostly water, once in a while a glass of milk'.[111] After breakfast, they worked cutting wood ('sometimes saws were dull'). The midday meal 'most of the time was fish, roasted fish in ovens, picked up two potatoes and a piece of bread'. Afterwards, the children worked and then went back to the classroom. Supper was a lighter meal, more like breakfast. Dinner at midday was the main meal. When children were disciplined, this included refusing to let them eat dinner.[112] Fish was central to school diets across the Mackenzie district, as it could be cheaply and readily provided – so long as there was a good fishery that year and the boats and nets were in good shape.[113] In the months prior to the Hay River tuberculosis outbreak in 1924–5, the principal D. A. B. Stoddart failed to secure essential supplies including wood, food, medicine, and clothing. He did not attend to the garden. Then, on top of this, the fish harvest failed and mice destroyed some of the stored food. Children were visibly malnourished during the outbreak.[114]

Schools also harvested vegetables, potatoes first and foremost, as well as cabbage, lettuce, turnips, oats, and other plants. Requests to expand and improve on fields and gardens were denied for lack of funds.[115] In the Yukon, the Carcross school had fields that produced potatoes, carrots, turnips, beets, cabbage, wild hay, rye, and cranberries. The school sold some of these to raise money until they had to stop because children had been going without.[116] In 1929, the doctor attending the children at the Carcross school recommended

110 George Sanderson, Albert Fabien in *That's the Way We Lived*, 22, 25.

111 MacKay interview Parker, 20 Sept. 1978. 112 MacKay interview Parker, 20 Sept. 1978.

113 Gabriel Breynat to D. C. Scott, n.d. [*c.* 1920], RG 10, vol. 6474, file 916–1, part 1, c-8790, LAC.

114 Vanast, 'Arctic Bodies', 330, 338, 349.

115 C. Bourget, 5 Mar. 1929, RG 10, vol. 6475, file 918–1, part 1, c-8791, LAC.

116 John Hawksley to J. D. McLean, 27 Oct. 1916, RG 10, vol. 6479, file 940–1, part 1, c-8794, LAC.

that they be given more meat; they were raised 'chiefly on a meat diet in their native homes and do not thrive so well on a largely farinaceous diet', wrote John Hawksley.[117] In 1930 and again in 1931, a 'strong rumour' was circulating 'among the white people and Indians ... that the pupils are insufficiently fed'.[118] Hawksley defended their diet, saying it was 'sufficient in quantity but very monotonous'. In 1931, the weekly menu was revised to have more variety, for example: 'Tuesday. Breakfast: Cream of Wheat, Jam and Tea; Dinner: Stew with Dumplings, Cornstarch; Supper: Soup, Fruit and Tea.' Yet complaints about food persisted at the Carcross school. In 1938, three children were expelled after complaining that there was not enough food and that they were fed floor sweepings and 'dog rice'. The principal, H. C. M. Grant, closed his letter on the incident writing peevishly, 'I feel that it would be only a just thing for their places to be filled by children who haven't such "wealthy" parents and who really need the food, clothing and attention the school provides'.[119] The attitude expressed here – of 'need' justifying whatever the school provided – speaks volumes about the governing mindset at Carcross and elsewhere. The following year 'an epidemic of stealing' included the theft of food. Children were punished. Parents upset about the incident argued that 'if the children were given enough to eat they would not steal'.[120]

The schools were tightly linked with southern, settler colonial Canada; in the economic downturn of the 1930s, they felt these reverberations particularly and experienced poverty in this period, more than any other part of northern society or economy.[121] In December 1930, Bishop Gabriel Breynat wrote to D. C. Scott: 'I respectfully beg to call your attention to the fact that, owing to tremendous rates we have to pay for the transportation of our annual outfit from railways terminals to our residential schools in the Mackenzie District, *we cannot give to our school children all the proper food and care they would need.*'[122] This was a rhetorical flourish on Breynat's part. He was not one to admit that the missionaries were failing in their care of the children; rather, Breynat used this dramatic phrasing to make the point that he needed more funding from the DIA. Transportation expenses were no minor issue in the North. The Carcross school returned children to the place where they had

117 John Hawksley, 'Report on the Carcross Indian Residential School', 9 Jul. 1929, RG 10, vol. 6479, file 940–1, part 1, c-8794, LAC.

118 John Hawksley, 'Report on the Carcross Indian Residential School', 22 Jul. 1930, RG 10, vol. 6479, file 940–1, part 1, c-8794, LAC.

119 H. C. M. Grant to G. Binning, 12 May 1938, RG 10, vol. 6481, file 940–10, part 4, c-8795, LAC; Coates in 'Betwixt and Between', 39 offers a different interpretation of this incident.

120 H. C. M. Grant to the Supt. Of Indian Affairs, 5 Feb. 1940, RG 10, vol. 6479, file 940–1, part 2, c-8794, LAC.

121 TRC, *Inuit and Northern Experience*, 18.

122 G. Breynat to D. C. Scott, 3 Dec. 1930, RG 10, vol. 6474, file 916–1, part 1, c-8790, LAC. Emphasis added.

been recruited, not to their parents in Fort McPherson, because it was cheaper.[123] In another instance, Carcross administrators admitted a child with a worrisome medical report because he had travelled so far it would be expensive to send him home. Parents sending their children to Hay River did not have to pay for transportation, if they agreed to keep their children enrolled for five years.[124] And, as Breynat pointed out in 1930, transportation costs affected the provision of food and the maintenance of infrastructure. But these transportation costs reflected explicit choices. D. C. Scott denied Breynat's request for additional funds. Yet in 1937, Mackenzie River Transport recorded the greatest tonnage in its history, thanks to mining activity at Yellowknife and on Lake Athabasca.[125] In 1938, the Northern Transportation Company carried supplies north for the Resolution school aboard the *Radium Queen*, so named because it supplied the mine on Great Bear Lake. Money was made in these transportation operations. And these vessels carried pitchblende ores, yellowcake, and gold bars from the mines and milling operations on the large lakes out to southern markets.

In 1944, Eden Corlett wrote to the Minister of Pensions and National Health about the Anglican residential school in Aklavik where she had worked. She described concerns with sanitary conditions, the children's diet, and the risk of fire. Corlett pointed out that of the annual government grant, $100 per child, only $20.42 was spent, per child, on food, as compared to the $162.19 expended on each staff member. 'That's a fact that can be proved', Corlett wrote emphatically. 'I studied all invoices and checked off the foods allotted to the children. This diet has been in force, since the school was established.' Corlett enclosed a copy of the menu served to the children, which she had eaten herself before concluding it was insufficient.[126] Aklavik faced even bigger challenges around food supply compared to the other schools, given the growing conditions at higher latitudes and the costs of transportation. By 1942, there was garden and greenhouse and parents supplied the school with meat and fish.[127] Nevertheless, Alice Masak French remembered a monotonous diet.[128] Leslie Livingstone was asked to respond to Corlett's letter. He deflected concerns about diet by suggesting that parents who had complained overstated the problem. He wrote, 'the natives themselves all claim that the children are better fed in the Roman Catholic School than in the

[123] H. C. M. Grant to Philip Phelan, 24 Aug. 1938, RG 10, vol. 6481, file 940–10, part 4, c-8795, LAC.

[124] Vanast, 'Arctic Bodies', 340.

[125] Piper, *Industrial Transformation*, 50; see also Allice Legat, *Walking the Land, Feeding the Fire: Knowledge and Stewardship among the Tlicho Dene* (Tuscon: University of Arizona Press, 2012), 112.

[126] Eden Corlett to I. A. MacKenzie, 18 Mar. 1944, RG 10, vol. 6476, file 919–1, part 1, c-8792, LAC.

[127] TRC, *Inuit and Northern Experience*, 38.

[128] TRC, *Inuit and Northern Experience*, 40.

Anglican school, and of course to these primitive people food is taken more into consideration than schooling, sanitary conditions or anything else'.[129] About Corlett herself, Livingstone was equally nasty, writing that he found the female staff in general suffered from 'neurosis, caused no doubt to [*sic*] environment and diet and I would suggest that the period of four years be cut down. I think two years here is long enough for any girl.'[130] The problem, in this mindset, was never the schools or those in charge – it was the wider environment, neurotic women, and 'primitive' parents.

A good diet was recognized as key to fighting tuberculosis infection in the 1920s and 1930s. Children may have been exposed to tuberculosis before or after they arrived at a school, but poor diets activated latent TB infections and made it harder for bodies to fight off the disease. Livingstone agreed that the school children could do with more fresh fruits, milk, cheese, and butter. Fresh milk in particular was seen as an important part of healthy diets for the school children.[131] Milk, cheese, and eggs were seen as therapeutic in fighting tuberculosis, and the schools kept cows and chickens to reduce costs (Figure 9.6).[132] But dairy cows could be infected with *Mycobacterium bovis*, which caused disease in animals and people. Residential schools across Canada routinely gave children unpasteurized milk.[133] In the 1920s and 1930s, *M. bovis* was specifically linked to tuberculosis of the glands (known as scrofula in the North before 1910), and the danger of infecting people through the consumption of milk from tubercular cows was recognized.

Achille Fournier ran a dairy farm with twenty head of cattle that supplied Dawson with milk and cream. In late summer 1928, RCMP Supt. R. Field received reports of children with 'gland troubles' thought to stem from drinking milk supplied by Fournier's herd. Field contacted the Medical Health Officer (MHO) W. E. Thompson, who refused to inspect the herd as 'he knew nothing about cattle'.[134] Territorial officials reached out to the federal Department of Agriculture, who advised that all milk needed to be pasteurized. But no one pasteurized their milk in the Yukon. The necessary equipment simply did not exist in the territory. As more children went south for operations on tubercular glands, the MHO sent milk samples out for testing, only to learn that the cows

129 For the menu at the Catholic school, see 'Extract from report of Mr. Mackay Meikle', 30 Jul. 1937.

130 Livingstone to McGill, 22 May 1944.

131 Urquhart, 'The Most Northerly Practice', 194–5.

132 E. E. Stockton to Deputy Superintendent General DIA, 29 Nov. 1912, RG 10, vol. 6479, file 940–1, part 1, c-8794, LAC; St Peter's Daily Journal, 7 Aug. 1919, 28 Mar. 1920.

133 J. S. Milloy, *'A National Crime': The Canadian Government and the Residential School System, 1879 to 1986*, foreword by M. J. L. McCallum (Winnipeg: University of Manitoba Press, 2017), 84.

134 R. Field to G. I. MacLean, 2 Aug. 1928, G. I. MacLean to O. S. Finnie, 3 Aug. 1928, GOV 1677, series 1, vol. 67, file 6, part 4, YA.

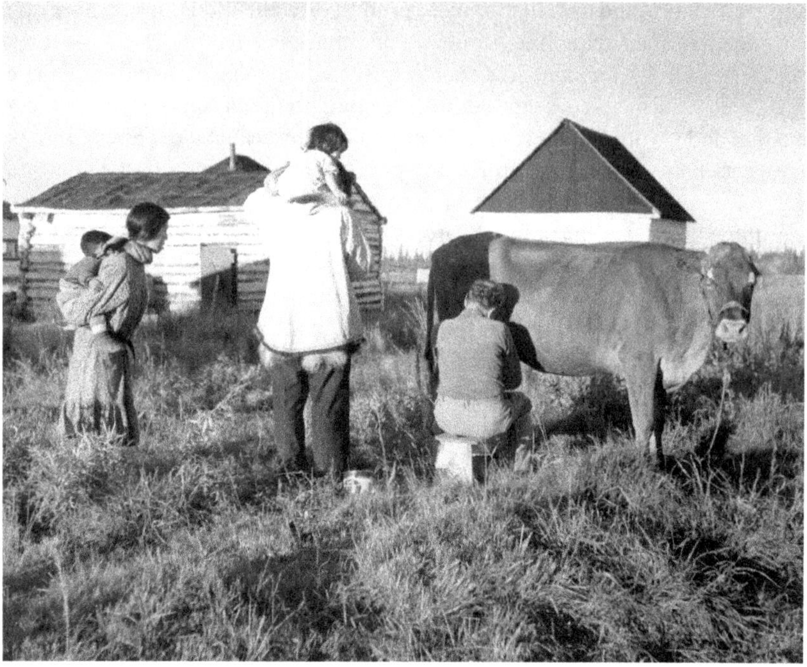

Figure 9.6 People watch as L. D. Livingstone milks his cow 'Clementine', Aklavik 1939. NWT Archives/©Richard Finnie/N-1979–063–0067.

needed to be tested, not the milk. University of British Columbia professor H. W. Hill wrote the MHO that even then 'from the Public Health standpoint, we are not interested in getting rid of Tuberculosis from cattle at all *provided the milk is not used in a raw state*, that is, *provided the milk from cattle is invariably boiled or pasteurized*'.[135]

Commissioner G. I. MacLean pressed O. S. Finnie to pay for regular cattle inspections across the Yukon in the interests of maintaining a safe local food supply. Finnie was little help, but a veterinary inspector from British Columbia, Graham Gillam, was found and arrived in October. Two of Fournier's cows tested positive and were slaughtered. Gillam wrote Finnie in 1929 and again in 1930 advising that the cattle should be retested and encouraging inspection of other cattle in the territory, specifically those at Mayo and at the 'Indian Mission at Carcross'.[136] Finnie forwarded the letter to MacLean, who replied

[135] H. W. Hill to W. E. Thompson, 20 Sept. 1928, GOV 1677, series 1, vol. 67, file 6, part 3, YA. Emphasis in original.

[136] W. Graham Gillam to O. S. Finnie, 23 Jun. 1930, GOV 1677, series 1, vol. 67, file 6, part 2, YA.

that as there had not been any cases of 'tubercular glands' in Dawson recently, he did not think any further test was necessary.[137] Meanwhile, in 1930, a seven-year-old boy at Champagne/Haines Junction, died of 'TB glands'.[138] This was one of forty-eight deaths from tuberculosis recorded in the Yukon between 1928 and 1932, at least half of whom were Indigenous children, including two pupils from the Chooutla Carcross school and four Métis children resident at the St Paul's hostel in Dawson, many of whom could have been exposed to milk from tubercular cattle. The four children sent south for medical treatment of their tubercular glands were all the children of settlers. White children in the Yukon and Mackenzie district received different care compared to their Indigenous counterparts.

In the Mackenzie district schools, children consumed fresh milk from cows, and there was never any mention of pasteurizing milk or testing cattle. Although pasteurization was commonplace in urban Canada, rural Canada was another matter altogether. Nevertheless, in the south, rural Canadians had access to herd testing and compensation from the Department of Agriculture. In late May 1935, the missionary at Hay River observed that, 'One of our milk cows now is showing a lump in the same vital spot. We have decided to use no more milk from the two affected Cows, although one of them appears to be better.'[139] The pause in milk consumption was temporary. If tuberculosis was widespread in cattle, as Hill had suggested, and given that the southern focus was on pasteurization or boiling milk not eliminating the disease, infected cattle could easily have been brought north. *M. bovis* also spread widely in northern bison herds between 1923 and the 1940s, introduced by the transfer of infected bison from Wainwright Park.[140] Bison could spread the disease to cattle and could have been a direct source of infection to children.[141] Those responsible for the schools and for protecting territorial food supplies made few efforts to protect the children in the schools from the known risks attached to drinking unpasteurized milk in the early twentieth century. Instead, fresh milk consumption was encouraged to benefit health.

Hospitals

Before the development of effective antibiotics, medical treatments for tuberculosis focused on surgeries to remove infected organs, as well as diet, light therapies, and rest. By the early twentieth century, northern Indigenous peoples had their own therapies for tuberculosis and its symptoms. Dene Elders

137 G. I. MacLean to O. S. Finnie, 23 Jul. 1930, GOV 1677, series 1, vol. 67, file 6, part 2, YA.

138 COD Database ID 1306. 139 St Peter's Daily Journal, 29 May 1935.

140 Sandlos, *Hunters at the Margin*, 56, 234; Gary Wobeser, 'Bovine Tuberculosis in Canadian Wildlife: An Updated History', *Canadian Veterinary Journal* 50, no. 11 (2009): 1169–76.

141 Bishop Breynat to W. W. Cory, 17 Nov. 1927, RG 10, vol. 6474 file 916–1, part 1, c-8790, LAC.

interviewed in the early 1990s spoke of the value of using bear bladder for coughing blood.[142] In August 1932, the missionary at Hay River had made the passing observation, 'The natives at present are using the gall of bear for TB'.[143] This was a rare missionary observation of Indigenous therapies, as plant and animal medicines were interwoven with traditional spirituality, and both were suppressed by colonial authorities. When Len Heron was diagnosed with TB at the age of twelve, 'The Doctor at the time in Fort Chip he said the only thing we could do was bed rest'. Heron was confined to bed for a year and a half. He recovered with the help of a medicine man. Heron believed 'those kind of people would've done a lot more for their own people but they were being watched by the police, by the doctors, they told them they couldn't practice their own medicine it was against the law'.[144] While people objected to the loss of autonomy enforced by doctors and police around traditional therapies, they also sought out medical expertise, often travelling long distances to see a doctor or go to a hospital, just as they travelled far to seek out medicine people.

As shown in Figure 9.7, tuberculosis created a major healthcare burden compared to other infectious diseases. Moreover, many of those hospitalized with tuberculosis spent weeks, months, or even years in the institution. Ruby McLeod was attending school in Aklavik when she was diagnosed with TB. She remembered being pulled to the hospital on a toboggan covered with a blanket. 'Here I just thought I was going in and was just going home the next day like you know. I keep saying when are we going home?' Ruby kept 'thinking we are going to go home any day but every time we ask they just say no, you are not ready to go home. Then they had no medication back then. All we had to do was bed rest, bed rest. Everyday.' In all that time, 'we weren't even allowed outside either in the summer. Not even allowed to go and [sit] outside.'[145] Rose Fabien remembered how people sick with TB in Fort Resolution in the 1920s and 1930s would go to the hospital in Fort Smith. 'Kids and lots of people died with TB. They would get sick for a long time and then die.' Fabien herself was in the hospital with TB for a year.[146]

With the construction of two hospitals in Aklavik, there were four hospitals across the Mackenzie district (one at Fort Smith and another at Fort Simpson) by the mid-1930s. Two more Catholic hospitals opened in 1939 and 1940, in response to the problem of tuberculosis: one at Fort Resolution (St Joseph's)

142 Rabesca, Romie, Johnson, and Ryan, *Traditional Dene Medicine*, part 2, section on 'Bleeding'.
143 St Peter's Daily Journal, 22 Aug. 1932.
144 Heron interview with Mercredi, pp. 6–7; Clara Frost, interview with Jennie Jack (and interpreter), 10 Jul. 1974, Old Crow, transcript p. 3, Yukon Women's Project Fonds, Series 13, tape 2, YA; Fred Dawson interview pp. 15–17.
145 Ruby McLeod, interview, GSCI, Gwich'in Elders' Biographies Research Project, tape 37.
146 Rose Fabien in *That's the Way We Lived*, 72.

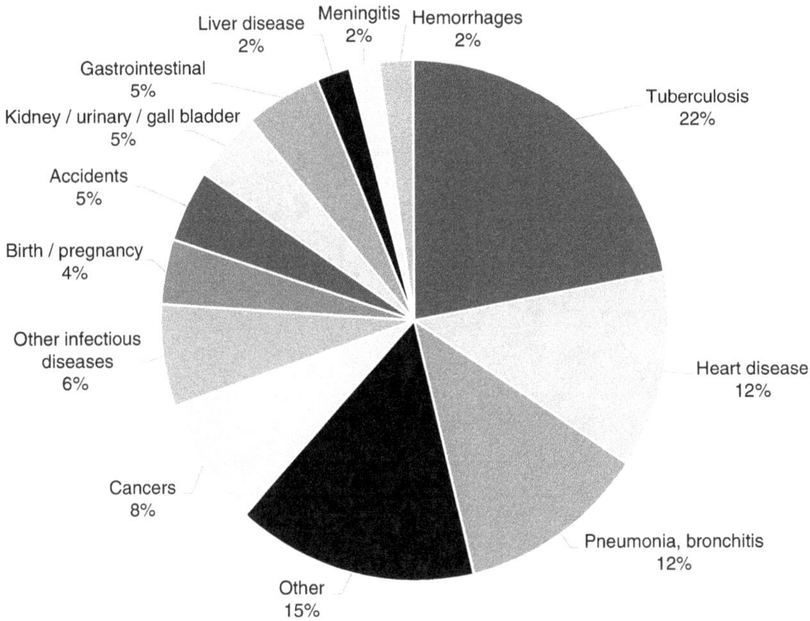

Figure 9.7 Deaths in hospital 1899–1950. Source: COD Database.

with twenty-four beds and the other at Behchokǫ̀ (Faraud) with thirty-five beds. Although denied permission to construct hospitals, the residential schools had medical services funded under the NWT hospital ordinance, which meant that they had nurses paid by the DIA.[147] At the Providence school, nursing sisters provided 'medication, dressings and consultation', and home visits for people in the community.[148] In the Yukon, there were three hospitals, at Dawson, Mayo, and Whitehorse. The Hudson Stuck Memorial Hospital in Fort Yukon, Alaska, treated Gwich'in from the Porcupine River area (Figure 9.8). Archie Linklater took his dying sixteen-year-old daughter, Emma, there in the winter of 1924–5. She was in hospital for a week before she passed away, 'I was with her to the very last minute', Linklater recorded in his diary.[149] The DIA paid for the treatment of Indigenous people from the Canadian side of the border who sought treatment at Hudson Stuck. When someone died at the hospital, Fort Yukon Chief Esias Loola paid for their coffin.[150] At Port Radium on Great Bear Lake, the government paid

[147] 'Nurses Employed in NWT', RG 85, vol. 191, file 554/119-1, part 2, LAC.
[148] Castonguay, *A Leap in Faith*, 202. [149] Linklater Diary, 6 Apr. 1925.
[150] Katherine Peter, *Khęhkwaii Zheh Gwiich'ì': Living in the Chief's House* (Fairbanks: Alaska Native Language Center, 2001), 35.

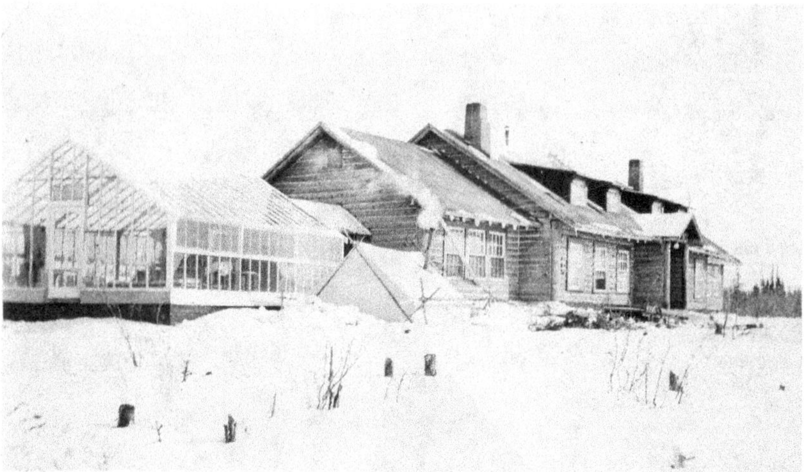

Figure 9.8 Hudson Stuck Memorial Hospital in Fort Yukon, Alaska. With sunroom to the left, c.1913–39. Dr. Ernest A. Cook Photograph Collection, UAF-2003–109–38, Alaska and Polar Regions Collections and Archives, University of Alaska Fairbanks.

for a doctor who also served as Medical Officer of Health but did not fund a hospital at the site.

Amid growing demands for medical care, as tuberculosis cases rose in the late 1920s and 1930s, government spending contracted in response to the Great Depression. In 1932, Yukon Indian Agent John Hawksley wrote to Dr Alfred Standfast at the Hudson Stuck hospital, noting that henceforth the DIA would only pay for care of acute cases of illness and accident, and asked Standfast to discharge any chronic or incurable cases. In a letter to D. C. Scott, Hawksley further advised that the new RCMP officer at Old Crow was expected to 'use more judgement in sending Indians to Fort Yukon for hospital treatment'.[151] In December 1934, the Department of the Interior turned its attention to 'chronic incurables', kept at Hay River. Lorne Turner tallied twenty-four patients who had been hospitalized for more than a year (the longest had been hospitalized for over a decade).[152] Confronted by these costs, calls for additional measures to address the tuberculosis problem went unheeded. In 1932, a meeting of the Anglican synod called for a comprehensive survey of Indigenous health in the Yukon.[153] John Hawksley spoke out firmly in opposition on the grounds that it

[151] J. Hawksley to A. Standfast and J. Hawksley to D.C. Scott, both 16 Mar. 1932, Gov 1619 1490 J file 2, YRG 1, series 1, vol. 9, YA.

[152] Vanast, 'Arctic Bodies', 245. [153] McMillen, *Discovering Tuberculosis*, 21.

was too expensive and too difficult, questioning whether the 'ends accomplished would justify the very heavy expenditures'.[154] In a 1934 meeting on northern medical services convened by the NWT and Yukon Branch, the question of establishing sanatoria for tuberculosis was on the agenda. However, the item was deferred to another time, citing the need to address other 'more pressing questions'.[155]

Soon enough, though, tuberculosis control and care became a central government concern. The problem of tuberculosis in the Yukon and Northwest Territories was already clear to the majority of northerners. It was clear to all those who had lost children, siblings, spouses, parents, or grandparents to the disease. It was clear to those lying in hospital beds for months or years wondering when they could go home. It was clear in budget reports showing the financial impacts of 'chronic incurables' in northern hospitals. It was clear to missionaries who delivered healthcare and to government doctors, like Fred Urquhart, who consistently supported the opening of more hospitals and the funding of more nurses.[156] In November 1937, the front page of the *Toronto Star* carried an article headlined, 'Tuberculosis Causing 50 [percent] Indian Deaths Flying Bishop Claims'. Gabriel Breynat, the 'flying bishop', had been making the case to the government for more northern health funding for years.

Breynat harnessed the cultural idea of the 'vanishing Indian' to push for greater government investment in northern health and social services.[157] Breynat has been praised for his compassion, his attention to the government failures to live up to their treaty responsibilities, and his calls to restrict white trappers in the North. However, as the bishop responsible for the major hospitals and residential schools in the Mackenzie district, his was a vested interest. Ignorant to the realities of life among northern Indigenous peoples, southern policymakers took Breynat at his word. They imagined the 'extinction' of 'the Indian population ... at the end of fifteen years' (Breynat's timeline) – ideas that pushed the deputy minister of Pensions and National Health, R. E. Wodehouse, to call for 'a check-up of all the Indians, with segregation of those found to be suffering from tuberculosis'.[158] Wodehouse continued, 'I fully appreciate the difficulty that is encountered in dealing with those suffering from tuberculosis and their reluctance to enter hospital, where

154 John Hawksley to A. F. Mackenzie, 12 Feb. 1932, Gov 1619 1490 J file 2, YRG 1, series 1, vol. 9, YA.

155 J. Lorne Turne to R. A. Gibson, 23 Nov. 1934, RG 85, vol. 191, file 554/119-1, part 2, LAC.

156 J. Lorne Turner to R. A. Gibson, 4 Dec. 1934, RG 85, vol. 191, file 554/119-1, part 2, LAC.

157 'Tuberculosis Causing 50 P.C. Indian Deaths Flying Bishop Claims', *Toronto Daily Star*, 25 Nov. 1937; Brian W. Dippie, *The Vanishing American: White Attitudes and U.S. Indian Policy* (Middletown: Wesleyan University Press, 1982).

158 'Fear Extinction' was the subtitle to the *Toronto Star* article; the other quotations are from R. E. Wodehouse to R. A. Gibson, 23 Dec. 1936, RG 85, vol. 1061, file 554/107, part 1, LAC.

they might receive adequate treatment'.[159] Couched in the language of reasonableness, we see here the ignorance among southern policymakers of the desire for medical care and the failures to provide the same in the North for decades.

Calls to do more to address tuberculosis in the Yukon and Mackenzie district intensified. In 1944, a Yukon doctor wrote to J. E. Gibben (who would soon become commissioner) to emphasize 'the lack of facilities in the Yukon Territory for the treatment of tuberculosis in the Indian population'. In his letter, the doctor emphasized 'There is a real need for some institution in the Yukon to treat suitable early cases of all types of tuberculosis, particularly pulmonary. This Territory is far behind the rest of Canada in this respect.' The doctor called for the kind of survey that the Anglican synod had suggested, which could be used to control and remove those who were infected with TB; according to him, 'These active ambulant cases are a danger to whites as well as other Indians'.[160] This doctor, Bishop Breynat, deputy minister of health Wodehouse – these were powerful voices articulating a shared, overlapping, and emergent understanding of the 'problem' of tuberculosis in the North.[161] These writings reveal the sentiment driving what would become a policy of coercive relocations to southern institutions. Having failed to attend to health needs in the North for years, tuberculosis was now major health crisis, amplified not eased within residential institutions, and one which, from the perspective of colonial authorities, justified significant interventions. At the same time, these colonial authorities denied liberal subjectivity to Indigenous peoples, denied Indigenous autonomy and awareness of what was in their own best interest, and believed paternalistically that Ottawa bureaucrats knew what was best.[162] When Clermont Bourget had tried to remove Catherine from the territory for reasons of public health, he failed – not because he lacked power and authority, not because he had nowhere to send her, but because she was one woman who was able to evade his grasp. When, in the 1940s and 1950s, the fuller resources of the southern state would be directed to health and schooling, with new tools for surveillance and relocations, the consequences were far broader and more profound.

There were always choices. In 1941, a young Gwich'in woman enrolled at Carcross asked to stay on at the school to get additional training so she could be a nurse. While the principal supported this and got approval for the young woman to stay on, the funds she needed to train as a nurse were denied.[163]

159 Wodehouse to Gibson, 23 Dec. 1936.

160 **** to Mr. J. Gibben, 26 May 1944, GOV 2206 file 7, severed file, YA.

161 Pat Sandiford Grygier, *A Long Way from Home: The Tuberculosis Epidemic among the Inuit* (Montreal: McGill-Queen's University Press, 1994), 55.

162 Lux, *Separate Beds*, 7.

163 Philip Phelan to H.C.M. Grant, 31 Dec. 1941, RG 10, vol. 6481, file 940–10, part 4, c-8795, LAC.

More hospitals could have been built in the North, as well as sanatoria or other facilities, to allow people to stay closer to their families while receiving treatment. As hospitals opened at Behchokǫ̀ and Fort Resolution, a hospital on Great Bear Lake never came to fruition, despite repeated requests, because neither the Catholic missionaries nor the federal state would pay for a building and equipment over which the mining company would exert control. The doctor stationed at Port Radium, whose salary was paid in part by Ottawa, served the needs of the white mining population, which in the 1930s was described as healthy, physically fit young men. Only when mining activity slowed did he turn attention to the local Dene and Métis population.[164] Even then, in 1936, the doctor suggested that treaty payments be moved from Tulita to Cameron Bay, at the far east end of the lake and the site of the main pitchblende mine. There the doctor could examine people without having to go to them.[165] When the mine was converted to a uranium operation and reopened in 1942, part of the supply chain for the US Manhattan Project, there was a plan to provide 'a suitable hospital' and a 'first class doctor' to serve the mine employees and their families.[166] No additional provision was made for Indigenous people, and, by 1950, company officials were writing to the government complaining that 'ours is a private hospital. While we are a Crown company we have no responsibility whatsoever with regards Indians. They have cost us a considerable amount of money in caring for their cases and also in extra work collecting for such cases.'[167] By this time, government officials focused on 'evacuating' people either to hospital in Yellowknife or Edmonton. Failures of care continued.

Conclusion

In his first book, *When the World Was New*, George Blondin wrote about health and medicine on Great Bear Lake in the 1940s and into the 1950s. He described the persistence of tuberculosis and how 'people were often sick, but the company doctor at Port Radium had a hard time treating us since we moved on the land all the time'.[168] Years before, George and his brother Frank had attended residential school together in Fort Providence, but when they came home (an expensive flight paid for by their father), Frank had tuberculosis. As children, George and Frank slept beside one another, 'until the day he died, so I was carrying TB. Finally it had caught up with me.' Blondin was sent to the

164 Extract from letter Maurice Thomson, 22 Dec. 1935, RG 85, vol. 1061, file 554/107, part 1, LAC.
165 R. A. Gibson to M. Thomson, 23 Dec. 1936, RG 85, vol. 1061, file 554/107, part 1, LAC.
166 R. A. Gibson to Mr. Cumming, 23 Jun. 1942, RG 85, vol. 1061, file 554/107, part 1, LAC.
167 E. B. Gillanders to W. L. Falconer, 28 Mar. 1950, RG 85, vol. 1061, file 554/107, part 1, LAC.
168 Blondin, *When the World Was New*, 241.

Charles Camsell Hospital in Edmonton, leaving behind a wife and four small children for nine months. When he returned to his family, Blondin was still weak and decided he 'couldn't live the old kind of life any more. Moving all around the country in cold weather wasn't good for me or my family. I'd already lost my oldest boy. I needed to live near a doctor and I wanted to be near the children's schools.'[169] Blondin moved with his family to Sǫ̀mbak'è (Yellowknife).

That tuberculosis was so widespread and severe in the Yukon and Mackenzie district in the 1920s and 1930s shows the diverse impacts of northern colonialism. From its early origins in the fur trade, the 'shifts in host ecology' that caused TB's amplification in the twentieth century can be tied most closely to the synergistic effects of major measles and influenza epidemics in those years, as well as the role of residential schools. In both these ways, tuberculosis had disproportionate impacts on young people such as Archie Linklater's daughter Emma, J. J. Van Bibber's sister Helen, Sarah Simon's daughter, or the children who survived the 1928 influenza, only to die of tuberculosis in the year that followed. Residential schools encouraged the spread of disease and failed to provide the necessary care. Blondin shows how tuberculosis did not in itself displace people from the land; nor was it a product of relocation to reserves or villages. Rather, without treatment and care available for people on the land, and with the sheer scale of tuberculosis infection in these years, the disease tore through the fabric of life, remaking social and environmental relations for decades to come.

[169] Blondin, *When the World Was New*, 243–4.

10 Epilogue and Conclusions

In the early 1940s, John F. Marchand was serving as medical officer for the US Public Roads Administration on the Alaska Highway. The highway was a defining wartime infrastructure project in the North, alongside the Canol pipeline, the Northwest Staging Route, and the reopening of the Eldorado mine on Great Bear Lake to extract uranium. One of three African American regiments, the 93rd, was tasked with building the section of highway through Teslin, just over the border from British Columbia and southeast of Whitehorse.[1] Marchand was their doctor. In December of 1943, Marchand published an article in the *Journal of the American Medical Association*, titled 'Tribal Epidemics in the Yukon'. In it, he described multiple outbreaks that appeared in Teslin beginning in September 1942 through the summer of 1943, including measles, dysentery, German measles, jaundice, mumps, whooping cough, and meningococcal meningitis. This last was the most serious and led to four deaths among children and young adults; measles also killed three people. Marchand emphasized in his brief report that these outbreaks 'can be attributed neither to insanitary living habits . . . nor to some supposed lack of resistance in disease in general on the part of the Indian'. Instead, Marchand highlighted the 'isolation' of the people of Teslin and others in 'remote regions of Alaska and Canada', in creating a 'serious hazard'.[2]

Marchand exaggerated the isolation and remoteness of the people of Teslin over the preceding half-century. He described that the villagers at Teslin Lake 'have had little intercourse with the white man for almost half a century'. 'Since the great gold rush of 1896', he wrote, there had been a long 'interval of isolation'.[3] On the one hand, this exaggeration appears benign. There were few settlers on Teslin Lake in this period. The new population centres were Dawson and Whitehorse and smaller communities such as Mayo. The Tlingit who spent their summers at Teslin Lake, like their many counterparts across

1 One of three African American regiments that made up about one-third of the total US presence. See William R. Morrison and Kenneth Coates, *Working the North : Labor and the Northwest Defense Projects, 1942–1946* (Fairbanks: University of Alaska Press, 1994).

2 John F. Marchand, 'Tribal Epidemics in the Yukon', *Journal of the American Medical Association* 123, no. 16 (1943): 1019–20.

3 Marchand, 'Tribal Epidemics', 1019.

northern lands, travelled widely, pursuing their seasonal rounds throughout the year.

On the other hand, through this exaggeration Marchand erased the colonial history of contact and interaction between Tlingit and settlers, including a history of disease. Erasure is integral to settler colonialism. Apparent in landscape art, the delineation of property, and, as a powerful recent example, in the removal of gravestones marking the deaths of children in residential schools, erasure works hand in hand with dispossession, replacement, and suppression of opposition – the key processes of settlement and domination.[4] The Anglican church established a mission on Teslin Lake in 1906 and ran a day school in the summer months from 1911 through 1939. As many as thirty-eight children attended the day school at the mission at one time. One inspector described that it 'must be rather crowded'.[5] By the 1940s, children from Teslin attended the Chooutla Residential School at Carcross. Anglican records describe people who were very sickly in 1917, as well as a serious influenza outbreak in 1932 that led to at least three deaths. There were deaths from tuberculosis noted in the burial registers in the 1930s.[6] Marchand himself mentioned a severe respiratory disease in 1936. The Tlingit who summered on Teslin Lake also interacted with other Indigenous peoples in the region. When he was interviewed at the age of seventy-four, Johnnie Johns told stories about Keish (Skookum Jim) travelling to Teslin country before the flu epidemic in 1920.[7] Good health arose not from isolation, as people maintained relationships with one another, with traders, RCMP officers, Indian Agents, and missionaries throughout this time. Good health arose from autonomy and independence, the persistence of ways of life dependent upon good hunts, successful fisheries, rich berry harvests, and access to plants for medicines. Good health was travelling far and the strength that came with life lived on the land.

The Second World War, like the gold rush before, brought serious illness and disruption to the people who lived in the Yukon and Mackenzie district. Marchand called attention to the diversity of pathogens (German measles, jaundice, meningitis) to underscore his point about northern Indigenous isolation from disease. These were cosmopolitan pathogens, like those that had circulated at the turn of the twentieth century. The most important cause of

4 Jonathan Bordo, 'Jack Pine: Wilderness Sublime or the Erasure of the Aboriginal Presence from the Landscape', *Journal of Canadian Studies* 27, no. 4 (1992–93): 98–128; Cole Harris, 'How Did Colonialism Dispossess? Comments from an Edge of Empire', *Annals of the Association of American Geographers* 94, no. 1 (2004): 165–82.

5 Stikine Agency Inspection Report No. 3, 31 Jul. 1935, COR 251 file 29, 'H.C.M. Grant', Series 1, Anglican Church of Canada, Diocese of Yukon, YA.

6 And described in 'Report on the Teslin Mission June–September 1933', COR 258, file 6, Series 1, Anglican Church of Canada, Diocese of Yukon, YA.

7 Johnnie Johns interview, Skookum Jim Oral History Project Fonds, COR 1096 (88/58R), YA.

death in this decade, however, was influenza in combination with widespread TB infection. Five years saw significant deaths from influenza – 1941, 1943, 1944, 1946, and 1949 (see Figure 8.2). In each of these years, at least ten deaths were recorded from influenza in outbreaks across the Yukon and Mackenzie district. In 1943, for instance, the deaths recorded were in Mayo and Tulita. In 1944, they were in Aklavik, Cambridge Bay, and Fort Selkirk. The total number of deaths that decade may have come close to the height of 1928; the absence of comparable reporting in these two periods makes precise comparison elusive. In Chapter 8, recall American physician Rufus Cole comparing the severity of flu in 1928 to the 1943–4 epidemic. What set influenza in the 1940s apart was the sheer frequency of severe outbreaks, reflecting the accelerated movement of workers, military personnel, and government employees as a result of the militarization of the North and the erection of what Philip Wight calls the 'Northwest Defense Complex'.[8] Where the 1928 influenza was defined by a single event, the 1940s epidemics were a series of repeated shocks taking place in the context of the Second World War. Daniel Sims, writing about the 1943 influenza among the Tsek'ehne to the south of the Yukon–NWT–BC border, emphasized that in Tsek'ehne histories, the influenza was part of the experience of the war and connected with the explosion of Japanese balloon bombs on their lands.[9] Yukon Elders, interviewed by Julie Cruikshank decades later, described the 1942–3 epidemics as part of a second 'rush', now focused on high-energy resources (uranium and oil) and strategic advantage.[10] Many of the influenza outbreaks took place in the spring, a shift (compared to the previous prevalence of influenza in the autumn and winter) that reflected the role of aviation in creating more fluid, year-round connections between the Mackenzie district, Yukon, and the south. Old rhythms and geographies were disrupted in this period, and so too the rhythms and geographies of infectious disease shifted.

In the Yukon, Cruikshank described the grief felt by families who lived through the epidemics and lost children and kin in these years.[11] Elders who were young children at the time later shared their experiences of influenza. Marka Bullock from Tsiigehtchic lost her new husband and her father in the 1944 outbreak:

> First it was my father who had passed away and I got married at that time. He wanted us to continue with our wedding. We were supposed to be married at Easter Sunday and he

[8] Wight, 'Hydrocarbon Frontier'. [9] Sims, 'Balloon Bombs', 124.

[10] Julie Cruikshank, 'The Gravel Magnet: Some Social Impacts of the Alaska Highway on Yukon Indians', in *The Alaska Highway: Papers of the 40th Anniversary Symposium*, ed. Kenneth Coates (Vancouver: University of British Columbia Press, 1985): 172–87 (p. 174).

[11] Cruikshank, 'Gravel Magnet', 182; see also Kenneth Coates, 'The Alaska Highway and the Indians of the Southern Yukon, 1942–50: A Study of Native Adaptation to Northern Development', in *The Alaska Highway*, ed. Coates, 151–71 (p. 158).

got sick couple of days before then. He couldn't attend the Church so he stayed home and we all went to Church and Francois and I got married. My father passed away that day and eight days later my husband, the young man that I just married passed away also. This was 1944, Easter time when the big flu that took many lives.[12]

Elders and younger people died that year, recalled Jim Vittrekwa. He himself was a healthy young man, but still 'I was very very sick'.[13] Pierre Benoit, husband of Annie, also lost his father in 1944. He remembered that there was influenza in Aklavik around Christmas time and then, 'around after Easter well they got it there too', in Tsiigehtchic and Aklavik as well.[14] Tom Thrasher, now a Tuktoyaktuk Elder, was a little boy in 1948 when flu hit his family living on the delta. He recalled isolation and quarantine measures. People were informed over the radio that if they got the flu, they were not to visit other camps in the area because of the risk of spreading the sickness. Because of these restrictions on movement, the government used aeroplanes to deliver food rations, 'so we don't have to travel anywhere to get them'.[15] Thrasher recalled the death of his stepbrother and the hard work, when weakened by the disease, of caring for others. Chief Julius Salu with Johnny Kyikavichik had signed Treaty 11 on behalf of the Gwich'in. Salu survived the 1928 epidemic but lost his eldest daughter to sickness in a residential school. He was an important leader at Fort McPherson who helped bring a nursing station and school to the community. Salu died in the influenza epidemic in 1948.

There were new tools with which to fight influenza. Most valuable were the new antibiotic drugs that found their way into northern hospitals and medical kits by the end of the decade. Antibiotics could not cure influenza, which is a viral infection. They could treat bacterial pneumonia, however, a common secondary infection and cause of death arising from influenza. The earliest record of penicillin use in the Northwest Territories came in a June 1945 requisition from the Fort Smith hospital, to treat sexually transmitted infections. As Roy A. Gibson wrote to the RCMP Commissioner in reference to the order request, 'this drug is reported to be very effective in cases of gonorrhea and during the first stages of syphilis'. Gibson continued by noting that, 'In fact all our doctors are being supplied with this drug and arrangements are being made to keep a stock available at all medical centres'.[16] Many physicians working in the North now had penicillin on hand for use in influenza outbreaks. Sulpha drugs, and specifically sulphadiazine, were approved for medical use in the United States in 1941 and were soon being used widely to treat colds,

[12] Marka Bullock, interview, GSCI, Gwich'in Elders' Biographies Research Project, tape 44.
[13] Jim Vittrekwa, interview, GSCI, Gwich'in Elders' Biographies Research Project, tape 40.
[14] Benoit interview, Gwich'in Elders' Biographies.
[15] CBC Radio 1 North, *Trailbreaker*, interview with Tuktoyaktuk Elder Tom Thrasher. Aired 6 Oct. 2009.
[16] R. A. Gibson to Commissioner, RCMP, 22 Jun. 1945, RG 85, vol. 987, file 15279, LAC.

influenza, and some pneumonias, as quinine had been in previous decades.[17] In the Northwest Territories, penicillin and sulpha drugs were used to treat pneumonia by the end of the 1940s.[18]

Thus, the bounty of southern pharmaceutical research made its way north during these years, as part of the larger militarization of the region. But the availability of new therapies and increased medical personnel remained piecemeal and incomplete. Money, resources, and feasibility continued to shape care. In July 1943, liaison officer C. K. LeCapelain reported to Roy Gibson about the Teslin epidemics. LeCapelain wrote that different bands in the Yukon had varying degrees of interaction with 'white people' over time and therefore had 'built up' different levels of 'immunity against the diseases of white people'. Relying on an old set of racist interpretations about the imminent annihilation of Indigenous peoples in the face of contact with civilization, LeCapelain wrote without a hint of irony, 'The new era is here to stay'.[19] In 1942–3, Tlingit from Teslin had spent the winter not out on the land but in the village, finding work alongside US Army soldiers and settlers in building the highway. In connecting this wage labour to the spread of disease, LeCapelain asked Gibson how the government should respond. 'Technically, I believe, the Indians are free agents and should be permitted the same opportunities of obtaining lucrative employment as white people and of associating with them', wrote LeCapelain. Then he continued:

> In practice this will be to their detriment if the majority of them die of disease within a few years. Consequently, I think every endeavour should be made to influence or persuade them to continue their ancestral and normal nomadic life of hunting and trapping and to avoid close association with white people.[20]

Historian Ken Coates has characterized sentiments such as these as a policy encapsulated in the title of his book, *Best Left as Indians*, which was pervasive in twentieth-century Yukon governance. But there is more to it than that. LeCapelain here embraced Indigenous peoples within a liberal order: 'Indians are free agents', he wrote, and should be left to their own devices. He then uses health to justify limiting the autonomy and freedom of this same population, should their own devices include waged industrial labour, for

[17] Howard A. Rusk and Arie C. van Ravenswaay, 'Sulfadiazine in Respiratory Tract Infections: Its Value in Treatment during Winter of 1942–1943 at Jefferson Barracks, Missouri', *Journal of the American Medical Association* 122, no. 8 (1943): 495–6.

[18] C. E. van Rooyen, L. McClelland, and E. K. Campbell, 'Influenza in Canada during 1949, including an Account of a Severe Epidemic at Cambridge Bay, Victoria Island, N.W.T.', p. 9, Interim Report to the Defence Research Board, RG 29, vol. 1192, file 311-J2-2, part 1, LAC.

[19] C. K. LeCapelain to R. A. Gibson, 17 Jul. 1943, Gov 1619 1490J, file 3, YRG 1, series 1, vol. 9, Central Registry Files, YA; also Shelagh Grant, *Sovereignty or Security? Government Policy in the Canadian North, 1936–1950* (Vancouver: UBC Press, 1988), 27.

[20] LeCapelain to Gibson, 17 Jul. 1943.

example. Moreover, LeCapelain was not especially concerned for the health of Indigenous peoples. His indifference resonates in his casual tone and in the remainder of his letter, where LeCapelain reveals his foremost concern: cost. LeCapelain continued: 'The necessity of providing greater medical care than has been necessary in the past, will thereby become an obligation upon the Department.' LeCapelain observed that military and civilian doctors and nurses were all overworked at that time and that the provision of proper care, 'is an almost insuperable problem'.[21] Ottawa's primary concern was not that increased settler, military, and resource activity in the Yukon would produce ill health, but the question of who would pay for the medical care that would then be required.

Into the antibiotic era, when penicillin could be supplied to posts preserved in oil, failures of care continued. Influenza broke out at Old Crow in March 1956. Neil McDonald remembered this sickness, as it was when three Elders, Rachel Cadzow (second wife of Dan Cadzow, the trader at Rampart House), Myra Edward, and Donald Fredson died. McDonald recalled,

> By that time, they had medicine, otherwise it would have killed more. The medicine came in time to save the others. The medicine came while Pete Lord was out in Crow Flats. He came in and they gave him medicine to take to people. By that time it was mostly over. As he went down, he went to Peter Charlie's place to give them medicine, and Mary Charlie, two more days and she would have been gone. He gave them medicine, told them how to drink lots of water. Peter was sick too. He was the one that saved them, with the medicine. The plane brought it in. The RCMP were the ones who went after the medicine. The minister here . . . he was the one that the Indian agent sent the medicine, Reverend Wheeler . . . No, not too long ago.[22]

The outbreak was reported in southern newspapers initially as an outbreak of an unknown respiratory disease, then a few days later dismissed in a short piece in the *Edmonton Journal* that opened: 'Three elderly Indians who died at Old Crow, an isolated northern Yukon community, were apparently victims of common colds, and not an epidemic of some more serious ailment as first indicated.'[23] The *Journal*'s reporting notwithstanding, the disease was influenza, not 'common colds', the deaths were from pneumonia, and a detailed RCMP report highlighted the course of the outbreak. Brought into the community by a plane carrying an RCMP inspector, two doctors, and other visitors from Aklavik ('What a price to pay for "orientation"!' read a marginal note), the sickness soon spread throughout the settlement. The three Elders were the only ones who died but, as Constable P. A. Robin with the Old Crow detachment noted, 'while it is true the three lives the present epidemic has claimed are all over 70 years of age, the writer is quite confident that had it not been for the

[21] LeCapelain to Gibson, 17 Jul. 1943. [22] Neil McDonald in *People of the Lakes*, 134.
[23] 'Find Colds Caused Deaths of 3 Indians', *The Edmonton Journal*, 5 May 1956, p. 12.

outbreak, several years of comfortable living could have been obtained by the deceased persons'.[24]

Robin placed much of the blame for deaths in this outbreak on the Anglican missionary, Rev. R. F. Wheeler, who had kept the day school open even while he himself was sick. As McDonald recalled, Wheeler was also the one who controlled medicines, now including sulphadiazine and penicillin. Wheeler had chosen not to dispense penicillin during his daily visits to the sick as he was concerned about depleting his stocks of medicine before the spring break-up. McDonald emphasized that it was Pete Lord who brought medicine to the people. From Robin's perspective, 'Wheeler is not capable or competent enough' to have responsibility for dispensing medicines, but Robin also reported that Wheeler had repeatedly requested additional supplies of penicillin 'from the Indian Department, only to have his order reduced by one half or not acknowledged at all'.[25] Robin's superior, Inspector W. G. Fraser, forwarded the report on, agreeing with some of Robin's conclusions and suggesting that the most the RCMP could do was discuss the matter with the Director of Indian Health Services in Ottawa. When outbreaks occurred, new therapies were now available, just not necessarily in the North.

Insufficient resources shaped access to tuberculosis treatment. The first antibiotic treatment for tuberculosis, streptomycin, was only developed in 1943 and not given to a patient until 1949. Effective antibiotics remained out of reach for northerners well into the 1950s. In the meantime, more northern physicians and hospitals had access to X-ray equipment. When St Mary's hospital in Dawson burned in January 1950, killing one elderly nursing sister, the surviving sisters salvaged a complete X-ray unit along with other essential equipment.[26] In Aklavik in the early 1940s, Dr Livingstone had access to an X-ray unit but had to forward the plates for interpretation by radiologists in Ottawa, creating enormous delays in diagnosis.[27] Livingstone's replacement, R. Hayward, complained that patients were kept in bed for weeks or months 'on suspicion of tuberculosis'.[28] By August 1946, the procedure had been changed to speed up diagnosis. Now northerners with tuberculosis 'in a curable condition', were sent south to the newly opened Charles Camsell Indian Hospital in Edmonton, the largest Indian Hospital in Canada.[29] Thereafter, northern hospitals treated people when the Camsell 'was filled', or those deemed unlikely to recover.[30]

24 Cst. P. A. Robin, RE: Epidemic of Influenza . . ., 17 May 1956, RG 29, vol. 2970, file 851-4-096, part 1, LAC.

25 All quotations, Robin, RE: Epidemic.

26 'St Mary's Hospital – Dawson YT', RG 85, vol. 742, file 554/201, LAC.

27 L. D. Livingstone to R. A. Gibson, 18 Dec. 1942, RG 85, vol. 178, file 552-1-1 [1], LAC.

28 Extract from letter of Dr Hayward, 12 Dec. 1944, RG 85, vol. 178, file 552-1-1 [1], LAC.

29 Extracts from Minutes of Special Meeting of the Northwest Territories Council, 22 Sept. 1949, RG 85, vol. 178, file 552-1-1 [1], LAC.

30 R. A. Gibson to M. Meikle, 16 Mar. 1949, RG 85, vol. 188, file 554/111, part 5, LAC; G. R. Davison to L. M. Riddell, 8 Mar. 1945, RG 85, vol. 178, file 552-1-1 [1], LAC.

Aviation gas produced at Norman Wells, from petroleum extracted on Treaty 11 lands, fuelled planes used across the Yukon and Mackenzie district for travel that was now cheaper and faster than by boat. Planes carried people to hospital, whether within the territories or south to Edmonton. They also carried medicines, like the penicillin sent to Old Crow in 1956. Marchand described evacuation by float plane in his article on the Teslin epidemics. William McNeill in his 1976 book *Plagues and Peoples* made reference to this in his passing mention of the epidemics, noting that despite the number of pathogens to which people were exposed in 1942–3, 'thanks to airlift into modern hospitals, only 7 of 130 individuals actually died'.[31] This was another common refrain, the importance of 'mercy flights' in the provision of 'modern' healthcare.[32] McNeill unwittingly highlighted their inadequacy to the people in Teslin: only three young people were flown out to the hospital in Whitehorse, and two died shortly after arrival. One received therapy and survived. More important was the use of sulphadiazine therapy to treat children and youth in the community during the meningitis outbreak. The proliferation of aeroplanes and increased road-building in the North made aviation a lower cost, faster healthcare alternative deemed more *feasible* by government officials than erecting a northern infrastructure of care with fully equipped hospitals, necessary medicines, and skilled staff.

The decision to systematically relocate those sick with tuberculosis came from the belated use of surveys in the 1940s to understand the scale and extent of TB infection in northern populations. The government chose not to invest in surveys until the wartime emergency, and the arrival of much larger numbers of southern personnel, created a sense of urgency. This was the case in the Northwest Territories, the Yukon, and in Alaska. Northern residents also called for surveys, as in Hay River, where parents were concerned about sending their children to the day school 'to be confined in a closed space with other children who may have active tuberculosis'.[33] Portable X-ray units were sent north, with physicians and other personnel. Encouraging participation was a key issue. Although the surveys focused on diagnosing tuberculosis, they were accompanied by other medical interventions including vaccinations and inoculations.[34] Teeth were pulled and the general health of the population recorded. Tess Lanzarotta writes about the mobile clinics used to survey the scale of tuberculosis disease in Alaska. Lanzarotta emphasizes that in Alaska these clinics were diagnostic, not therapeutic, producing a 'form of colonial biopolitics' in which people were informed that they had tuberculosis or some

[31] McNeill, *Plagues and Peoples*, 181. [32] Piper, 'Diphtheria Antitoxin', 305–8

[33] Extracts F. Fraser's letter 20 Jan. 1949, RG 85, vol. 178, file 552-1-1 [1], LAC.

[34] See also Lanzarotta, 'Disappearing Clinic', 262; J. C. Callaghan, Medical Officer, Aklavik, 'Report X-Ray Survey Trip Western Arctic Coast April 1949', 1 May 1949, RG 85, vol. 178, file 552-1-1 [1], LAC.

other illness, but the therapies needed to get well – to heal – were not provided before the mobile clinic moved on.[35] In the Yukon and Northwest Territories, therapies were offered but at the cost of relocation – away from family, language, culture, and the land – for months or years at a time.

The TB surveys also created research opportunities at a time when 'isolated' and 'pristine' Indigenous populations were perceived as unique sources of biomedical data. During the 1949 western Arctic survey, J. C. Callaghan, Medical Officer from Aklavik, found a major influenza outbreak underway among the Inuit of Cambridge Bay and the surrounding region. After unloading the X-ray equipment at Cambridge Bay and having some dinner, the RCMP informed Callaghan that many people were sick and several had died. The seriousness of the situation soon became clear. Fourteen people had died in recent days, and many others were very sick with pneumonia. Notwithstanding the diagnostic purposes of the survey, Callaghan and the survey crew immediately shifted to care for the people of Cambridge Bay. With the assistance of the RCMP, the survey crew set up an emergency hospital using Jamesway huts ('wartime buildings about 16' by 16' with five beds and an oil heater already in them').[36] The sick were brought to the temporary hospital by snowmobile and given bedding and penicillin. The survey crew nonetheless continued their TB work and taking X-rays, but 'if the individual showed any signs of the illness as evidenced by malaise, temperature elevation and/or chest signs they were given 300,000 units of penicillin at once and admitted to hospital'. In total, forty-two people were admitted to hospital, and seventeen people died.[37] Many recovered after treatment with penicillin. Callaghan noted that he had 'great supplies of that drug in oil', sufficient to meet the needs of the outbreak because he was supposed to distribute the drug at each post for emergency use. He concluded, 'It certainly served its purpose well and certainly justified its expenditure'.[38] The survey continued on after the outbreak, X-raying just over a thousand people. Twenty-nine cases of active tuberculosis were identified, in addition to inactive, healed, and 'suspect' tuberculosis. Seventeen of these people were then sent to hospital for treatment. Eleven, aged one to forty-four, were sent south to the Charles Camsell Hospital in Edmonton, while another six people, the youngest aged three and the oldest sixty, were sent to the Aklavik hospital. This 1949 survey and outbreak reverberated in the lives of those who lost loved ones, those who went to hospital and their families, for years to come.

The survey and the influenza outbreak also reverberated in the south where it almost immediately became the subject of federal research looking at virus strains and immunity. 'Following notification of the outbreak', Dr Percy

35 Lanzarotta, 'Disappearing Clinic', 259, 264.
36 All quotations this paragraph, Callaghan, 'Report X-Ray Survey Trip'.
37 Van Rooyen, McClelland, and Campbell, p. 5; Callaghan, 'Report X-Ray Survey Trip'.
38 Callaghan, 'Report X-Ray Survey Trip', 7.

Moore, with the DIA and J. Gibbard, Director of the Dominion Laboratory of Hygiene in Ottawa 'made arrangements for the collection of specimens'.[39] Dr Fred P. Nagler, a federal government researcher, and Dr J. H. Sturdy, a pathologist at the Royal Alexandra Hospital in Edmonton, flew to Cambridge Bay to secure samples. They took 'post mortem tissue' from three people and 'nose and throat washings were procured from 12 patients'.[40] These were then sent by air to the Connaught Medical Research Laboratories in Toronto. They travelled south around the same time as samples taken from a poliomyelitis outbreak among Inuit at Chesterfield Inlet, while John Paul collected frozen blood samples to the west in Alaska, and while people from Cambridge Bay and Chesterfield Inlet were on route to southern hospitals for treatment.[41] The war and then the Cold War brought an enormous increase in scientific research that viewed Arctic environments as field laboratories and Indigenous peoples as laboratory subjects. But the coincidence here was much more precise than the shared context of intensified scientific research in the Cold War. The main players in this were part of an interwoven network of virologists in the 1940s and 1950s who perceived northern Indigenous peoples, and Inuit in particular, as essential subjects for study. As Joanna Radin has shown, while questions of immunity were an immediate source of interest, the goals of collecting and freezing samples were much larger and imagined these tissue samples as a form of 'latent life'. Paul and others with the World Health Organization 'envisioned an explicit program of accumulating blood from populations living in distinctive environments', with the intention that 'the various known and not-yet-known entities within the blood would be able to be accessed by multiple scientific constituencies, again and again'.[42]

The Canadian researchers were influential in their fields of study. Fred Nagler was a virologist with the department of National Health and Welfare's Laboratory of Hygiene in Ottawa. C. E. Van Rooyen was the first author on the initial 1949 report from Cambridge Bay as well as an article published in the *Canadian Journal of Public Health* in November of that same year and was also the co-author of a major virology textbook, *Virus Diseases of Man*, described as 'possibly the most exhaustive and valuable that has yet been published' and, in a later review, as 'an essential part of the equipment of the virus worker'.[43] His textbook co-author, A. J. Rhodes, was leading the

[39] Van Rooyen, McClelland, and Campbell, p. 5.

[40] Van Rooyen, McClelland, and Campbell, p. 5; for autopsies, see Jennifer Fraser, 'Rendering Inuit Cancer "Visible": Geography, Pathology, and Nosology in Arctic Cancer Research'. *Science in Context* 33, no. 3 (2020): 195–225.

[41] L. Piper, 'Chesterfield Inlet, 1949 and the Ecology of Epidemic Polio', *Environmental History* 20, no. 4 (2015): 671–98.

[42] Radin, *Life on Ice*, 56.

[43] Chas. F. Craig, Book Review, *American Journal of Tropical Medicine and Hygiene* s1-21, no. 2 (1941), 352, https://doi.org/10.4269/ajtmh.1941.s1-21.352; Keith Dumbell, Review of

research into the Chesterfield poliomyelitis outbreak. Dr Ronald Hare and Dr Laurella McClelland directed influenza virus studies at Connaught Laboratories, a centre for research on influenza virus strains.[44] Hare had written to Roy Gibson, then director of the NWT and Yukon Branch, in March 1942 asking for information on the 1928 influenza outbreak. McClelland was Van Rooyen's co-author on the Cambridge Bay research. The war, the tuberculosis surveys, and the general expansion of government interest and activity in the Yukon and Mackenzie district created opportunities for surveillance harnessed by researchers who viewed northern populations as potential sources of unique insight – like Ruggles with his race science two decades earlier.

Work on polio and influenza in the 1940s was united by research questions involving immunity. Van Rooyen, McClelland, and E. K. Campbell used the samples from Cambridge Bay to better understand the diversity of virus strains circulating in Canada in 1949. They drew on samples taken from Inuit at Southampton Island in 1947 to compare the antibodies in Inuit to those from a 'similar adult group' drawn from 'University of Toronto personnel'.[45] In their discussion of antibodies, the authors described 'Southampton Island and Victoria Island are about 500 miles apart, but both are lonely outposts of humanity … It is probable that sera gathered from Southampton Island in 1947 were representative specimens indicative of the prevailing low level of antibodies to influenza virus among the local Arctic inhabitants.'[46] This research fed directly into the 'virgin soil' model, the idea that northern Indigenous populations were exemplars of 'pristine', 'island populations' disproportionately vulnerable to disease because of their exceptional isolation. Nagler would go on to publish more research on immunity, isolation, and 'virgin soils', including in a paper on a 1952 measles outbreak co-authored with Arthur Peart cited repeatedly by Alfred Crosby in his 1976 article, 'Virgin Soil Epidemics as a Factor in the Aboriginal Depopulation in America'. Beyond its immediate influence, biomedical research from the 1940s and 1950s would go on to have many afterlives, circulating in ideas about contact-era epidemics for years to come.

Virology, by A. J. Rhodes and C. E. van Rooyen, *The British Medical Journal* 2, no. 4897 (1954): 1151–2.

44 Christopher J. Rutty, 'Connaught Labs, World War II & Biotech Innovation', *Connaught History Series*, https://connaught.research.utoronto.ca/history/article6/.

45 Van Rooyen, McClelland, and Campbell, p. 8.

46 C. E. van Rooyen, L. McClelland, and E. K. Campbell, 'Influenza in Canada during 1949: Including Studies on Eskimos', *Canadian Journal of Public Health / Revue Canadienne de Santé Publique* 40, no. 11 (1949): 447–56 (p. 452); in the same issue this article appeared: F. P. Nagler, C. E. van Rooyen, and J. H. Sturdy, 'An Influenza Virus Epidemic at Victoria Island, N.W.T., Canada', pp. 457–65.

In rooting his interpretation in geography and time, not race, John Marchand's 1944 interpretation of 'tribal epidemics' arising from isolation appealed to post-war researchers such as Alfred Crosby for whom 'race' was no longer an acceptable category of analysis. Crosby emphasized environments, ecologies, and geography more so than genetics in his interpretation of ecological imperialism and the role of disease.[47] Moreover, where he engaged source materials in detail, Crosby's analyses were nuanced and valuable, as for instance in his work on the influenza pandemic in Alaska in 1918–19. But it is not so simple as to sequester ideas of geography from those of race in late twentieth-century biomedical or historical research. That tissues and blood samples from Arctic Indigenous people were used to advance the study of influenza, poliomyelitis, and immunology arose out of – and then reinforced – prevailing ideas about pristine northern environments, 'protected by distance', in the words of Stephen Bocking, 'a perspective inspired by the historical notion of the north as remote, unknown, and unspoiled'.[48] And as Donna Haraway reflected, in her analysis of scientific culture in the United States in the 1980s – in the context of the emergent HIV/AIDS pandemic – 'the immune system is an elaborate icon for principal systems of symbolic and material "difference" in late capitalism'.[49] The model of 'virgin soils' helped elide 'difference' and 'race', a phenomenon observed by David S. Jones in his assessment of Jared Diamond's popular work on 'virgin soil epidemics'. As Jones wrote in 2003: 'The ability of a racial theory of disease susceptibility to slip unnoticed into Diamond's explicitly antiracist theory of history hints at how deeply embedded such theories are in the stories we tell about post-Columbian America.'[50] The preceding chapters have built on Jones's work about these old stories to show how they were articulated in northern contexts and with what consequences. Specifically, how they served to justify coercive interventions, inadequate infrastructure, and failures of care. More broadly, scholars have shown how the purported shift in scientific research away from biological race to populations and genetics was less transformative than is generally assumed. Similar to how racial arguments were transposed into cultural ones after 1945, as Osagie Obasogie and others write, work preoccupied with identifying '"pure" or isolated racial/ethnic group[s]' may have involved shifts in discourse and areas of focus, but biological theories of

[47] Jones, 'Virgin Soils Revisited', 704.

[48] Stephen Bocking, 'Toxic Surprises: Contaminants and Knowledge in the Northern Environment', in *Ice Blink: Navigating Northern Environmental History*, ed. Stephen Bocking and Brad Martin (Calgary: University of Calgary Press, 2017): 421–64 (p. 423).

[49] Donna J. Haraway, 'The Biopolitics of Postmodern Bodies: Constitutions of Self in Immune System Discourse', in *Simians, Cyborgs, and Women: The Reinvention of Nature* (New York: Routledge, 1991): 203–30 (p. 204).

[50] Jones, 'Virgin Soils Revisited', 710.

race persist.[51] These ideas haunt northern histories while continuing to shape northern and Indigenous healthcare in Canada.

Major changes came to the Yukon and Mackenzie district after 1940. Some were a result of the intensified military and scientific work of the war and Cold War era and the increased involvement of the federal government. The ineptitude of Rev. Wheeler in Old Crow in 1956 can be seen as a statement about the continued inadequacies of healthcare. But Constable Robin's criticism of Wheeler's role was a common view among secular personnel, that missionaries were not suited as colonial authorities in the 'New North', ideas that heralded the end of the 'mission era' in schooling and healthcare and greater federal government involvement.[52] The burial registers show a marked change in the latter half of the twentieth century. In the years from 1940 to 1970, automobile accidents, cancers, and suicides appear far more commonly, while infectious diseases decline as causes of death.[53] The new ways of life after 1940 are coming to be better understood within the historical literature through the important work of Crystal Fraser on residential schooling, Stephen Bocking on science, Jennifer Fraser and Tess Lanzarotta on biomedicine, John Sandlos and Arn Keeling on resource industries, and many others. New nursing stations and hospitals were built, while some of the smaller hospitals closed down. Indigenous political entities exerted greater power, after the 1970s especially. Inequities and failures of care persisted, sometimes a result of people making bad decisions rooted in stubbornly persistent ideas about the superiority of southern, colonial institutions, sometimes a result of underfunding, ignorance, and the fact that communities did not share the same priorities as federal bureaucrats or others with power. Relocations to southern hospitals endured as a key feature of northern healthcare. Public health remained a site of surveillance and control.

The foremost dynamic shaping the history of epidemic disease between 1860 and 1940 was the distinctive, northern form of colonialism that took shape among settlers, sojourners, and northern Indigenous peoples who spent some of their time in the very small communities along Dehcho, the Yukon river, the tributaries, and the coast, and the rest out on the water, travelling to and through the mountains, and out on the land. Colonial ecologies were formed by divergent knowledge and understandings of health and how to ease sickness, by

[51] Osagie K. Obasogie, Julie N. Harris-Wai, Katherine Darling, Carolyn Keagy, and Michael Levesque, 'Race in the Life Sciences: An Empirical Assessment, 1950–2000', *Fordham Law Review* 83, no. 6 (2015): 3089–114 (p. 3101); for the shift from 'race' to 'culture', see Sangster citing Malik in *Iconic North*, 18.

[52] A. Stuhl, 'The Politics of the 'New North': Putting History and Geography at Stake in Arctic Futures', *Polar Journal* 3, no. 1: 94–119.

[53] Tanacross Athabaskan Elder Kenny Thomas Sr., interview with Marilyn Jensen and Percy Henry, Tanacross, AK, 31 Jul. 1997, Tape/Transcript #97–05 A&B, Tr'ondëk Hwëch'in Heritage Department.

great gulfs of expertise in living with the land and in relationship to other-than-human nature in the North, by power inequities, assertions of control, and racist ideologies, and by encounters with cosmopolitan pathogens over time. Through all of this, people in the North suffered great loss in successive epidemics, often referred to as 'flus' because of the defining role of influenza as a colonial pathogen. Philip Simba spoke to this before the Berger Inquiry in 1976 in the statement that opened this book. Elders reflected on the historical changes they had witnessed before 1940 and since, and their memories, knowledge, and interpretations are essential to understanding this history. Through all of this change, Gwich'in, Dene, Inuvialuit, Métis, Tutchone, Tr'ondëk Hwëch'in, Tlingit, Tagish, and others showed strength, resilience, and the importance of relationships of care. As the land changes, in the face of global heating and its impacts at high latitudes, these relationships of care – our responsibilities to one another and to the rest of nature – will become ever more important to sustain communities and health in the North.

Appendix: Cause of Death Database

In the absence of early health statistics for the Northwest Territories and Yukon, I constructed a Cause of Death (COD) database using available burial registers to better understand the character of historical outbreaks and epidemics in relationship to other causes of death. The database holds 7,005 unique entries. Of these, 5,767 are drawn from parish (Anglican (n=4,569)) or (Roman Catholic (n=1,198)) burial registers. The St Mary's Hospital (Dawson) register and the Dawson City Funerals records account for another 1,238 entries. The distinction between parish and other records was considered in the analysis. The records in the database were anonymized (a condition of access) and assigned a unique ID. References to the database are apparent where I discuss causes of death quantitatively in the text and in the figures illustrating key findings. Information that was drawn from the registers included: age (both in years or described, e.g. 'very old'), gender, occupation, family relationships ('son of Chief'), class ('indigent'), religion, cause of death, physician, hospitalization, days in hospital, date of death, date of burial, place of birth, place of residence, place of death, place of burial, and funeral. There were also comment fields that sometimes gave additional information about the person, their relations, and their death. Date of death and date of burial were used interchangeably in the analysis. For the most part, the database was used to organize information about deaths by place and time. Intensely quantitative analysis was eschewed in favour of drawing on subsets of the database to inform the discussion.

Figure A.1 shows the geographic and temporal coverage of records. Given that registers were not secured from every community nor were the registers consistently kept over time, the COD database is best understood as a sample of the larger population, comprising detailed evidence from specific places at certain times. The database has the most comprehensive coverage for the period for 1890 to 1950. Before 1900, the majority of deaths do not have a cause assigned. Of course, as other scholars of disease have noted, burial registers as sources of information about 'cause of death' present unique

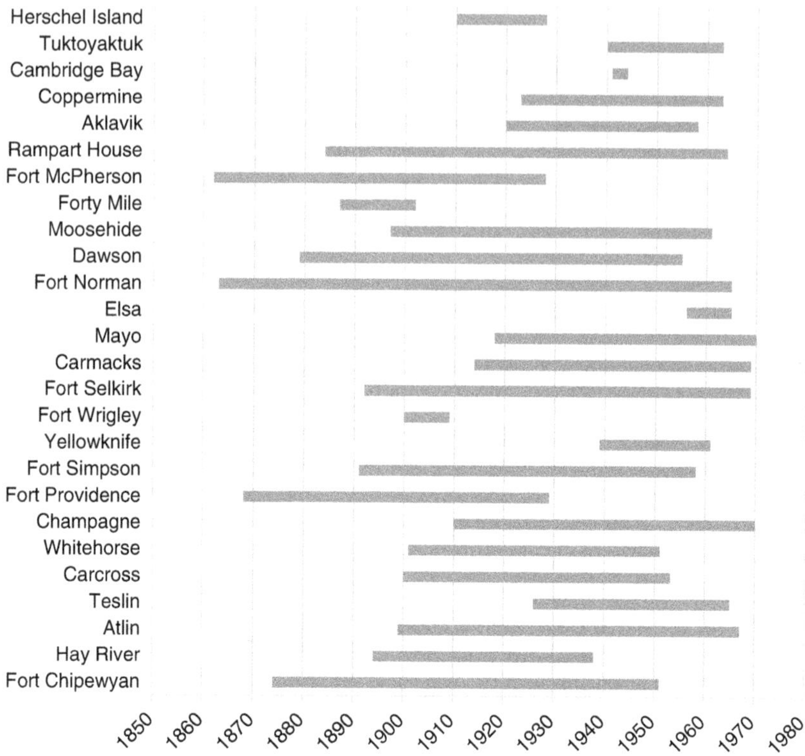

Figure A.1 Coverage of records in Cause of Death Database. Note: Herschel Island registers include 'Eskimo Deaths'; Champagne registers include Haines Junction; Rampart House registers include Old Crow.

contextual challenges.[1] The parish burial registers used here were completed by Anglican and Roman Catholic missionaries, with varying degrees of medical expertise as is discussed in Chapters 2 and 3. While they sometimes had recourse to a physician's diagnosis, as the records from St Mary's Hospital obviously did, most of these assigned 'causes of death' reflected what these observers thought to have caused the death of the person in question, rather than a laboratory or biomedical diagnosis. Causes of death were grouped for analytical purposes. The 'TB Deaths' in Figure 9.5, for instance, include deaths recorded as consumption, scrofula, tuberculosis, phthisis, and TB. Some of

[1] R. Munkhoff, 'Searchers of the Dead: Authority, Marginality, and the Interpretation of Plague in England, 1574–1665', *Gender and History* 11, no. 1 (1999): 1–29; J. C. Robertson, 'Reckoning with London: Interpreting the 'Bills of Mortality' before John Graunt', *Urban History* 23, no. 3 (1996): 325–50, www.jstor.org/stable/44612835.

the registers only came into being during outbreaks or epidemics. While this makes them useful source materials for studying these same events, the registers must also be understood as efforts by Christian missionaries to keep a record of their work among Indigenous populations, proselytizing and converting people to Christianity. By the 1910s, most northern Indigenous peoples had converted to Christianity or were considered as belonging to either the Anglican or Roman Catholic religion.[2] The use of parish records can therefore be seen as a reasonably accurate sample of the population as a whole.

The one marked peculiarity to the records collected in the COD database is that they disproportionately represent the deaths of males over females. Within the dataset, there are 6,431 records where gender was identified; of these, 2,287 were female and 4,144 were male. The Dawson records skew the total when it comes to gender (see pp. 96). Adult men made up the vast majority of residents in Dawson at the turn of the twentieth century, and many of them died, from accidents and violence as well as infectious disease, in the Yukon. However, even when all Dawson records are excluded, females still only make up approximately 40 percent of the records where gender is known. A similar distortion is apparent in the HBC censuses from 1858 and 1871 and has been interpreted as evidence of female infanticide among Dene populations.[3] However, there is no evidence that female infanticide was practised into the twentieth century, and this practice cannot account for the persistent gender imbalance in the burial records. In the end, this gender imbalance highlights the extent to which the burial registers are records kept by a patriarchal settler colonial society predicated on the disappearance of Indigenous women, in life and in death.[4]

[2] Nagy, *Yukon North Slope*, 105; Asen Balikci, *Vunta Kutchin Social Change: A Study of the People of Old Crow, Yukon Territory* (Ottawa: Northern Co-ordination and Research Centre, 1963), 51–2; McCarthy, *Great River*.

[3] Helm, 'Female Infanticide', 259–85; Able, *Drum Songs*, 21.

[4] Audra Simpson, 'The State Is a Man: Theresa Spence, Loretta Saunders, and the Gender of Settler Sovereignty', *Theory & Event* 19, no. 4 (2016), https://muse.jhu.edu/article/633280; *Reclaiming Power and Place: The Final Report of the National Inquiry into Missing and Murdered Indigenous Women and Girls*. [Privy Council Office], 2019.

Select Bibliography

Oral History Collections, Transcripts, Testimony, and Publications

Arrowmaker, Alexis, Madeline Judas, Pierre Judas, et al. *We Know and Love Tłįchǫ̀ Ndè: Comments and Concerns from the Dechılaot'ı Elders to the Environmental Assessment Review Panel, February 1996*. Yellowknife: Dene Cultural Institute, 1996.

Blondin, George. *Trail of the Spirit: The Mysteries of Medicine Power Revealed*. Edmonton: NeWest Press, 2006.

Blondin, George. *When the World Was New: Stories of the Sahtu Dene*. Yellowknife: Outcrop, 1990.

Blondin, George. *Yamoria the Lawmaker: Stories of the Dene*. Edmonton: NeWest Press, 1997.

Canada. Mackenzie Valley Pipeline Inquiry. 'Proceedings at Inquiry, April 22, 1974–June 8, 1976'. 67 vols. Burnaby: Allwest Reporting Ltd., 2003. Electronic version.

Cockney, Cathy. *Kitigaaryuit Oral Traditions Research Project 1996*. Inuvik: Inuvialuit Social Development Program, 1997.

Cockney, Cathy. *Kitigaaryuit Oral Traditions Research Project 1997*. Inuvik: Inuvialuit Social Development Program, 1998.

'Federal Environmental Assessment Panel Review of BHP Diamonds Inc. Northwest Territories Diamonds Project'. Public Hearing, Dettah, NWT, 3 Feb. 1996. English transcript.

Fort Resolution Elders. *That's the Way We Lived. An Oral History of the Fort Resolution Elders*. Yellowknife: Northwest Territories Culture and Communications, 1987.

'Gwich'in COPE stories.' Fort McPherson: Gwich'in Social and Cultural Institute, 2010.

Gwich'in Elders. *Nành' Kak Geenjit Gwich'in Ginjik / Gwich'in Words about the Land*. Inuvik: Gwich'in Renewable Resource Board, 1997.

Gwich'in Social and Cultural Institute. Interview Transcripts. Gwich'in Elders' Biographies Research Project and GLC Files.

Heine, Michael, Alestine Andre, Ingrid Kritsch, Alma Cardinal, and the Elders of Tsiigehtshik. *Gwichya Gwich'in Googwandak. The History and Stories of the Gwichya Gwich'in, as Told by the Elders of Tsiigehtshik*. Tsiigehtshik: Gwich'in Social and Cultural Institute, 2007.

Life Histories of Elders. Gwich'in Social and Cultural Institute, GTC Department of Culture and Heritage. https://gwichin.ca/elders-biographies.

Metis Heritage Association Fonds. NWTA.

Nagy, Murielle, ed. *Aulavik Oral History Project: English Translations and Transcriptions of Interviews 3 to 30*. Inuvik: Inuvialuit Social Development Program, 1999.

Nagy, Murielle, ed. *Yukon North Slope Cultural Resources Survey*. Books 1 and 2. Inuvik: Inuvialuit Social Development Program, 1994.

Nagy, Murielle, ed. *Qikiqtaqruk (Herschel Island) Cultural Study*. Inuvik: Inuvialuit Social Development Program, 1994.

Nagy, Murielle Ida. *Yukon North Slope Inuvialuit Oral History*. [Whitehorse]: Yukon Tourism Heritage Branch, 1994.

Parks Canada. *Paulatuuq Oral History Project: Inuvialuit Elders Share Their Stories*. Inuvik: Parks Canada Western Arctic Field Unit, 2004.

Rabesca, Marie Adele, Diane Romie, Martha Johnson, and Joan Ryan. *Traditional Dene Medicine*. 2 parts. Lac La Martre: [Gov't of the Northwest Territories], 1994.

Rampart House: Stories Told by Our Elders. Old Crow: Te'sek Gehtr'oonatun Zzeh College, 1993.

Salt River Settlement Oral History Project. Transcripts. N-1997–009. NWTA.

Sherry, Erin and Vuntut Gwitchin First Nation. *Jii Nành Tth'aih Hèe Gıinkhii / The Land Still Speaks: Gwitchin Words About Life in Dempster Country*. Lead translator: Jane Montgomery. Lead interpreter: Annie Lord. Lead Community Researcher: Ruby Charlie. Old Crow: Vuntut Gwitchin First Nation, 1999.

Skookum Jim Oral History Project Fonds. YA.

Thom, Margaret M. and Ethel Blondin-Townsend, eds., with Tessa Macintosh Wah-See (photographer). *Nahecho keh/Our Elders*. Fort Providence: Slavey Research Project, 1987.

Tr'ondëk Hwëch'in Heritage Department. Interview Transcripts. Dawson, YT.

Vuntut Gwitchin First Nation and Shirleen Smith. *People of the Lakes: Stories of Our Van Tat Gwich'in Elders*. Edmonton: University of Alberta Press, 2009.

Yukon College. *Moosehide (Èdhä Dädhëchan Kek'èt): An Oral History*. Dawson City: Yukon College, 1994.

Yukon Territory. Heritage Branch. *Fort Selkirk Elders Oral History Project*. Whitehorse: Yukon Heritage Branch, 1987.

Yukon Territory. Heritage Branch. *Fort Selkirk Oral History 1984*. Whitehorse: Yukon Heritage Branch, 1987.

Yukon Women's Project Fonds. YA.

Archival Sources

Anglican Church of Canada, Diocese of the Arctic. YA.

Anglican Diocese of Athabasca. PAA.

Anglican Diocese of the Arctic Collection. GSA.

Archibald Lang Fleming Fonds. GSA.

Archibald (Archie) Linklater Fonds. YA.

Central Registry Files (Yukon Record Group Series 1 and 2). YA.

Claude and Mary Tidd Fonds. YA.

Codex Historicus (Fort Chipewyan, Fort Good Hope, Fort Norman, Arctic Red River, Fort Resolution), OMI. PAA.

Frank Foster Fonds. YA.

Hudson's Bay Company. Fort Liard Account Books. HBCA.
Hudson's Bay Company. Fort Simpson Correspondence Books. 1860–1892. HBCA.
Hudson's Bay Company. Reports on Districts. 1892. Fort Good Hope, Fort Liard, Fort Rae, Fort Resolution, Peel River, Providence. HBCA.
James Fyfe Fonds. YA.
James M. Parker Fonds. UAA.
June Helm Fonds. NWTA.
Paul Nieman Fonds. YA.
Records of the Department of Indian Affairs (RG 10). LAC.
Records of the Department of National Health and Welfare (RG 29). LAC.
Records of the Northern Affairs Program (RG 85). LAC.
Records of the North West Mounted Police and the Royal Canadian Mounted Police (RG 18). LAC.
René Fumoleau Fonds. NWTA.
Robert McDonald Fonds. YA.
Séguin, Jean. Correspondence. OMI. PAA.

Published Primary Sources

Alunik, Ishmael. *Call Me Ishmael: Memories of Ishmael Alunik*. Inuvik: Kolausok Ublaaq Enterprises, 1998.
Back, George. *Narrative of the Arctic Land Expedition: To the Mouth of the Great Fish River and along the Shores of the Arctic Ocean, in the Years 1833, 1834, and 1835*. Edmonton: M.G. Hurtig, 1970, first published 1836.
Baker, Peter. *Memoirs of an Arctic Arab: A Free Trader in the Canadian North: The Years 1907–1927*. Yellowknife: Yellowknife Pub. Co., 1976.
Blue, Archibald. *Fourth Census of Canada 1901: Instructions to Chief Officers, Commissioners, and Enumerators*. Ottawa: Government Printing Bureau, 1901.
Bourget, Clermont. *Douze ans chez les sauvages au Grand-Lac Des Esclaves, comme médecin et Agent des Indiens (1923–1935)*. Ste-Anne-de-Beaupré: En vente chez l'auteur, 1938.
Breynat, Gabriel. *Bishop of the Winds: Fifty Years in the Arctic Regions*. Translated by A. G. Smith. New York: P. J. Kenedy, 1955.
Bryce, Peter Henderson. *Report on the Indian Schools of Manitoba and the North-West Territories*. Ottawa: Government Printing Bureau, 1907.
Camsell, Charles. *Son of the North*. Toronto: The Ryerson Press, 1954.
Canada. *Fourth Census of Canada 1901*. Vol. 1 Population. Ottawa: S. E. Dawson, 1902.
Canada. *Sixth Census of Canada, 1921*. Vol. 1 Population. Ottawa: F. A. Acland, printer, 1924.
Canada. Parliament. *Sessional Papers*. 'Report of the Commissioner of the North-West Mounted Police', 1890–1903. Ottawa, 1891–1904.
Canada. Parliament. *Sessional Papers*. 'Report of the Royal North-West Mounted Police', 1904–1919. Ottawa 1905–20.
Canada. Parliament. *Sessional Papers*. 'Report of the Royal Canadian Mounted Police', 1920–1935. Ottawa 1921–36.
Cody, Hiram Alfred. *An Apostle of the North: Memoirs of the Right Reverend William Carpenter Bompas, D.D.* London: Seeley and Co., 1908.

Dall, William H. *Alaska and Its Resources*. Boston: Lee and Shepherd, 1870.

Franklin, John. *Narrative of a Second Expedition to the Shores of the Polar Sea, in the Years 1825, 1826, and 1827, including an Account of the Progress of a Detachment to the Eastward by John Richardson*. London: J. Murray, 1828.

Gates, R. Ruggles. 'Blood Groups of Canadian Indians and Eskimos'. *American Journal of Physical Anthropology* 12, no. 3 (1929): 475–85.

Godsell, Jean Walker. *I Was No Lady; I Followed the Call of the Wild*. Toronto: Ryerson Press, 1959.

Godsell, Philip H. *Arctic Trader: The Account of Twenty Years with the Hudson's Bay Company*. New ed. London: Travel Book Club, [1950?].

Hearne, Samuel. *A Journey from Prince of Wales's Fort in Hudson's Bay to the Northern Ocean: Undertaken by Order of the Hudson's Bay Company, for the Discovery of Copper Mines, a North West Passage, &c. in the Years 1769, 1770, 1771, & 1772*. London: A. Strahan and T. Cadell, 1795.

Ingstad, Helge. *The Land of Feast and Famine*. Montreal: McGill-Queen's University Press, 1992.

Keith, Lloyd, ed. *North of Athabasca: Slave Lake and Mackenzie River Documents of the North West Company, 1800–1821*. Montreal: McGill-Queen's University Press, 2001.

Kemp, Vernon A. M. *Without Fear, Favour or Affection: Thirty-Five Years with the Royal Canadian Mounted Police*. Toronto: Longmans, Green and Company, 1958.

King, Richard. *Narrative of a Journey to the Shores of the Arctic Ocean in 1833, 1834 and 1835, under the Command of Capt. Back, R.N.* London: R. Bentley, 1836.

Mair, Charles. *Through the Mackenzie Basin: A Narrative of the Athabasca and Peace River Treaty Expedition of 1899*. Toronto: William Briggs, 1908.

Marchand, John F. 'Tribal Epidemics in the Yukon'. *Journal of the American Medical Association* 123, no. 16 (1943): 1019–20.

McIlroy Mills, Thora. 'Gold Rush Nurse'. *north/nord* 20, no. 5 (1973): 10–13.

Missions de la Congrégation des Missionnaires Oblats de Marie Immaculée. Vols. 6–9. Paris: Hennuyer, 1869–83.

Murray, Alexander H. *Journal of the Yukon 1847–48*. Edited by L. J. Burpee. Ottawa: Publications of the Canadian Archives No. 4, 1910.

Nuligak [Cockney, Bob]. *I, Nuligak*, transl. by M. Métayer. Toronto: P. Martin Associates, 1966.

Okpik, Abraham. *We Call It Survival: The Life Story of Abraham Okpik*. Edited by Louis McComber. Iqaluit: Nunavut Arctic College, 2005.

Petitot, Émile. *Autour du Grand Lac des Esclaves*. Paris: Albert Savine, 1891.

Petitot, Émile. *Exploration de la région du Grand Lac des Ours*. Paris: Téqui, 1893.

Petitot, Émile. *Les grands Esquimaux*. Paris: E. Plon, Nourrit et Cie., 1887.

Petitot, Émile. *Quinze ans sous le Cercle Polaire: Mackenzie, Anderson, Youkon*. Paris: E. Dentu, 1889.

Petrone, Penny, ed. *Northern Voices: Inuit Writings in English*. Toronto: University of Toronto Press, 1992.

Report of Commissioners for Treaty No. 8, 22 Sept. 1899. Online 'Treaty Texts: Treaty No. 8', www.rcaanc-cirnac.gc.ca/eng/1100100028813/1581293624572/.

Report of the Select Committee of the Senate Appointed to Enquire into the Resources of the Great Mackenzie Basin. Ottawa: Brown Chamberlin, 1888.

Simon, Sarah. *Fort McPherson, N.W.T.: A Pictorial Account of Family, Church, and Community*. Whitehorse: Yukon Native Language Centre, 1982.

Simpson, Sir George and E. E. Rich. *Journal of Occurrences in the Athabasca Department by George Simpson, 1820 and 1821, and Report*. Toronto: Champlain Society, 1938.

Stefansson, Vilhjalmur. *Hunters of the Great North*. New York: AMS Press, 1922.

Stefansson, Vilhjalmur. *The Stefansson–Anderson Arctic Expedition of the American Museum: Preliminary Ethnological Report*. Anthropological Papers of the American Museum of Natural History. Vol. 14. Part 1. New York: Published by Order of the Trustees, 1914.

The Church Missionary Intelligencer. Vol. 4. London: Church Missionary Society, 1868.

Thrasher, Anthony Apakark. *Thrasher ... Skid Row Eskimo*. Edited by Gerald Deagle and Alan Mettrick. Toronto: Griffin, 1976.

Urquhart, James Alfred. 'The Most Northerly Practice in Canada'. *Canadian Medical Association Journal* 33, no. 2 (1935): 193–6.

Van Bibber, John James. *I Was Born under a Spruce Tree*. Compiled by Niall Fink. Illustrations by Shane Van Bibber. Vancouver: Talus Publishing, 2012.

Van Rooyen, Clennel Evelyn and Andrew James Rhodes. *Virus Diseases of Man*. London: Oxford University Press, 1940.

Vyvyan, Clara. *The Ladies, the Gwich'in, and the Rat: Travels on the Athabasca, Mackenzie, Rat, Porcupine, and Yukon Rivers in 1926*. Edited by I. S. MacLaren and Lisa N. LaFramboise. Edmonton: University of Alberta Press, 1998.

Whittaker, Charles Edward. *Arctic Eskimo: A Record of Fifty Years' Experience & Observation among the Eskimo*. London: Seeley, Service & Co., 1937.

Secondary Sources

Abel, Kerry. *Drum Songs: Glimpses of Dene History*. Montreal: McGill-Queen's University Press, 1993.

Alchon, Suzanne Austin. *A Pest in the Land: New World Epidemics in a Global Perspective*. Albuquerque: University of New Mexico Press, 2003.

Alexie, Elaine. '"*Nakhwanh Gwich'in Khehłok Iidilii* – We Are Our Own People": Teetł'it Gwich'in Practices of Indigeneity: Connection to Land, Traditional Self-Governance, and Elements of Self Determination'. MA thesis, University of Victoria, 2011.

Alunik, Ishmael, Eddie D. Kolausok, and David Morrison. *Across Time and Tundra: The Inuvialuit of the Western Arctic*. Vancouver: Raincoast Books; Seattle: University of Washington Press; Gatineau: Canadian Museum of Civilization, 2003.

Anderson, Warwick. *Colonial Pathologies: American Tropical Medicine, Race, and Hygiene in the Philippines*. Durham, NC: Duke University Press, 2006.

Andre, Alestine and Alan Fehr. *Gwich'in Ethnobotany: Plants Used by the Gwich'in for Food, Medicine, Shelter and Tools*. Tsiigehtchic: Gwich'in Social and Cultural Institute, 2001.

Arndt, Katherine Louise. 'Dynamics of the Fur Trade on the Middle Yukon River, Alaska, 1839–1868'. PhD diss., University of Alaska, 1996.

Arnold, Charles, Wendy Stephenson, Bob Simpson, and Zoe Ho, eds. *Taimani – At That Time: Inuvialuit Timeline Visual Guide*. Inuvik: Inuvialuit Regional Corporation, 2011.

Arnold, David. *Colonizing the Body: State Medicine and Epidemic Disease in Nineteenth-Century India*. Berkeley: University of California Press, 1993.

Asch, Michael. 'On the Land Cession Provisions in Treaty 11'. *Ethnohistory* 60, no. 3 (2013): 451–67.

Auld, James and Robert Kershaw. *The Sahtu Atlas: Maps and Stories from the Sahtu Settlement Area in Canada's Northwest Territories*. Norman Wells: Sahtu GIS Project, 2005.

Backhouse, Constance. *Colour-Coded: A Legal History of Racism in Canada, 1900–1950*. Toronto: Osgood Society for Canadian Legal History, 1999.

Backhouse, Constance B. 'Nineteenth-Century Canadian Prostitution Law: Reflection of a Discriminatory Society'. *Histoire sociale/Social History* 18, no. 36 (1985): 387–423.

Backhouse, Constance. *Petticoats and Prejudice: Women and Law in Nineteenth-Century Canada*. Toronto: Women's Press, 1991.

Balikci, Asen. *Vunta Kutchin Social Change: A Study of the People of Old Crow, Yukon Territory*. Ottawa: Northern Co-ordination and Research Centre, 1963.

Barkan, Elazar. *The Retreat of Scientific Racism: Changing Concepts of Race in Britain and the United States between the World Wars*. Cambridge: Cambridge University Press, 1992.

Bashford, Alison. *Imperial Hygiene: A Critical History of Colonialism, Nationalism, and Public Health*. New York: Palgrave Macmillan, 2004.

Bashford, Alison and Carolyn Strange. 'Isolation and Exclusion in the Modern World: An Introductory Essay'. In *Isolation: Places and Practices of Exclusion*, ed. Carolyn Strange and Alison Bashford, 1–18. Routledge Studies in Modern History. London: Routledge, 2003.

Beairsto, Shelagh Marie. 'Dinjii Kat Chih Ahaa: Gwich'in Notions of Leadership'. MEd thesis, University of Manitoba, 1999.

Beaumont, Susan. *Jijuu, Who Are My Grandparents? Where Are They From?* Fort McPherson: Gwich'in Enrolment Board, 1998.

Binnema, Theodore. *Common and Contested Ground: A Human and Environmental History of the Northwestern Plains*. Toronto: University of Toronto Press, 2004.

Binnema, Ted. *Enlightened Zeal: The Hudson's Bay Company and Scientific Networks, 1670–1870*. Toronto: University of Toronto Press, 2014.

Binnema, Ted. '"With Tears, Shrieks, and Howlings of Despair": The Smallpox Epidemic of 1781–82'. In *Alberta Formed, Alberta Transformed*, vol. 1, ed. Michael Payne, Donald Wetherell, and Catherine Cavanaugh, 110–31. Edmonton: University of Alberta Press, 2006.

Black-Rogers, Mary. 'Varieties of "Starving": Semantics and Survival in the Subarctic Fur Trade, 1750–1850'. *Ethnohistory* 33, no. 4 (1986): 353–83.

Bliss, Michael. *Plague: A Story of Smallpox in Montreal*. Toronto: Harper Collins, 1991.

Bocking, Stephen and Brad Martin, eds. *Ice Blink: Navigating Northern Environmental History*. Calgary: University of Calgary Press, 2017.

Boyd, Robert. *The Coming of the Spirit of Pestilence: Introduced Infectious Diseases and Population Decline among Northwest Coast Indians, 1774–1874*. Vancouver: UBC Press, 1999.

Burch, Ernest S., Igor Krupnik, and Jim Dau. *Caribou Herds of Northwest Alaska, 1850–2000*. Fairbanks: University of Alaska Press, 2012.

Cameron, Catherine M., Paul Kelton, and Alan C. Swedlund, eds. *Beyond Germs: Native Depopulation in North America*. Tucson: The University of Arizona Press, 2015.

Cameron, Emilie. *Far Off Metal River: Inuit Lands, Settler Stories, and the Making of the Contemporary Arctic*. Vancouver: UBC Press, 2015.

Carlos, Ann M. and Frank Lewis. 'Smallpox and Native American Mortality: The 1780s Epidemic in the Hudson Bay Region'. *Explorations in Economic History* 49, no. 3 (2012): 277–90. http://doi.org/10.1016/j.eeh.2012.04.003.

Carter, Sarah. *Capturing Women: The Manipulation of Cultural Imagery in Canada's Prairie West*. Montreal: McGill-Queen's University Press, 1997.

Castenbrandt, Helene. 'A Forgotten Plague: Dysentery in Sweden, 1750–1900'. *Scandinavian Journal of History* 39, no. 5 (2014): 612–39. http://doi.org/10.1080/03468755.2014.953199.

Castonguay, Thérèse. *A Leap in Faith: The Grey Nuns Ministries in Western and Northern Canada*. 2 vols. Edmonton: Grey Nuns of Alberta, 1999.

Choquette, Robert. *The Oblate Assault on Canada's Northwest*. Ottawa: University of Ottawa Press, 1995.

Coates, Ken. 'Asking for All Sorts of Favours: The Anglican Church, the Federal Government, and the Natives of the Yukon Territory, 1891–1909'. In *The Anglican Church and the World of Western Canada, 1820–1970*, ed. Barry Ferguson, 126–42. Regina: Canadian Plains Research Centre, 1987.

Coates, Kenneth. *Best Left As Indians: Native–White Relations In the Yukon Territory, 1840–1973*. Montreal: McGill-Queen's University Press, 1993.

Coates, Kenneth. '"Betwixt and Between": The Anglican Church and the Children of the Carcross (Chooutla) Residential School, 1911–1954'. *BC Studies* 64 (1984): 27–47.

Coates, Kenneth. *Canada's Colonies: A History of the Yukon and Northwest Territories*. Toronto: Lorimer, 1985.

Coates, Kenneth, ed. *The Alaska Highway: Papers of the 40th Anniversary Symposium*. Vancouver: University of British Columbia Press, 1985.

Colpitts, George. *Pemmican Empire: Food, Trade, and the Last Bison Hunts in the North American Plains, 1780–1882*. Cambridge: Cambridge University Press, 2015.

Coulthard, Glen Sean. *Red Skin White Masks: Rejecting the Colonial Politics of Recognition*. Minneapolis: University of Minnesota Press, 2014.

Crosby, Alfred W. *America's Forgotten Pandemic: The Influenza of 1918*. New York: Cambridge University Press, 1989.

Crosby, Alfred W. *Ecological Imperialism: The Biological Expansion of Europe, 900–1900*. Cambridge: Cambridge University Press, 1986.

Crosby, Alfred W. 'Virgin Soil Epidemics as a Factor in the Aboriginal Depopulation in America'. *The William and Mary Quarterly* 33, no. 2 (1976): 289–99.

Cruikshank, Julie. *Do Glaciers Listen? Local Knowledge, Colonial Encounters, and Social Imagination*. Vancouver: UBC Press, 2005.

Cruikshank, Julie. 'Images of Society in Klondike Gold Rush Narratives: Skookum Jim and the Discovery of Gold'. *Ethnohistory* 29, no. 1 (1992): 20–41.

Cruikshank, Julie. 'Oral Traditions and Written Accounts: An Incident from the Klondike Gold Rush'. *Culture* 9, no. 2 (1989): 25–34.

Dákeyi Teaching Guide. Dákeyi Athapaskan Language Course: Southern Tutchone Place Names. Whitehorse: Yukon Native Language Centre, 1997. https://yukonplacenames.ca/dakeyi/.

Daschuk, James. *Clearing the Plains: Disease, Politics of Starvation, and the Loss of Aboriginal Life*. Regina: University of Regina Press, 2013.

Davenport, Romola, Leonard Schwarz, and Jeremy Boulton, 'The Decline of Adult Smallpox in Eighteenth-Century London'. *Economic History Review* 64, no. 4 (2011): 1289–314.

Decker, Jody F. 'Depopulation of the Northern Plains Natives'. *Social Science & Medicine* 33, no. 4 (1991): 381–93.

Decker, Jody F. 'The York Factory Medical Journals, 1846–52'. *Canadian Bulletin of Medical History/ Bulletin canadien d'histoire de la médecine* 14, no. 1 (1997): 107–31.

Decker, Jody F. 'Tracing Historical Diffusion Patterns: The Case of the 1780–82 Smallpox Epidemic among the Indians of Western Canada'. *Native Studies Review* 4, nos. 1 &2 (1988): 1–24.

Dehner, George. *Influenza: A Century of Science and Public Health Response*. Pittsburgh: University of Pittsburgh Press, 2012.

Dippie, Brian W. *The Vanishing American: White Attitudes and U.S. Indian Policy*. Middletown: Wesleyan University Press, 1982.

Dobrowolsky, Helene and Thomas J. Hammer. *Tr'ochëk: The Archaeology and History of a Hän Fish Camp*. [Dawson City, Yukon]: Tr'ondëk Hwëch'in, 2001.

Duchaussois, R. P. *Aux glaces polaires, Indiens et Esquimaux*. Lyons: Oeuvre Apostolique de Marie Immaculée; Ville La Salle: Noviciat des Oblats, 1921.

Duchaussois, R. P. *The Grey Nuns in the Far North*. Toronto: McClelland and Stewart, 1919.

Duffy, John. *The Sanitarians: A History of American Public Health*. Urbana: University of Illinois Press, 1990.

Duggan, Ana T., Maria F. Perdomo, Dario Piombino-Mascali, et al. '17th Century Variola Virus Reveals the Recent History of Smallpox'. *Current Biology* 26 (Dec. 2016): 3407–12. http://doi.org/10.1016/j.cub.2016.10.061.

Easton, Norman Alexander. 'King George Got Diarrhea: The Yukon-Alaska Boundary Survey, Bill Rupe, and the Scottie Creek Dineh'. *Alaska Journal of Anthropology* 5, no. 1 (2007): 95–118.

Edwards, Keri. *Dictionary of Tlingit*. First ed. Juneau: Sealaska Heritage Institute, 2009.

Fafard, Mélanie and Ingrid Kritsch. *Yeenoo Daì' Gwatsat Teetł'it Zheh Googwandak: The History and Archaeology of Fort McPherson*. Tsiigehtchic: Gwich'in Social and Cultural Institute, 2005.

Fenn, Elizabeth A. *Pox Americana: The Great Smallpox Epidemic of 1775–82*. New York: Hill and Wang, 2001.

Fortuine, Robert. *Chills and Fever: Health and Disease in the Early History of Alaska*. Fairbanks: University of Alaska Press, 1992.

Fortuine, Robert. *'Must We All Die?': Alaska's Enduring Struggle with Tuberculosis*. Fairbanks: University of Alaska Press, 2005.

Fraser, Crystal. 'T'aih k'ìighe' tth'aih zhit dìidìch'ùh (By Strength, We Are Still Here): Indigenous Northerners Confronting Hierarchies of Power at Day and Residential Schools in Nanhkak Thak (the Inuvik Region, Northwest Territories), 1959–1982'. PhD diss., University of Alberta, 2018.

Friesen, T. Max. *When Worlds Collide: Hunter-Gatherer World-System Change in the Nineteenth-Century Canadian Arctic*. Tucson: University of Arizona Press, 2013.

Fumoleau, René. *As Long as This Land Shall Last: A History of Treaty 8 and Treaty 11, 1870–1939*. Calgary: University of Calgary Press, 2004.

Gagnon, Alain, Matthew S. Miller, Stacey A. Hallman, et al. 'Age-Specific Mortality during the 1918 Influenza Pandemic: Unravelling the Mystery of High Young Adult Mortality'. *PLoS ONE* 8, no. 8 (2013). http://doi.org/10.1371/journal.pone.0069586.

Gates, Michael. 'How the Yukon was Spared the Influenza Pandemic of 1918.' *Yukon News*, 26 Mar. 2020.

Grant, Shelagh. *Sovereignty or Security? Government Policy in the Canadian North, 1936–1950*. Vancouver: UBC Press, 1988.

Green, Heather. 'The Tr'ondëk Hwëch'in and the Great Upheaval: Mining, Colonialism, and Environmental Change in the Klondike, 1890–1940'. PhD diss., University of Alberta, 2018.

Gwich'in Social and Cultural Institute. *Gwich'in Place Names Atlas*. http://atlas.gwichin.ca.

Hackett, Paul. 'Averting Disaster: The Hudson's Bay Company and Smallpox in Western Canada during the Late Eighteenth and Early Nineteenth Centuries'. *Bulletin of the History of Medicine* 78, no. 3 (2004): 575–609.

Hackett, Paul. *'A Very Remarkable Sickness': Epidemics in the Petit Nord, 1670–1846*. Winnipeg: University of Manitoba Press, 2002.

Hamilton, Michelle A. '"Anyone Not on the List Might as Well Be Dead": Aboriginal Peoples and the Censuses of Canada, 1851–1916'. *Journal of the Canadian Historical Association* 18, no. 1 (2007): 57–79.

Hammer, Thomas J. and Christian D. Thomas. *Archaeology at Forty Mile / Ch'ëdä Dëk*. [Whitehorse]: Yukon Tourism and Culture, 2006.

Hardy, Anne. *The Epidemic Streets: Infectious Disease and the Rise of Preventive Medicine, 1856–1900*. Oxford: Clarendon Press, 1993.

Hare, Greg and Ruth Gotthardt. *A Look Back in Time: The Archaeology of Fort Selkirk*. [Yukon]: Selkirk First Nation, 1996.

Harris, Cole. 'How Did Colonialism Dispossess? Comments from an Edge of Empire'. *Annals of the Association of American Geographers* 94, no. 1 (2004): 165–82.

Hayden, Shannon. 'One Land, Many People: Archaeology, Agency, and Landscape at Old Fort Rae, Northwest Territories'. MA thesis, University of Leicester, 2010.

Helm, June. 'Bilaterality in the Socio-territorial Organization of the Arctic Drainage Dene'. *Ethnology* 4 (1965): 361–85.

Helm, June. 'Female Infanticide, European Diseases, and Population Levels among the Mackenzie Dene'. *American Ethnologist* 7 (1980): 259–85.

Helm, June, ed. *Handbook of North American Indians*. Vol. 6. *Subarctic*. Washington: Smithsonian Institution, 1981.

Helm, June. *The People of Denendeh*. Montreal: McGill-Queen's University Press, 2000.

Highet, Megan J. 'Catching Gold Fever: A Social History of Typhoid Fever among the Klondike Gold Rushers, 1896–1904'. *Alaska Journal of Anthropology* 15, nos. 1 &2 (2017): 141–57.

Highet, Megan J. 'Gold Fever: Death and Disease During the Klondike Gold Rush, 1898–1904.' MA thesis, University of Manitoba, 2008.

Houston, C. Stuart and Stan Houston. 'The First Smallpox Epidemic on the Canadian Plains: In the Fur-Traders' Words'. *Canadian Journal of Infectious Diseases* 11, no. 2 (March/April 2000): 112–15.

Humphries, Mark Osborne. *The Last Plague: Spanish Influenza and the Politics of Public Health in Canada*. Toronto: University of Toronto Press, 2013.

Ingram, Rob and Helene Dobrowolsky. *Waves upon the Shore: An Historical Profile of Herschel Island*. [Whitehorse]: Yukon Tourism Heritage Branch, 1989.

Innis, Harold A. *The Fur Trade in Canada*. With a new introduction by Arthur J. Ray. Toronto: University of Toronto Press, 1999.

Inuvialuit Elders with Robert W. Bandringa. *Inuvialuit Nautchiangit: Relationships between People and Plants*. Inuvik: Inuvialuit Cultural Resource Centre, 2010.

Jones, David S. *Rationalizing Epidemics: Meanings and Uses of American Indian Mortality since 1600*. Cambridge: Harvard University Press, 2004.

Jones, David S. 'Virgin Soils Revisited'. *The William and Mary Quarterly* 60, no. 4 (2003): 703–42.

Jones, Esyllt W. *Influenza 1918: Disease, Death and Struggle in Winnipeg*. Toronto: University of Toronto Press, 2007.

Jones-Imhotep, Edward and Tina Adcock, eds. *Made Modern: Science and Technology in Canadian History*. Vancouver: UBC Press, 2018.

Jørgensen, Dolly, and Sverker Sörlin. *Northscapes: History, Technology, and the Making of Northern Environments*. Vancouver: UBC Press, 2013.

Katz, Alan R. and David M. Morens. 'Severe Streptococcal Infections in Historical Perspective'. *Clinical Infectious Diseases* 14 (1992): 298–307.

Kelm, Mary-Ellen. *Colonizing Bodies: Aboriginal Health and Healing in British Columbia, 1900–50*. Vancouver: UBC Press, 1998.

Kelton, Paul. *Cherokee Medicine, Colonial Germs: An Indigenous Nation's Fight against Smallpox, 1518–1824*. Norman: University of Oklahoma Press, 2015.

Kelton, Paul. *Epidemics and Enslavement: Biological Catastrophe in the Native Southeast, 1492–1715*. Lincoln: University of Nebraska Press, 2007.

Krech, III, Shepard. 'Disease, Starvation, and Northern Athapaskan Social Organization'. *American Ethnologist* 5 (1978): 710–32.

Krech, III, Shepard. 'The Influence of Disease and the Fur Trade on Arctic Drainage Lowlands Dene, 1800–1850'. *Journal of Anthropological Research* 39, no. 1 (1983): 123–46.

Kritsch, Ingrid. *Gwich'in Territorial Park (Campbell Lake) Oral History Project Final Report: prepared for Dept. of Economic Development and Tourism (GNWT)*. Tsiigehtchic: Gwich'in Social and Cultural Institute, 1994.

Lampard, Robert. *Alberta's Medical History: Young, Lusty, and Full of Life*. Red Deer: R. Lampard, 2008.

Lanzarotta, Tess. 'Ethics in Retrospect: Biomedical Research, Colonial Violence, and Iñupiat Sovereignty in the Alaskan Arctic'. *Social Studies of Science* 5, no. 5 (2020): 778–801.

Lanzarotta, Tess. 'The Disappearing Clinic'. *Modern American History* 2 (2019): 257–64.

Lee, Chang-Hoon, E. G. Lee, J. Y. Lee, et al. 'The Incidence of Tuberculosis after a Measles Outbreak'. *Clinical Infectious Diseases* 46, no. 6 (2008): 902–4.

Legat, Allice. *Walking the Land, Feeding the Fire: Knowledge and Stewardship among the Tlicho Dene*. Foreword by Joanne Barnaby. Tucson: University of Arizona Press, 2012.

Longley, Hereward. 'Bitumen Exploration and the Southern Re-inscription of Northeastern Alberta: 1875–1967'. *RCC Perspectives* 4 (2016): 17–24.

Lux, Maureen. 'Disease and the Growth of Dawson City: The Seamy Underside of a Legend'. *Northern Review* 3/4 (1989): 96–117.

Lux, Maureen K. *Medicine That Walks: Disease, Medicine and Canadian Plains Native People, 1880–1940*. Toronto: University of Toronto Press, 2012.

Lux, Maureen K. *Separate Beds: A History of Indian Hospitals in Canada, 1920s–1980s*. Toronto: University of Toronto Press, 2016.

Lyons, Natasha. 'Quliaq tohongniaq tuunga (Making Histories): Towards a Critical Inuvialuit Archaeology in the Canadian Western Arctic'. PhD diss., University of Calgary, 2007.

Madill, Dennis F. K. 'Treaty Research Report Treaty Eight (1899)'. Prepared for Treaties and Historical Research Centre Indian and Northern Affairs Canada, 1986. www.rcaanc-cirnac.gc.ca/eng/1100100028809/1564415096517.

Mamelund, Svenn-Erik. 'Geography May Explain Adult Mortality from the 1918–20 Influenza Pandemic'. *Epidemics* 3 (2011): 46–60.

Mamelund, Svenn-Erik, Lisa Sattenspiel, and Jessica Dimka. 'Influenza-Associated Mortality during the 1918–1919 Influenza Pandemic in Alaska and Labrador: A Comparison'. *Social Science History* 37, no. 2 (2013): 177–229.

Marles, Robin James. *Aboriginal Plant Use in Canada's Northwest Boreal Forest*. Vancouver: UBC Press, 2009.

Mathews, John D., Joanne M. Chesson, James M. McCaw, and Jodie McVernon. 'Understanding Influenza Transmission, Immunity and Pandemic Threats'. *Influenza and Other Respiratory Viruses* 3, no. 4 (2009): 143–9.

McCallum, Mary Jane Logan. 'Starvation, Experimentation, Segregation, and Trauma: Words for Reading Indigenous Health History'. *Canadian Historical Review* 98, no. 1 (2017): 96–113.

McCallum, Mary Jane. 'This Last Frontier: "Isolation" and Aboriginal Health'. *Canadian Bulletin of Medical History/ Bulletin canadien d'histoire de la médecine* 22, no. 1 (2005): 103–20.

McCallum, Mary Jane Logan and Adele Perry. *Structures of Indifference: An Indigenous Life and Death in a Canadian City*. Winnipeg: University of Manitoba Press, 2018.

McCarthy, Martha. *From the Great River to the Ends of the Earth: Oblate Missions to the Dene, 1847–1921*. Edmonton: University of Alberta Press, 1995.

McCormack, Patricia. *Fort Chipewyan and the Shaping of Canadian History, 1788–1920s: 'We Like to Be Free in This Country'*. Vancouver: UBC Press, 2010.

McCormack, Patricia. 'The Athabasca Influenza Epidemic of 1835'. *Issues in the North* 1 (1996): 33–42.

McMillen, Christian W. *Discovering Tuberculosis: A Global History, 1900 to the Present*. New Haven: Yale University Press, 2016.

McNeill, John R. *Mosquito Empires: Ecology and War in the Greater Caribbean 1620–1914*. New York: Cambridge University Press, 2010.

McNeill, William. *Plagues and Peoples*. Garden City: Anchor Press, 1976.

Meijer Drees, Laurie. *Healing Histories: Stories from Canada's Indian Hospitals*. Edmonton: University of Alberta Press, 2013.

Mina, Michael J., T. Kula, Y. Leng, et al. 'Measles Virus Infection Diminishes Preexisting Antibodies That Offer Protection from Other Pathogens'. *Science* 366, no. 6465 (2019): 599–606.

Mishler, Craig. 'Missionaries in Collision: Anglicans and Oblates among the Gwich'in, 1861–65'. *Arctic* 43, no. 2 (1990): 121–6.

Mishler, Craig. *The Crooked Stovepipe: Athapaskan Fiddle Music and Square Dancing in Northeast Alaska and Northwest Canada*. Urbana: University of Illinois Press, 1993.

Mishler, Craig and William E. Simeone. *Han People of the River*. Fairbanks: University of Alaska Press, 2004.

Möller, Marlo, Craig J. Kinnear, Marianna Orlova, et al. 'Genetic Resistance to *Mycobacterium tuberculosis* Infection and Disease'. *Frontiers in Immunology* 9 (September 2018). http://doi.org/10.3389/fimmu.2018.02219.

Mooney, Graham. *Intrusive Interventions: Public Health, Domestic Space, and Infectious Disease Surveillance in England, 1840–1914*. Rochester: University of Rochester Press, 2015.

Moore, Patrick. 'Archdeacon Robert McDonald and Gwich'in Literacy'. *Anthropological Linguistics* 49, no. 1 (2007): 27–53.

Morens, David M. and Jeffery K. Taubenberger. 'A Forgotten Epidemic that Changed Medicine: Measles in the US Army, 1917–18'. *Lancet Infectious Diseases* 15, no. 7 (2015): 852–61.

Morrison, William R. *Showing the Flag: The Mounted Police and Canadian Sovereignty in the North, 1894–1925*. Vancouver: University of British Columbia Press, 1985.

Morse, Kathryn Taylor. *The Nature of Gold: An Environmental History of the Klondike Gold Rush*. Seattle: University of Washington Press, 2003.

Nadasdy, Paul. *Hunters and Bureaucrats: Power, Knowledge, and Aboriginal-State Relations in the Southwest Yukon*. Vancouver: UBC Press, 2003.

Nash, Linda. *Inescapable Ecologies: A History of Environment, Disease, and Knowledge*. Berkeley: University of California Press, 2006.

Nettelbeck, Amanda. 'On the Side of Law and Order: Indigenous Aides to the Mounted Police on the Settler Frontiers of Australia and Canada'. *Journal of Colonialism and Colonial History* 15, no. 2 (2014). http://doi.org/10.1353/cch.2014.0031.

Newfield, Timothy P. 'Syndemics and the History of Disease: Towards a New Engagement'. *Social Science & Medicine* 295 (2022). http://doi.org/10.1016/j.socscimed.2021.114454.

Njamkepo, Elisabeth, Nizar Fawal, Alicia Tran-Dien, et al., 'Global Phylogeography and Evolutionary History of *Shigella dysenteriae* Type 1'. *Nature Microbiology* 1 (21 Mar. 2016). http://doi.org/10.1038/nmicrobiol.2016.27.

Ó Gráda, Cormac. 'Making Famine History'. *Journal of Economic Literature* 45, no. 1 (2007): 5–38.

Osgood, Cornelius. *Contributions to the Ethnography of the Kutchin*. Reprint ed. New Haven: Human Relations Area Files Press, 1970.

Osgood, Cornelius. 'Kutchin Tribal Distribution and Synonymy'. *American Anthropologist* 36, no. 2 (1934): 168–79.

Parlee, Brenda L. and Ken J. Caine. *When the Caribou Do Not Come: Indigenous Knowledge and Adaptive Management in the Western Arctic*. Vancouver: UBC Press, 2018.

Peake, Frank A. 'Robert McDonald (1829–1913): The Great Unknown Missionary of the Northwest'. *Journal of the Canadian Church Historical Society* 17, no. 3 (1975): 54–72.

Peake, Frank A. *The Bishop Who Ate His Boots: A Biography of Isaac O. Stringer*. Toronto: Anglican Church of Canada, 1966.

Pepin, Jacques. *The Origins of AIDS*. Cambridge: University of Cambridge Press, 2011.

Pepperell, Caitlin S., Julie M. Granka, David C. Alexander, et al. 'Dispersal of *Mycobacterium tuberculosis* via the Canadian Fur Trade'. *PNAS* 108, no. 16 (2011): 6526–31.

Perry, Adele. *Colonial Relations: The Douglas-Connolly Family and the Nineteenth-Century Imperial World*. New York: Cambridge University Press, 2015.

Perry, Adele. *On the Edge of Empire : Gender, Race, and the Making of British Columbia, 1849–1871*. Toronto: University of Toronto Press, 2001.

Piper, Liza. 'Diphtheria Antitoxin and Tales of Mercy in Northern Health Care'. *Canadian Bulletin of Medical History/ Bulletin canadien d'histoire de la médecine* 38, no. 2 (2021): 285–319.

Piper, Liza. *The Industrial Transformation of Subarctic Canada*. Vancouver: UBC Press, 2009.

Podruchny, Carolyn. *Making the Voyageur World: Travelers and Traders in the North American Fur Trade*. Lincoln: University of Nebraska Press, 2006.

Porsild, Charlene. *Gamblers and Dreamers: Women, Men, and Community in the Klondike*. Vancouver: UBC Press, 1998.

Porsild, Charlene. 'Klondike Family Life'. *BC Studies* 123 (Autumn 1999): 59–68.

Porter, Roy. *The Greatest Benefit to Mankind: A Medical History of Humanity*. New York: W.W. Norton, 1998.

Price, Richard, ed. *The Spirit of the Alberta Indian Treaties*. 3rd ed. Edmonton: University of Alberta Press, 1999.

Prince of Wales Northern Heritage Centre. *Northwest Territories Official Community Names and Pronunciation Guide*. www.pwnhc.ca/cultural-places/geographic-names/community-names/.

Raibmon, Paige. *Authentic Indians: Episodes of Encounter from the Late-Nineteenth-Century Northwest Coast*. Durham: Duke University Press, 2005.

Radin, Joanna. 'Latent Life: Concepts and Practices of Human Tissue Preservation in the International Biological Program'. *Social Studies of Science* 43, no. 4 (2013): 484–508.

Radin, Joanna. *Life on Ice: A History of New Uses for Cold Blood*. Chicago: University of Chicago Press, 2017.

Rampart House Historic Site, Lapierre House Historic Site Management Plan. Prepared for the Vuntut Gwitchin First Nation and the Government of the Yukon. March 1999.

Ray, Arthur J. 'Diffusion of Diseases in the Western Interior of Canada, 1830–1850'. *Geographical Review* 66, no. 2 (1976): 139–57.

Ray, Arthur J. *Indians in the Fur Trade: Their Role as Trappers, Hunters, and Middlemen in the Lands Southwest of Hudson Bay, 1660–1870*. Toronto: University of Toronto Press, 1974.

Ray, Arthur J. *The Canadian Fur Trade in the Industrial Age*. Toronto: University of Toronto Press, 1990.

Reardon, Jenny and Kim TallBear. '"Your DNA Is *Our* History": Genomics, Anthropology, and the Construction of Whiteness as Property'. *Current Anthropology* 53, suppl. 5 (2012): S233–45.

Rich, Edwin Ernest. 'The Fur Traders: Their Diet and Drugs'. *The Beaver* (Summer 1976): 43–53.

Roberts, Peder and Adrian Howkins, eds. *Cambridge History of the Polar Regions*. Cambridge: Cambridge University Press, 2023.

Rutherdale, Myra. *Women and the White Man's God: Gender and Race in the Canadian Mission Field*. Vancouver: UBC Press, 2002.

Sahtúot'ı̨ne Gokedé: Sahtúot'ı̨ne Dictionary Délı̨ne Kədə́ / Dialect of the North Slavey Language. [Norman Wells]: Sahtú Divisional Education Council, 2012.

Sandlos, John. *Hunters at the Margin: Native People and Wildlife Conservation in the Northwest Territories*. Vancouver: UBC Press, 2007.

Sangster, Joan. *The Iconic North: Cultural Constructions of Aboriginal Life in Postwar Canada*. Vancouver: UBC Press, 2016.

Sax, Lee and Effie Linklater. *Gikhyi: One Who Speaks the Word of God*. Whitehorse: Diocese of Yukon, 1990.

Scott, Susan and Christopher J. Duncan. *Human Demography and Disease*. Cambridge: Cambridge University Press, 1998.

Shanks, G. Dennis and John F. Brundage. 'Pacific Islands Which Escaped the 1918–1919 Influenza Pandemic and Their Subsequent Mortality Experiences'. *Epidemiology & Infection* 141 (2013): 353–6.

Shanks, G. Dennis and John F. Brundage. 'Pathogenic Responses among Young Adults during the 1918 Influenza Pandemic'. *Emerging Infectious Diseases*, 18, no. 2 (2012): 201–7.

Shanks, G. Dennis, Zheng Hu, Michael Waller, et al. 'Measles Epidemics of Variable Lethality in the Early 20th Century'. *American Journal of Epidemiology* 179, no. 4 (2014): 413–22.

Sims, Daniel Chester Forest. 'Balloon Bombs, the Alaska Highway, and Influenza: Tsek'ehne Perspectives on the 1943 Flu Epidemic'. *BC Studies* 203 (2019): 111–30.

Smith, David M. *Moose-Deer Island House People: A History of the Native People of Fort Resolution*. Ottawa: National Museums of Canada, 1982.

South Slave Divisional Education Council. *Dene Yatié K'ę́ę́ Ahsíi Yats'uuzi Gha Edı̨htł'éh Kátł'odehche / South Slavey Topical Dictionary Kátł'odehche Dialect*. Fort Smith: South Slave Divisional Education Council, 2009.

South Slave Divisional Education Council. *Dëne Dédlıné Yatıé: ʔerehtł'ischo Denínu Kuę́ Yatıé / Chipewyan Dictionary*. Fort Smith: South Slave Divisional Education Council, 2012.

Stager, John K. 'Fort Anderson: The First Post for Trade in the Western Arctic'. *Geographical Bulletin* 9, no. 1 (1967): 45–56.

Stevenson, Lisa. *Life beside Itself: Imagining Care in the Canadian Arctic*. Oakland: University of California Press, 2014.

Stuhl, Andrew. *Unfreezing the Arctic: Science, Colonialism, and the Transformation of Inuit Lands*. Chicago: University of Chicago Press, 2017.

Taubenberger, Jeffery K. and David M. Morens. '1918 Influenza: The Mother of All Pandemics'. *Emerging Infectious Diseases* 12, no. 1 (2006): 15–22.

Tester, Frank J. and Peter Kulchyski. *Tammarniit (Mistakes): Inuit Relocation in the Eastern Arctic*. Vancouver: UBC Press, 1994.

Tester, Frank James and Paule McNicoll. 'Why Don't They Get It? Talk of Medicine as Science. St Luke's Hospital, Panniqtuuq, Baffin Island'. *Social History of Medicine* 19 (2006): 87–106.

Tough, Frank. *'As Their Natural Resources Fail': Native Peoples and the Economic History of Northern Manitoba, 1870–1930*. Vancouver: UBC Press, 1996.

Tricoire, Damien, ed. *Enlightened Colonialism: Civilization Narratives and Imperial Politics in the Age of Reason*. Cham: Palgrave Macmillan, 2017.

Truth and Reconciliation Commission of Canada. *Canada's Residential Schools*. Vols. 2 and 3. Montreal: McGill-Queen's University Press, 2015.

Tuck, Eve and K. Wayne Yang. 'Decolonization Is Not a Metaphor'. *Decolonization: Indigeneity, Education & Society* 1, no. 1 (2012): 1–40.

Usher, Peter J. *Fur Trade Posts of the Northwest Territories 1870–1970*. Ottawa: Northern Science Research Group, Dept. of Indian Affairs and Northern Development, 1971.

Usher, Peter. 'The Canadian Western Arctic: A Century of Change'. *Anthropologica*. New Series, 13, no. 1/2, 'Pilot, Not Commander: Essays in Memory of Diamond Jenness' (1971): 169–83.

Vanast, Walter J. '"Arctic Bodies; Frontier Souls": Missionaries and Medical Care in the Canadian North 1896–1926'. PhD diss. University of Wisconsin–Madison, 1996.

Vanast, Walter. '"Hastening the Day of Extinction": Canada, Québec, and the Medical Care of Ungava's Inuit, 1867–1967'. *Études/Inuit/Studies* 15, no. 2 (1991): 55–84.

Vijgen, Leen, Els Keyaerts, Elien Moës, et al. 'Complete Genomic Sequence of Human Coronavirus OC43: Molecular Clock Analysis Suggests a Relatively Recent Zoonotic Coronavirus Transmission Event'. *Journal of Virology* 79, no. 3 (2005): 1595–604.

Waldram, James B., D. Ann Herring, and T. Kue Young, *Aboriginal Health in Canada: Historical, Cultural, and Epidemiological Perspectives*. Toronto: University of Toronto Press, 1995.

Wight, Philip A. 'The Militarized "Hydrocarbon Frontier": Petroleum Development and the State in Arctic North America, 1919–1977', in *Cambridge History of the Polar Regions*, ed. P. Roberts and A. Howkins, 593–620. Cambridge: Cambridge University Press, 2023.

Wolfe, Patrick. 'Settler Colonialism and the Elimination of the Native'. *Journal of Genocide Research* 8, no. 4 (2006): 387–409.

Wolfe, Robert J. 'Alaska's Great Sickness, 1900: An Epidemic of Measles and Influenza in a Virgin Soil Population'. *Proceedings of the American Philosophical Society* 126, no. 2 (1982): 91–121.

Worboys, Michael. 'Was There a Bacteriological Revolution in Late Nineteenth-Century Medicine?' *Studies in History and Philosophy of Biological and Biomedical Sciences* 38 (2007): 20–42.

Wright, Allen A. *Prelude to Bonanza: The Discovery and Exploration of the Yukon*. Sidney: Gray's Publishing, 1976.

Yellowknives Dene First Nation and Prince of Wales Northern Heritage Centre. *This Land Is Our Home: Wìilìideh Yellowknives Dene*. Yellowknife: Prince of Wales Northern Heritage Centre, 2015. www.nwtexhibits.ca/navigator/ykdene/index-en.html.

Yerbury, John Collin. *The Subarctic Indians and the Fur Trade, 1680–1860*. Vancouver: University of British Columbia Press, 1986.

Yukon Tourism and Culture. *Gazetteer of Yukon*. Whitehorse: Yukon Geographical Names Program, 2022. https://yukon.ca/sites/yukon.ca/files/tc/tc-gazetteer-of-yukon.pdf.

Yukon Tourism and Culture. *Rampart House*. Whitehorse: Yukon Historic Sites, 2010.

Zaslow, Morris. *The Opening of the Canadian North 1870–1914*. Toronto: McClelland and Stewart, 1971.

Index

For EU product safety concerns, contact us at Calle de José Abascal, 56–1°,
28003 Madrid, Spain or eugpsr@cambridge.org.

www.ingramcontent.com/pod-product-compliance
Lightning Source LLC
LaVergne TN
LVHW011703200926
848484LV00004B/1058
* 9 7 8 1 0 0 9 3 2 0 8 7 0 *